Molecular and Cellular Advances in Endometriosis Research

Molecular and Cellular Advances in Endometriosis Research

Editor

Antonio Simone Laganà

MDPI • Basel • Beijing • Wuhan • Barcelona • Belgrade • Manchester • Tokyo • Cluj • Tianjin

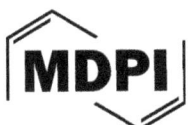

Editor
Antonio Simone Laganà
Department of Obstetrics
and Gynecology
"Filippo Del Ponte" Hospital
University of Insubria
Varese
Italy

Editorial Office
MDPI
St. Alban-Anlage 66
4052 Basel, Switzerland

This is a reprint of articles from the Special Issue published online in the open access journal *International Journal of Molecular Sciences* (ISSN 1422-0067) (available at: www.mdpi.com/journal/ijms/special_issues/endometriosis_research2).

For citation purposes, cite each article independently as indicated on the article page online and as indicated below:

LastName, A.A.; LastName, B.B.; LastName, C.C. Article Title. *Journal Name* **Year**, *Volume Number*, Page Range.

ISBN 978-3-0365-2803-8 (Hbk)
ISBN 978-3-0365-2802-1 (PDF)

© 2022 by the authors. Articles in this book are Open Access and distributed under the Creative Commons Attribution (CC BY) license, which allows users to download, copy and build upon published articles, as long as the author and publisher are properly credited, which ensures maximum dissemination and a wider impact of our publications.

The book as a whole is distributed by MDPI under the terms and conditions of the Creative Commons license CC BY-NC-ND.

Contents

About the Editor vii

Milan Terzic, Gulzhanat Aimagambetova, Jeannette Kunz, Gauri Bapayeva, Botagoz Aitbayeva and Sanja Terzic et al.
Molecular Basis of Endometriosis and Endometrial Cancer: Current Knowledge and Future Perspectives
Reprinted from: *Int. J. Mol. Sci.* **2021**, *22*, 9274, doi:10.3390/ijms22179274 1

Quanah J. Hudson, Katharina Proestling, Alexandra Perricos, Lorenz Kuessel, Heinrich Husslein and René Wenzl et al.
The Role of Long Non-Coding RNAs in Endometriosis
Reprinted from: *Int. J. Mol. Sci.* **2021**, *22*, 11425, doi:10.3390/ijms222111425 25

Xiyin Wang, Luca Parodi and Shannon M. Hawkins
Translational Applications of Linear and Circular Long Noncoding RNAs in Endometriosis
Reprinted from: *Int. J. Mol. Sci.* **2021**, *22*, 10626, doi:10.3390/ijms221910626 43

Chiara Sabbadin, Alessandra Andrisani, Gabriella Donà, Elena Tibaldi, Anna Maria Brunati and Stefano Dall'Acqua et al.
Endometriosis Susceptibility to Dapsone-Hydroxylamine-Induced Alterations Can Be Prevented by Licorice Intake: In Vivo and In Vitro Study
Reprinted from: *Int. J. Mol. Sci.* **2021**, *22*, 8476, doi:10.3390/ijms22168476 61

Iveta Yotova, Quanah J. Hudson, Florian M. Pauler, Katharina Proestling, Isabella Haslinger and Lorenz Kuessel et al.
LINC01133 Inhibits Invasion and Promotes Proliferation in an Endometriosis Epithelial Cell Line
Reprinted from: *Int. J. Mol. Sci.* **2021**, *22*, 8385, doi:10.3390/ijms22168385 75

Joanna Olkowska-Truchanowicz, Agata Białoszewska, Aneta Zwierzchowska, Alicja Sztokfisz-Ignasiak, Izabela Janiuk and Filip Dabrowski et al.
Peritoneal Fluid from Patients with Ovarian Endometriosis Displays Immunosuppressive Potential and Stimulates Th2 Response
Reprinted from: *Int. J. Mol. Sci.* **2021**, *22*, 8134, doi:10.3390/ijms22158134 95

Ludmila Lozneanu, Raluca Anca Balan, Ioana Păvăleanu, Simona Eliza Giușcă, Irina-Draga Căruntu and Cornelia Amalinei
BMI-1 Expression Heterogeneity in Endometriosis-Related and Non-Endometriotic Ovarian Carcinoma
Reprinted from: *Int. J. Mol. Sci.* **2021**, *22*, 6082, doi:10.3390/ijms22116082 109

Cássia de Fáveri, Paula M. Poeta Fermino, Anna P. Piovezan and Lia K. Volpato
The Inflammatory Role of Pro-Resolving Mediators in Endometriosis: An Integrative Review
Reprinted from: *Int. J. Mol. Sci.* **2021**, *22*, 4370, doi:10.3390/ijms22094370 123

Renata Voltolini Velho, Eliane Taube, Jalid Sehouli and Sylvia Mechsner
Neurogenic Inflammation in the Context of Endometriosis—What Do We Know?
Reprinted from: *Int. J. Mol. Sci.* **2021**, *22*, 13102, doi:10.3390/ijms222313102 133

Sarah Brunty, Kristeena Ray Wright, Brenda Mitchell and Nalini Santanam
Peritoneal Modulators of EZH2-miR-155 Cross-Talk in Endometriosis
Reprinted from: *Int. J. Mol. Sci.* **2021**, *22*, 3492, doi:10.3390/ijms22073492 145

About the Editor

Antonio Simone Laganà

Medical Doctor at the Department of Obstetrics and Gynecology, "Filippo Del Ponte" Hospital, University of Insubria, Varese, Italy.

Antonio Simone Laganà was born in Reggio Calabria (Italy) on 8th May 1986. He is Deputy of the Special Interest Group for Endometriosis & Endometrial Disorders (SIGEED) of the European Society of Human Reproduction and Embryology (ESHRE) and Ambassador of the World Endometriosis Society (WES).

His research interests include endometriosis, reproductive immunology, infertility, gynaecological endocrinology, laparoscopy, and hysteroscopy. He is the author of more than 300 papers published in PubMed-indexed international peer-reviewed journals, and his presence is often requested as an invited speaker at international congresses. He is currently an editor of high-impact journals, including Scientific Reports, PLOS One, Journal of Minimally Invasive Gynecology, Journal of Ovarian Research, Gynecologic and Obstetric Investigation, and many others.

He is habilitated as Associate Professor in Italy for Gynecology and Obstetrics.

Review

Molecular Basis of Endometriosis and Endometrial Cancer: Current Knowledge and Future Perspectives

Milan Terzic [1,2,3], Gulzhanat Aimagambetova [4,*], Jeannette Kunz [4], Gauri Bapayeva [2], Botagoz Aitbayeva [2], Sanja Terzic [1] and Antonio Simone Laganà [5]

1. Department of Medicine, School of Medicine, Nazarbayev University, Kabanbay Batyr Avenue 53, Nur-Sultan 010000, Kazakhstan; milan.terzic@nu.edu.kz or terzicmm@pitt.edu (M.T.); sanja.terzic@nu.edu.kz (S.T.)
2. National Research Center for Maternal and Child Health, Clinical Academic Department of Women's Health, University Medical Center, Turan Avenue 32, Nur-Sultan 010000, Kazakhstan; gauri.bapaeva@gmail.com (G.B.); aitbayeva_botagoz@inbox.ru (B.A.)
3. Department of Obstetrics, Gynecology and Reproductive Sciences, University of Pittsburgh School of Medicine, 300 Halket Street, Pittsburgh, PA 15213, USA
4. Department of Biomedical Sciences, School of Medicine, Nazarbayev University, Kabanbay Batyr Avenue 53, Nur-Sultan 010000, Kazakhstan; jeannette.kunz@nu.edu.kz
5. Department of Obstetrics and Gynecology, "Filippo Del Ponte" Hospital, University of Insubria, 21100 Varese, Italy; antoniosimone.lagana@uninsubria.it
* Correspondence: gulzhanat.aimagambetova@nu.edu.kz

Abstract: The human endometrium is a unique tissue undergoing important changes through the menstrual cycle. Under the exposure of different risk factors in a woman's lifetime, normal endometrial tissue can give rise to multiple pathologic conditions, including endometriosis and endometrial cancer. Etiology and pathophysiologic changes behind such conditions remain largely unclear. This review summarizes the current knowledge of the pathophysiology of endometriosis and its potential role in the development of endometrial cancer from a molecular perspective. A better understanding of the molecular basis of endometriosis and its role in the development of endometrial pathology will improve the approach to clinical management.

Keywords: endometriosis; endometrial cancer; ovarian cancer; molecular basis of endometriosis

1. Morphological Features of the Human Endometrium

The uterine endometrium is an inner mucosal layer of the uterine cavity with the unique ability to regenerate or shed depending on the phases of the menstrual cycle and hormonal levels [1,2]. The human endometrium consists of two layers: functional (stratum functionalis) and basal (stratum basalis). The endometrium undergoes structural modification and changes in specialized cells in response to fluctuations of estrogen and progesterone during the menstrual cycle [3]. The basal layer of the endometrium is responsible for the regeneration of functional layer during the proliferative phase [4–6]. A hypothesis on the regeneration process of the endometrium suggests that the functional layer quality depends on endometrial progenitors/stem cells located in the basal layer [7–9]. However, understanding of the regenerative mechanism of the endometrium during the menstrual cycle and the location of endometrial progenitor/stem cells have not been fully elucidated [10–12]. The traditional morphological theory of the endometrium describes it as two-dimensional (2D) histological structure [13–15]. However, due to the complexity of the morphology of the endometrial glands, the technical characteristics of 2D histopathological imaging have been found to be insufficient [4].

It was hypothesized that clonal genomic alterations in histologically normal endometrial glands may change the stereoscopic structure of the endometrial glands. Three-dimensional (3D) pathological morphology of tissue affected by adenomyosis and 3D morphology of the normal endometrial glands was compared using 3D full-thickness images of the human uterine endometrium with microscopy [4]. 3D imaging revealed a more complex network of endometrial glands in human endometrium than was observed with traditional 2-dimensional (2D) imaging [4]. Using 3D imaging, Yamaguchi and co-authors (2021) found specific morphological features of human endometrial glands, including occluded glands, the plexus of the basal glands, and the gland-sharing plexus with other glands, which were not observed in the past using 2D histological methods [4]. The 3D analysis of the endometrial layers clarified that the plexus structure of the glands expanded horizontally along the muscular layer. Furthermore, these morphological features were detected regardless of age or phase of the menstrual cycle, suggesting that they are basic components of the normal human endometrium [4]. These novel findings suggest that 2D histology, which has been in use for more than 100 years, does not adequately depict the morphology of the endometrium. A clearer picture of the structure of the human could develop our understanding of various endometrial conditions and the etiology of endometriosis and endometrial cancer (EC). These diseases significantly affect reproductive age women and impact their quality of life [16–18]. Understanding the pathogenesis, immunohistochemical and molecular mechanisms of these conditions could improve the management of patients with endometriosis and EC [19–22].

2. Endometriosis
2.1. Definition, Epidemiology and Classification

Endometriosis is an estrogen-dependent inflammatory disorder of the endometrium that is characterized by the presence of functionally active endometrial tissue, stroma and glands outside the uterine cavity [21,23–26]. This condition estimated to affect up to 11% of women in reproductive age (or ∼200 million women) worldwide and up to 50% of women with pelvic pain or infertility [21,24,25,27,28]. The etiology of endometriosis is largely unknown. Previous research has shown that endometriosis is prevalent after menarche and dramatically drops after menopause, which has led researchers to believe that the disorder is estrogen- and progesterone-dependent [26,27,29].

There are different classifications of endometriosis based on staging and types (Table 1) [30]. According to the revised American Society for Reproductive Medicine (ASRM) scoring system [31,32], endometriosis is classified into four stages based on the localization and extension of the implants. The disease is classified as peritoneal, ovarian, or deep infiltrating endometriosis, which can be roughly described as the presence of endometrial tissue expanding to a depth of more than 5 mm below the peritoneum [22,32,33]. The classification includes four stages based on the severity, quantity, location, depth, and size of growths, those stages being stage I (minimal disease), stage II (mild disease), stage III (moderate disease), and stage IV (severe disease) [26,33,34]. This classification, however, has not been shown to be a reliable predictor of clinical outcomes.

As the supplement to the ASRM classification, and in order to provide a morphologically descriptive classification of deep infiltrating endometriosis, the ENZIAN classification was developed (Table 1) [30]. It takes into account retroperitoneal structures.

The Endometriosis Fertility Index (EFI) is another attempt to improve the endometriosis classification (Table 1). The EFI aims to predict pregnancy rates in patients with surgically documented endometriosis who attempt non-IVF conception. The EFI classification is a scoring system that includes assessment of factors related to a patient's history at the time of surgery, of adnexal function at conclusion of surgery, and of the extension of endometriosis [30].

Table 1. Classification of endometriosis.

Classification			
American Society for Reproductive Medicine (ASRM)			
Staging	Points		
Stage 1—Minimal Endometriosis	1–5		
Stage 2—Mild Endometriosis	6–15		
Stage 3—Moderate Endometriosis	16–40		
Stage 4—Severe Endometriosis	>40		
ENZIAN (supplement to ASRM)			
Compartments			
Compartment A: vagina, recto-vaginal septum;			
Compartment B: uterosacral ligaments to the pelvic wall (BB: bilateral involvement);			
Compartment C: rectum and sigmoid colon.			
		Disease severity	Invasion
		Grade 1:	<1 cm
		Grade 2:	1–3 cm
		Grade 3:	>3 cm
			Deep endometriosis invasion beyond the pelvis
			FA: adenomyosis
			FB: bladder invasion
			FU: intrinsic ureteral endometriosis;
			FI: bowel disease cranial to the sigmoid colon
			FO: other locations
The Endometriosis Fertility Index (EFI)			
Historical factor	Years	Points	
Patient age	≤35	2	
	36–39	1	
	≥40	0	
Duration of infertility	≤3	1	
	>3	0	
Prior pregnancy	Yes	1	
	No	0	
		Score	Description
		4	Normal
		3	Mild
		2	Moderate
		1	Severe
		0	Absent or nonfunctional

Following another classification, endometriosis is subdivided into three types: superficial peritoneal disease, ovarian endometrioma, and deep endometriotic lesions [35,36]. Adenomyosis, as "internal" uterine endometriosis, is characterized by the presence of endometrial glands and stromas within the myometrium that causes myometrial inflammation and hypertrophy [35,37,38]. Adenomyosis can be classified in several different subtypes: (a) intrinsic adenomyosis, (b) extrinsic adenomyosis, (c) adenomyosis externa, and (d) focal adenomyosis located in the outer myometrium [35,37,38]. Although there are many studies supporting this new classification, international consensus has not yet been achieved [35].

A major disadvantage of all existing classifications is that no one of them links the severity of the pain with the findings (imaging, laparoscopic) [39]. Some patients who are classified as "severe" by ASRM experience little pain but have associated infertility. Others, with only superficial red and blue lesions and minor adhesions, may experience severe pain and consequently a low quality of life [39–41].

Abrao and Miller recently proposed a new classification system [42]. They propose that a classification should (1) clearly describe the sites and extent of disease; (2) provide a close correlation with the symptoms of endometriosis; (3) reflect the surgical difficulty encountered relative to the disease location; (4) be user-friendly with tools that are conducive to support a surgeon's busy practice by enabling completion of documentation immediately upon procedure conclusion; (5) be validated for both pain and infertility; (6) create a comprehensive universal language that is meaningful for clinical practitioners and researchers [39,42].

2.2. Risk Factors of Endometriosis

A number of modifiable and non-modifiable risk factors have been reported to be both positively and negatively associated with the development of endometriosis (Figure 1) [27,28,43,44]. Non-modifiable risk factors known to be associated with endometriosis are the following: genetic, endocrine, immunological, and ethnicity [21,45]. There are also modifiable factors, the effect of which could be decreased substantially by lifestyle changes. Those factors are microbiotic, environmental factors (exposure to endocrine-disrupting chemicals), alcohol/caffeine intake, smoking, and physical activity [27]. Those factors may influence estrogen levels and contribute to the development of endometriosis [27].

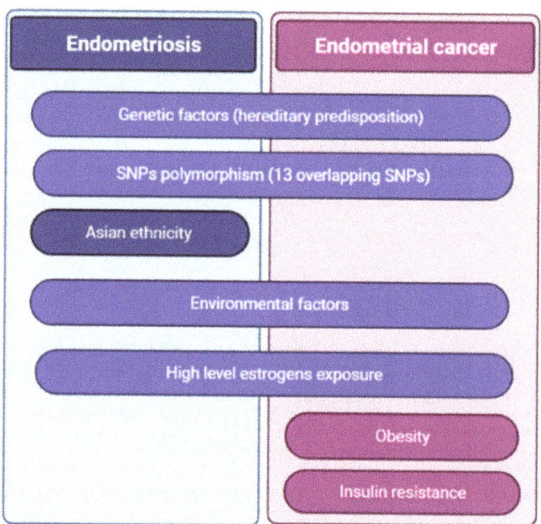

Figure 1. Risk factors for endometriosis and endometrial cancer. Created at BioRender.com (accessed on 15 July 2021).

The risk of endometriosis has been strongly linked to ethnicity. Many researchers have reported a nine-fold increase in risk of endometriosis development among women of Asian ethnicity if compared with the European-American Caucasian female population [27,43,46]. Among other factors, prolonged estrogen exposure (e.g., early age at menarche, shorter menstrual cycles, nulliparity) [47], low body mass index, and uterine outlet obstruction [48] have been suggested as predisposing to endometriosis.

It is well known that endometriosis has a strong genetic predisposition [25,43]. The evidence for an association between genetic polymorphisms and risk of endometriosis is robust [43]. Together with the strong link to hereditary factors, development of endometriosis is also affected by environmental exposures [26]. Environmental factors such as elevated levels of phthalate esters, persistent organochlorine pollutants, perfluorochemicals, and exposure to cigarette smoke can increase risk of developing endometriosis by inducing oxidative stress, altering hormonal homeostasis, or by changing immune responses [43]. Maternal exposure to diethylstilbestrol (DES) has been associated with a greater risk of endometriosis in female offspring [28].

Modifiable risk factors such as caffeine intake have been hypothesized to be influential in the pathology of gynecological disease due to its ability to influence estradiol levels [27,49]. Much like caffeine, alcohol intake and tobacco smoking are hypothesized to alter reproductive hormones due to the activation of aromatases leading to increased conversion of testosterone to estrogens [27]. Moreover, tobacco smoking may also increase the inflammatory response. Physical activity has been shown to reduce the risk of developing many gynecological diseases [27,50]. Other risk factors, such as the presence of lower genital tract infections, have also been proposed as risk factors. [43,51].

Some genetic factors have been found to serve as risk factors for endometriosis. Genome-wide association studies have, to date, identified 19 independent single-nucleotide polymorphisms (SNPs) as being significantly associated with endometriosis [52]. Moreover, the authors found a significant genetic overlap between endometriosis and EC in a genetic correlation analysis, which found 13 SNPs that appeared to be involved in development of both conditions [52].

2.3. Pathophysiology of Endometriosis

To date, the etiology and pathogenesis of endometriosis remains controversial. Multiple theories have been proposed to explain the pathogenesis of endometriosis [24,25,38]. Among the most recognized and reasonable are retrograde menstrual blood flow, coelomic metaplasia, and Müllerian remnants theories [21,24,39,53,54]. Amongst the various hypotheses, the one that has the greatest consensus is Sampsons' retrograde menstruation. Retrograde menstruation is the process in which endometrial cells and fragments of the tissue shed during menstrual bleeding and are transported into the peritoneal cavity due to the retroperistaltic movements of the fallopian tubes [21,24,53]. Implantation of these particles and subsequent proliferation during the menstrual cycle leads to the damage of pelvic organs at positions of implantation [21]. However, the hypothesis about the retrograde menstruation as a potential cause of endometriosis does not explain localization of endometrial tissue that can be found in rare cases of extragonadal endometriosis and endometriosis in male patients [26]. Another theory suggests that endometriosis develops due to endometrial cells transferred through the lymphatic system to other parts of the body, where they further grow and proliferate [21,24,26]. Additionally, it has been proposed that circulating blood cells originating from bone marrow differentiate into endometriotic tissue at various body sites [24,55]. Distant organ endometriosis, such as lung and brain endometriosis, is very rarely described and might be explained by vascular spread [21,24].

Meyer's hypothesis about coelomic metaplasia suggests development of endometriosis from the visceral epithelium, which can be converted to endometrial tissue by metaplastic processes [21,39].

More recent studies suggest that endometriosis is a pelvic inflammatory condition, so called "peritonitis without germs" [39,53]. This is based on the fact that the peritoneal fluid has an increased concentration of activated macrophages and an inflammatory profile in the cytokine/chemokine axis [39,56]. Cousins and Gargett in 2018 proposed that the human endometrium regenerates cyclically every month mediated by endometrial stem/progenitor cells such as CD140b+, CD146+, or SUSD2+ endometrial mesenchymal stem cells (eMSCs) [57]. N-cadherin + endometrial epithelial progenitor cells and side population cells may also contribute to the pathogenesis of the disease. They hypothesized that the eMSCs may have a role in the generation of progesterone-resistant phenotype endometrial stromal fibroblasts [39,57]. According to the other recent theories, deregulation of genes and the Wingless-related integration site (Wnt)/β-catenin signaling pathway would produce an aberration and the axial extension of the identity of the anterior-posterior patterning, whilst a deregulation of Hox genes and cofactor pre-B-cell leukemia homeobox 1 (Pbx1) produces an aberration in the segmentation of the mesoderm [21]. This may cause aberrant placement of stem cells with endometrial phenotype and maintain them in a quiescent niche. Transcriptional activity induces the expression of vascular endothelial growth factor (VEGF) that stimulates the vascular endothelial cell. On the other hand, Müllerian inhibiting factor (MIF) induces endometrial cell mitosis, whose survival is supported by the activation of antiapoptotic gene B-cell lymphoma 2 (Bcl-2), by the degradation of the extracellular matrix by matrix metalloproteinases (MMPs) via intercellular adhesion molecule 1 (ICAM-1) and vascular cell adhesion protein 1 (VCAM-1), creating the conditions for differentiation, adhesion, proliferation, and survival of ectopic endometrial cells [21]. This will lead to decreased apoptosis of ectopic endometrial-like cells [58–60], which escape from immune surveillance, and subsequently implant and proliferate. According to a recent review by Patel and colleagues, there is growing evidence that hormonal and immune factors create a pro-inflammatory microenvironment that support the persistence of endometriosis [61]. It is clear there is still much to learn about the nature and pathophysiology of endometriosis, and development of these theories could contribute to a greater understanding of the disease.

2.4. Clinical Presentation and Diagnostic Tools

Endometriosis is difficult to diagnose for many reasons: lack of clear understanding of etiologic factors, diversity of hypotheses for pathogenesis, different clinical presentation of the disease, and existence of asymptomatic cases [62]. Careful patient interview including family history, detailed examination, and additional imaging work-up are required for diagnosis [63,64].

Most women diagnosed with endometriosis present with multiple diverse symptoms [25]. Commonly reported complaints include chronic pelvic pain, dysmenorrhea, dyspareunia, dyschezia, and infertility/subfertility [25,33,39].

Chronic pelvic pain accounts for 10% of outpatient gynecologic visits, while local pain or tenderness on pelvic examination is associated with pelvic disease in 97% of patients and with endometriosis in 66% of patients [65]. Dysmenorrhea and general pelvic pain are common symptoms of endometriosis, regardless of age at diagnosis [66]. Pelvic pain due to endometriosis is usually chronic (lasting ≥6 months) and is associated with dysmenorrhea (in 50 to 90% of cases), dyspareunia, deep pelvic pain, and lower abdominal pain with or without back and loin pain [65]. Most women experience pain of different severity: from mild or moderate pain (pain usually requiring medication) to severe pain (pain requiring medications and bed rest) during menses over the lifetime [66]. Pain in endometriosis has a complex mechanism. Increased systemic and local proinflammatory cytokines and growth factors due to the chronic inflammation in endometriosis contribute to the mechanism of chronic pain development through persistent noxious stimulation, chronic inflammation, and nerve injury, which will alter pain processing and result in central sensitization [25,62]. Surgical treatment in many cases increases central sensitization, and patients often report worsening of symptoms after surgery [25,67]. The severity of pain is often associated with the depth of endometriotic infiltration rather than the size of the lesion or cyst [25,62,68]. Dyspareunia is another common symptom that is closely related to pain and nerve sensitization [25].

Some patients may experience gastrointestinal (nausea and vomiting, more frequent bowel movements accompanying pelvic pain) and urinary (frequent urination when experiencing menstrual pain) symptoms [65,66].

Infertility and subfertility are other important issues related to endometriosis. In cases of severe and deep infiltrating endometriosis [22,33,69], the mechanism of infertility is the alteration of normal anatomy of the reproductive organs [25]. However, in cases of a small ectopic endometrial implants/lesions, the mechanism of infertility is not clear yet. The authors suggested an endometrial defect as the explanation of implantation impairment in endometriosis. This hypothesis is supported by numerous studies showing decreased expression of several biomarkers of implantation [25,69].

Following the key steps during the initial clinical examination in the diagnosis of women with endometriosis, imaging investigations should be done in order to confirm the condition. Some biological tests invented currently have little or no merit in the diagnosis of endometriosis, and no biomarker tests have been identified to be conclusive [26,62,70,71]. In contrast, imaging techniques led to substantial improvements in the diagnosis of endometriosis [25,62,72]. The most helpful tools are transvaginal ultrasound (TVUS) [73,74] and MRI [62,72]. In addition, sigmoid, ileocecal, and urological lesions can be detected with supplementary radiological techniques such as transrectal sonography (TRS), rectal endoscopic sonography (RES) [75,76], multidetector CT scan with retrograde colonic opacification and late urography, and/or uro-MRI [62,77]. However, a recent Cochrane meta-analysis reported inconclusive data from TRS and RES studies [77]. If using these methods, it is important to remember that TRS (5 MHz frequency) enables a limited analysis of the rectosigmoid colon, whereas RES (7.5–12 MHz) provides an overview of the whole sigmoid and rectosigmoid colon with higher spatial resolution [72].

3. Endometrial Cancer
3.1. Definition, Epidemiology and Classification

Endometrial cancer is a malignant disease of the inner layer of the uterus (endometrium) [3,78]. It is one of the most common gynecological malignant tumors in developed countries [3,78–80]. In 2012, 527,600 women worldwide were diagnosed with EC, and the mortality rate was 1.7 to 2.4 per 100,000 women [81]. According to the American Cancer Society (ACS), in 2021, there will be an estimated 66,570 new cases of the uterine body cancer diagnosed in the United States and more than 12,940 deaths [82]. These calculations include both EC and uterine sarcomas. Up to 10% of uterine body cancers are sarcomas, so the actual numbers for EC cases and deaths are slightly lower than these estimates [82].

Nowadays, worldwide, EC is the seventh most common malignant disorder, but incidence varies among regions [3]. In less developed countries, risk factors are less common and EC is rare, although specific mortality is higher. Uterine corpus cancer is the 6th leading cause of cancer death among women in the United States and the 8th leading cause of cancer-related death amongst European women [83]. The incidence is ten times higher in North America and Europe than in less developed countries; in these regions, this cancer is the most common of the female genital organs and the 4th most common site after breast, lung, and colorectal cancers [3,83].

During the past two decades, the incidence and mortality rate for EC has increased by more than 100% [80,84,85]. Moreover, the incidence varies ~10-fold worldwide, with estimated age-standardized rates of 15 per 100,000 women and higher in 2018 in Europe and North America (developed countries) [84,85].

EC affects mainly post-menopausal women [86]. The average age of women diagnosed with EC is 60. It is uncommon in women under the age of 45 [82].

ECs are classified into various histological subtypes, including endometrioid EC, serous EC, clear-cell EC, mixed EC, and uterine carcinosarcoma (UCS), which differ in their frequency, clinical presentation, prognosis, and associated epidemiological risk factors [82,83].

Most EC are adenocarcinomas, and endometrioid cancer is the most common type of adenocarcinoma [82]. Endometrioid cancers arise from the glandular cells of the endometrium, and they look like the normal endometrium. There are many variants (or sub-types) of endometrioid cancers including adenocarcinoma (with squamous differentiation), adenoacanthoma, adenosquamous (or mixed cell), secretory carcinoma, ciliated carcinoma, and villoglandular adenocarcinoma [82].

Endometrioid ECs constitute more than 80% of newly diagnosed EC cases [83]. These cancers with its subtypes are generally estrogen-dependent and have a mean age at diagnosis of 62 years [83]. In contrast, serous ECs and clear-cell ECs are relatively uncommon, accounting for ~10% and 3% of newly diagnosed ECs, are generally estrogen-independent, and are diagnosed later in life (mean of 66.5 and 65.6 years, respectively) [82,83].

The prognosis for most newly diagnosed EC patients is good, with a relative 5-year survival rate of 81.1% (2008–2014) [83,87]. The generally high survival rate for EC is largely driven by the frequent early detection of endometrioid ECs, coupled with the effectiveness of surgery for treating many early-stage, low-grade EECs.

3.2. Risk and Protective Factors of Endometrial Cancer

Multiple genetic (non-modifiable) and non-genetic (modifiable) risk factors have been associated with the development of EC (Figure 1) [78,88,89]. Genome-wide association studies have found nine independent SNPs being significantly associated with EC [52].

Race is a non-modifiable, genetic factor that plays an important role in the development of EC, as rates are highest in North America and northern Europe, lower in eastern Europe and Latin America, and the lowest in Asia and Africa [79,84,90]. Age is another non-modifiable risk factor. It is well-documented that EC primarily affects postmenopausal women, with the average age of 60 at the time of diagnosis [90]. The peak age-specific incidence is from 75 to 79 years, with 85% of cases occurring after the age of 50 and only 5% before the age of 40 [90]. Young, premenopausal women diagnosed with EC usually have other factors, contributing to the risk of the disease.

Several non-genetic risk factors are linked with an increased risk of EC, particularly for the most prevalent histological subtype of endometrioid EC [78]. These include obesity, physical inactivity, excess of endogenous estrogens, insulin resistance, and polycystic ovary syndrome [3,78,79,84,88]. In addition, conditions involving excess of exogenous estrogens due to hormone replacement with unopposed estrogen (i.e., estrogen therapy without progesterone) predispose women to endometrial cancer [88,90].

Tamoxifen (selective estrogen receptor modulator (SERM)) used for breast cancer treatment approximately doubles the risk of both endometrioid and non-endometrioid types of EC if administered for 5 years and longer [78,88]. The mechanism behind is antiestrogenic effects in the breast and proestrogenic effects in the uterus [88,91].

The recent systematic review studying risk factors of EC concluded the presence of strong evidence associating increased body mass index (BMI) and obesity with the risk of EC development [78,85,90,92]. According to the US statistics, 57% of all ECs are attributable to obesity [76,80,86]. In the United Kingdom (UK) almost half of all ECs are attributed to overweight (BMI $\geq$ 25 kg/m^2) and obesity (BMI $\geq$ 30 kg/m^2) [93]. If compared with all other cancers, EC has the strongest association with obesity [78,88,93]. Women with a normal BMI have a much lower lifetime risk of EC (up to 3%), but for every 5-unit increase in BMI, the risk of EC increases by more than 50% [88,93,94]. Although the average age at diagnosis is 63 years, EC incidence is increasing among young obese women [88]. Specific lipid metabolites, including phospholipids and sphingolipids (sphingomyelins), demonstrated good accuracy for the detection of EC [93]. The underling mechanisms of the association of obesity with EC are not fully understood; however, they likely include higher estrogen levels in postmenopausal women due to aromatase activity and adipose tissue conversion of androgens into estrogens, hyperinsulinemia, and chronic inflammation [78,95,96].

As a condition closely associated with insulin resistance and obesity, highly suggestive evidence that diabetes mellitus increases the risk of EC was reported in recent systematic reviews [78,97]. Hyperinsulinemia, which is a common phenomenon prior to diabetes onset, likely has a causal association with EC through direct mitogenic effects or by increasing the levels of bioavailable estrogen through a reduction in sex hormone binding globulin levels [78,98].

However, there are some factors that have protective effect against EC [3,78,88]. Those factors include parity (with an inverse association between parity and the risk of endometrial cancer) and oral contraceptive pills [88]. The recent systematic review studying risk factors of EC found strong evidence for a 40% reduction in endometrial cancer incidence among parous compared to nulliparous women [78]. Hormonal changes during pregnancy may explain this association, usually featured by increased progesterone production with protective effects on the endometrium [78].

Oral contraceptive use reduces the risk of endometrial cancer up to 40%. Moreover, the longer the administration, the stronger the protective effect, which can persist even decades after cessation [88,99]. Additionally, coffee consumption has been shown to be inversely associated with EC [78,100,101].

Some researchers reported evidence that smoking reduced the risk of EC in cohort studies, although the evidence became strong when case–control studies were included [78,101]. The majority of the published cohort studies showed a reduction in risk of endometrial cancer among current or former smokers compared to never smokers [78,92,102,103]. A mechanism behind the link between decreased incidence of EC and smoking is the possible anti-estrogenic effect of nicotine; however, it has limited direct evidence and requires further investigations [78].

3.3. Pathophysiology of Endometrial Cancer

Based on epidemiology, histopathology, prognosis, and treatment, EC can appear as type 1 (endometrioid), affecting approximately 80% of patients, and type 2 (non-endometrioid), affecting approximately 20% of patients [78,85,88]. Type 1 tumors develop from atypical glandular hyperplasia. This type is related to long-lasting unopposed estrogen stimulation and often preceded by endometrial hyperplasia [3,90]. The molecular basis of this process is not clear yet [3].

Carcinomas of type 1 are associated with significant incidences of *CTNNB1*, *KRAS*, and *POLE* oncogene mutations; phosphatase and tensin homolog (*PTEN*) tumor suppressor gene; defects in deoxyribonucleic acid (DNA) mismatch repair; and near-diploid karyotype (Table 2) [3,88,104]. From a molecular point of view, ECs resemble proliferative rather than secretory endometrium [3,78]. Specific tumor suppressor gene, *PTEN* that is expressed most highly in an estrogen-rich environment, could be responsible for the disease development. Progestogens affect *PTEN* expression and promote involution of *PTEN*-mutated endometrial cells in various histopathological settings [3,78]. This hypothesis can explain therapeutic effect of progestogens in EC cases.

Table 2. Molecular mechanisms of endometrial cancer development.

Endometrial Cancer Type	Molecular Factors/Genes	Changes in Function Leading to Endometrial Cancer
	Type 1	
	CTNNB1	Mutation
	POLE	Mutation
	KRAS	Mutation
	PTEN	Loss
	AKT	Up-regulation
	PI3KSA	Up-regulation
	G_1/S cell cycle phase	Progression
	Bcl-2	Loss of down-regulation
	MLH1/MSH6	Instability
	DNA	Mismatch
	Type 2	
	TP53	Mutation
	ERBB-2 (HER2/neu)	Overexpression
	p-16	Inactivation
	E-cadherin	Reduction

Type 2 tumors include predominantly unspecified EC, clear-cell, carcinosarcoma and high-grade EC, and mixed (typically endometrioid and a high-grade non-endometrioid pattern) variants [103]. Type 2 tumors are associated with mutations in TP53 and *ERBB-2* (*HER2/neu*) overexpression (Table 2) [3]. The features of endometrial serous carcinomas are the following: presence of *TP53* mutations, an overall low mutation rate, and frequent copy-number alterations [88].

For the majority of EC cases, sporadic mutations are responsible; however, approximately 5% of EC cases are caused by inherited genetic mutations. EC caused by genetic predispositions typically occur 10 to 20 years before sporadic EC [90]. The following syndromes are known to predispose to EC:

1. Lynch syndrome (LS), an autosomal dominant syndrome, results from a germline mutation in one of four DNA mismatch repair genes—*MLH1*, *MSH2*, *MSH6*, or *PMS2* [90]. It is associated with significantly increased lifetime risk of colorectal, ECs and some other cancers [90,105].
2. Cowden syndrome: Cowden syndrome is an autosomal dominant syndrome characterized by *PTEN* mutations. It is associated with a 19% to 28% risk of EC by age 70 [90].

Currently, there is no approved effective screening program for EC. However, for patients with genetic syndromes, because of the significantly increased risk of the disease onset in reproductive age, the ACS recommends annual EC screening with endometrial biopsies starting at age 35 [85,90,105].

3.4. Clinical Presentation and Diagnostic Tools

Nowadays, for the general population there are no approved screening programs for the early detection of EC [90].

Patients' evaluation should include thorough history taking, especially focusing on family history and possible risk factors [90]. Symptoms of EC are non-specific; thus, diagnosis of the condition is challenging in some cases. Abnormal uterine bleeding (AUB) is the most common symptom of endometrial cancer and is present in 90% of affected patients [3,84,85,90,106,107]. However, this symptom appears to be present in many other female genital disorders. Furthermore, as AUB can also be a sign of EC in premenopausal women, who comprise 20% of cases of EC, the approach to a patient with abnormal uterine bleeding will depend on the age group this patient belongs to (reproductive or postmenopausal) [79,84,85]. All postmenopausal women with AUB, especially if any of the risk factors discussed above are present [108,109], should undergo endometrial biopsy [3,79,84]. The risk of EC in postmenopausal women with uterine bleeding is up to 10% [3,84,90].

Women may also present with vague complaints of increased vaginal discharge or an incidental finding of a thickened endometrium on imaging [90]. Patients with advanced stages of the disease may complain of pelvic pain, abdominal distension, early satiety, changes in bowel or bladder function, pain during intercourse, and dyspnea because of pleural effusion [90]. However, it is important to keep in mind that up to 5% of patients with EC are asymptomatic [3,90].

Transvaginal ultrasound (TVUS) is a widely used approach for further investigations in patients suffering from AUB [3,85]. After the thorough investigation via sonography, the vast majority will undergo endometrial sampling [110,111]. The most useful approach to diagnose and confirm EC is endometrial sampling with histological examination [3,84,106,107].

The strategy with TVUS, followed by endometrial biopsy if an abnormality is detected, is the most cost-effective; therefore, TVUS is considered as the first step in any woman presenting with AUB [3,85,112,113].

Endometrial biopsy could be performed using different devices [84]. However, the most popular are the following methods: dilation and curettage (D&C), Pipelle sampling (Pipelle de Cornier prototype), and hysteroscopy with targeted biopsy. Histological examination reports may include presence of endometrial cells, atypical glandular cell of uncertain significance, or adenocarcinoma in situ [3,85,90].

4. Molecular Basis of Endometriosis and Endometrial Pathology
4.1. Genetic and Epigenetic Changes in Endometriosis
4.1.1. Genetic Association and Meta-Analyses Studies

Endometriosis is a complex disease with multiple genetic and environmental factors contributing to disease pathology [114,115]. First evidence for the presence of a heritable component contributing to endometriosis came from studies published as early as the 1950s [116] that demonstrated familial clustering of endometriosis [117–119]. These studies showed that first-degree relatives of affected women have a five to seven times higher risk of being diagnosed with endometriosis [117,118]. Familial endometriosis was further shown to be associated with earlier age of symptom onset and a more severe disease course [120]. The genetic predisposition to endometriosis was corroborated by twin studies that showed an increased disease risk in monozygotic versus dizygotic twins, and the estimated contribution of genetic factors to endometriosis was up to 51% [121].

Large-scale genetic linkage and meta-analyses represented an important means to identify endometriosis susceptibility loci [122]. Most notable, family-based linkage studies of endometriosis conducted by the International Endogene Consortium in two combined cohorts of Australian and UK families identified two linkage regions that likely harbor rare causal variants, one on chromosome 10q26 [123] and one on chromosome 7p13-15 [124]. A third region of suggestive linkage identified by Treloar et al. is located on chromosome 20p13 [123]. Chromosome 10q26 contains two genes that were previously implicated in candidate gene mapping studies as potential endometriosis risk loci, *EMX2* [125], which encodes a transcription factor required for reproductive-tract development [126], and the tumor suppressor gene *PTEN*, which encodes a phosphatidylinositol-3,4,5-triphosphate 3-phosphatase [88].

Both *EMX2* and *PTEN* were previously reported to be aberrantly expressed in endometrial lesions [125,127–130]. However, systematic resequencing of the region could not confirm either gene as an endometriosis risk locus [131]. Instead, *CYP2C19* (Cytochrome P450 Family 2 Subfamily C Member 19), a nearby gene, was found to be weakly associated with endometriosis [132,133]. *CYP2C19* is a member of the cytochrome p450 family and encodes an aromatase associated with the metabolism of drugs and estrogen [134,135]. The linkage peak on chromosome 7p13-15 may represent a susceptibility allele with high penetrance for more severe forms of endometriosis [123], but the involved allele remains elusive.

Other genome-wide association studies conducted in women of European ancestry led to the identification of two new genomic regions associated with a significant risk of endometriosis. The first locus with significant disease association was located to chromosome 7p15.2 [135]; this region may regulate expression levels of nearby gene(s) involved in the development of the uterus and endometrium [136]. A second genetic variant was mapped to chromosome 1p36.12 near the *WNT4* gene [136], which is implicated in the development and function of the female reproductive tract and sex hormone metabolism. Both risk loci were independently confirmed in Japanese and European cohorts [137,138].

Genome-wide studies identified additional susceptibility loci for endometriosis [139–142]. Several candidate genes were mapped that exhibit varying degrees of disease association including genes involved in hormone signaling (*GREB1*), cell proliferation and differentiation (*ID4, CDKN2PAS*), as well as cell migration and invasion (*FN1, VEZT*) [137,138,143]. However, most polymorphisms identified by genome-wide association studies to date are located in non-coding regions, suggesting they affect the expression of nearby genes [137,138].

In conclusion, genome-wide association studies, with few exceptions, failed to confirm a clear association between endometriosis and specific risk loci. This may indicate that there are many genetic variants, each of which has a weak impact on endometriosis development, yet in combination they can significantly increase the likelihood of endometriosis and, thus, represent true endometriosis risk loci [144–146]. Detection of weak effects of gene variants influencing a complex trait such as endometriosis, therefore, requires datasets of significant size.

4.1.2. Genome Mapping Studies and Targeted Gene Sequencing

In addition to genome-wide association studies, candidate gene approaches were used to test the association of specific genes with endometriosis. These studies focused on systematic sequencing of identified risk loci or used genetic mapping where variants of a gene of interest with an inferred pathophysiological relevance are tested for association with the disease in samples of endometriosis cases and controls. These approaches identified genes involved in sex hormone metabolism and signaling, growth factor signaling, cell adhesion, apoptosis, cell-cycle regulation, detoxification, and inflammation [138]. Several studies also reported genetic aberrations in tumor suppression genes, such as TP53 and PTEN, in endometriotic tissues [88]. However, most associations identified by targeted gene mapping approaches suffered from low statistical power and lack of replication [145,146].

4.1.3. Genome-Wide Sequencing Studies

Endometriosis is characterized by the growth of ectopic endometrial-like epithelium and stroma [40,41] with neoplastic characteristics that shares striking similarities with malignancy [147]. Indeed, endometriosis shares many of the key hallmarks of cancer including resistance to apoptosis, stimulation of angiogenesis, invasion, and inflammation [148]. Moreover, endometriosis is well-established as the precursor of clear cell and endometrioid ovarian carcinomas [149]. A plausible link between benign endometriosis and endometriosis associated cancer was provided by several recent next-generation sequencing approaches [121–124]. These studies also offered important insight into the molecular basis of cancer development.

Anglesio et al. were the first to report on the genome-wide identification of somatic cancer driver mutations in deep infiltrating endometriosis [150]. Deep endometriosis represents a subtype of endometriosis that occurs under the peritoneum [40] and rarely undergoes a malignant transformation. The cited authors identified somatic mutations in *PIK3CA*, *KRAS*, and *PPP2R1A*, which encodes a regulatory subunit of protein phosphatase 2. In addition, frequent loss of function mutations in AT-rich interactive domain 1A (*ARID1A*) were detected, altogether affecting approximately one-quarter of patients subjected to comprehensive genomic analysis [150]. Targeted sequencing of a subpopulation of patients further identified *KRAS* activating mutations in one-quarter of deep endometriosis patient samples [150]. Overall, of the 24 women taking part in the study, 19 had one or more driver mutations in their endometriosis tissue that were not present in their normal tissue [151,152]. Notably, cancer-associated mutations were found only in laser microdissected epithelial cells of ovarian and extraovarian pelvic endometriotic tissues, but not in stromal cells of the same tissue. These findings suggest that the occurrence of driver mutations in the epithelium is clonal and contributes to endometriosis development independently of stroma [152].

Besides *ARID1A*, *PIK3CA*, *KRAS*, and *PPP2R1A*, several other cancer-associated genes, such as *PTEN*, *PIK3R1*, *TP53*, *FBXW7*, and *CTNNB1*, were recurrently mutated in both endometriotic and uterine endometrial epithelium samples. In particular, *KRAS* and *ARID1* are frequently mutated in the endometriotic epithelium, although these epithelia were histologically benign and normal [153,154]. All of these mutations are well characterized cancer driver mutations that are known for controlling cell proliferation and survival, angiogenesis, invasion, and DNA damage repair. Importantly, besides deep endometriosis [150], other types of endometriosis also contained somatic cancer driver mutations, including endometriotic cysts, iatrogenic endometriosis as a rare complication associated with laparoscopic supracervical hysterectomy (LASH), and eutopic normal endometrial epithelium [151,155].

How precisely cancer driver mutations affect endometriosis in histologically normal tissue is still an outstanding question. The presence of these mutations in benign endometriotic lesions is clearly non-random. However, affected epithelial cells only carried one to two somatic mutations, which is not sufficient for malignant transformation [156]. Given the known roles of driver mutations in cancer progression, one can speculate that these mutations are necessary for driving the growth of endometriotic tissue in other regions of the body. Only accumulation of additional driver mutations in combination with microenvironmental factors, such as chronic estrogen exposure and/or inflammation, may then lead to cancer development.

4.2. Endometrial Stem Cells in Pathogenesis of Endometrial Pathology

There are several theories to account for the origin of endometriosis and to explain how tissue can be scattered throughout the abdominal cavity. However, there is no single theory that can explain all clinical presentations and pathological features observed in endometriosis, and several mechanisms may in fact contribute.

The stem cell origin theory of endometriosis has gained considerable attention in recent years following the advances in molecular and genetic findings. There are two main models that are differentiated based on the tissue origin of the stem cells: stem cells arising from the regenerating uterine endometrium or stem cells originating from the bone marrow. The uterus in women is the only organ that undergoes repeated cycles of physiological damage, repair, and regeneration following menstrual shedding [114–116]. Menstrual shedding, and the subsequent repair of the endometrial functionalis, is a process unique to humans and higher-order primates [117–119]. These approximately 400 cycles of shedding and regeneration occur over a woman's lifetime. This significant regenerative capacity is thought to be driven by stem cells that reside in the terminal ends of the basalis glands at the endometrial/myometrial interface, also termed endometrial functionalis layer, which persists after menstruation and regenerates the epithelium during the proliferative phase in response to estrogen [9]. The first model proposes that circulating epithelial progenitor or stem cells intended to regenerate the uterine endometrium are shed with menstruation and may become aberrantly activated and trapped outside the uterus, thus giving rise to ectopic lesions after retrograde menstruation and trans-tubal migration in to the pelvic cavity [157].

Irrespective of the site of stem cell origin, the growth of the ectopic tissue, which retains hormone responsiveness, is further influenced by sex hormones and other factors present in the microenvironment. These factors collectively control the adhesion, proliferation, angiogenesis, and invasion of the trapped progenitor cells. The ectopic tissue, in turn, induces the recruitment of immune cells leading to local inflammation and the formation of a dysregulated inflammation–hormonal autoregulatory loop. The trapped progenitor cells thereby may form nascent glands in the epithelium through clonal expansion leading to the establishment of deep infiltrating endometriosis.

However, more studies for a better understanding of endometrial epithelial stem cell function and regulation are required to understand the eventual changes behind the endometrial pathologies.

4.3. Endometriosis as a Risk Factor for Endometrial Cancer

With respect to endometriosis itself as a risk factor for other conditions, women with endometriosis have a higher risk of infection, allergy, autoimmune disease, psychiatric conditions, preterm birth, metabolic syndrome, coronary heart disease, and cancer, especially ovarian [158] and breast cancers, and melanoma [159].

A history of endometriosis has been recognized as a precursor lesion of several types of malignancies and endometriosis-associated carcinoma [160,161].

Some investigations suggested no association between endometriosis and EC [28,149, 160,162–164]. One of the recent systematic reviews performed to search for evidence on the association of endometriosis with gynecological cancers also reported no clear association between endometriosis and EC [165]. On the other hand, some studies have reported an association between endometriosis and EC reflecting overlapping risk factors between the two conditions, including endogenous or exogenous hyperestrogenism and ovulatory dysfunction [160,166]. Another recent epidemiologic study on the association of endometriosis with malignancy reported that patients with endometriosis were significantly more likely to be diagnosed with EC at a younger age than those without endometriosis (mean age at EC diagnosis 57 years vs. 62 years; $p = 5.0 \times 10^{-11}$) [167]. Moreover, two population-based studies have shown associations between endometriosis and EC [52,168,169].

If we analyze the role of risk factors in the development of endometriosis and EC, some overlapping genetic factors (Figure 1) are worth highlighting. Genetic correlation analyses by Painter et al. (2018) revealed the presence of "weak to moderate, but significant" genetic overlap between endometriosis and EC [52,144]. Namely, in the cross-disease meta-analysis the authors found 13 SNPs that appeared to be involved in replication. These SNPs are the following: rs2475335, rs9865110, rs2278868, rs12303900, rs9349553, rs10008492, rs9530566, rs10459129, rs2198894, rs7042500, rs17693745, rs7515106, and rs1755833 [52,144]. SNP rs2475335, which is located on chromosome 9p23, was most significantly associated with both diseases ($p = 4.9 \times 10^{-8}$) [52].

To conclude about the link between endometriosis and EC, epidemiological studies have reported conflicting data for an association between the diagnosis of endometriosis and risk of EC [52]. More large-scale investigations are required in order to confirm or refute the link between endometriosis and risk of EC development.

5. Clinical Applications of Current Knowledge and Directions for Future Research

5.1. Molecular Basis for a Specific Therapeutic Approach

Collectively, studies performed over the last decade shed new light on the pathophysiology of endometriosis. Linkage and sequencing studies have identified genes and pathways important for endometriosis development and have highlighted potential causal links between endometriosis and endometriosis-associated cancer. The identification of women with endometriosis who are at risk of cancer development provides a basis for improved diagnosis and prognosis and is likely to aid in improved cancer surveillance of patients at risk.

As treatment of endometrial cancer was based on histological characteristics and staging [170,171], prognosis was not promising, especially if the stage is advanced [172–174]. Therefore, in the last couple of years, efforts have been directed to molecular aberrations within the specific tumor, as a novel biological targeted therapy with promising outcomes in clinical trials [175].

Various biomarkers [176], such as *mTOR* pathway disruptions, loss of estrogen and progesterone nuclear expression, TP53 mutation, changes in Wnt-signaling, or *L1CAM* expression, were identified as a link to endometrial cancer development [177]. All these mutations were associated with poor prognosis, but their clinical utilization is still questionable.

Preclinical investigations related to molecular-targeted therapies in ECs enabled deeper understanding of underlying mechanisms and highlighted different approaches to EC patients.

According to genomic characteristics of 373 endometrial carcinomas, The Cancer Genome Atlas (TCGA) classified EC into four molecular subtypes [178,179], which differ a lot from the molecular point, underlying risk factors, clinical and pathological features, treatment modalities, and prognosis [180–182]. These four distinct prognostic groups are *POLE* ultramutated, microsatellite instability/hypermutated, copy number-low microsatellite stable, and copy number-high/serous like.

Compared with other subtypes of tumors, prognosis for the copy number-high/serous-like group of patients is poor [183]. Poor prognosis is related to the loss of tumor suppressor *TP53* resulting in a high degree of genomic instability and rapid tumor progression and invasion [184,185]. As one-quarter of serous-like tumors have ERBB2 overexpression, there is a need to investigate the role of human epidermal growth factor receptor 2 (HER2)-targeted inhibitors [186–188]. Considering molecular similarities between high-grade endometrioid and serous carcinomas, patients of this subtype may benefit from treatment as if their tumor was serous. Moreover, specific mutations and overexpression of molecular targets in these tumors could tailor treatment in both the primary and recurrent setting.

From the clinical point of view, there is a need to create an integrated molecular risk profile for endometrial cancer. For that purpose, these four molecular subgroups were combined with additional molecular markers. Integrated molecular and clinico-pathologic risk assessment was based on a multivariate analysis of four molecular subgroups, clinical and histopathological characteristics of tumors, and various molecular classifiers. Molecular markers involved were *TP53* expression, *MSI*, *POLE* mutation, protein expression of *L1CAM, ARID1a, PTEN, ER/PR*, as well as analysis of 13 genes found to have variable expression in the TCGA classification groups (*BRAF, CDKNA2, CTNNB1, FBXW7, FGFR2, FGFR3, FOXL2, HRAS, KRAS, NRAS, PIK3CA, PPP2R1A*, and *PTEN*). This integrated model for prediction of endometrial cancer recurrence was confirmed to be more reliable than the traditional one relying on clinical and pathologic factors [189]. Moreover, this classification system enhances risk stratification of endometrial cancers. Importance for molecular subtyping was confirmed in clinical practice, as sorting of patients into molecular subgroups was confirmed to predict response rates to conventional, targeted systemic and radiotherapy [190,191]. For clinicians, molecular subtype stratification could be used in both preoperative evaluation (whether to prepare the whole set up for lymph node dissection or not) and postoperative treatment (the need for eventual adjuvant therapy). Moreover, molecular subtyping was confirmed to be very important for targeted therapy in patients with recurrent and metastatic diseases [175,177,192–194]. Thus, once the diagnosis of endometrial cancer has been established, there is a need to perform molecular subtyping, which will enable proper therapeutic approach.

5.2. Prognostic Biomarkers for Endometrial Cancer

There is no screening method for EC for the general population. Women with LS and their first-degree relatives are offered annual screening with TVUS and endometrial biopsy from the age of 35 years [90,105].

There are several types of biomarkers: gene-based biomarkers, proteins biomarkers, and hormonal biomarkers [105]. Gene-based biomarkers include the following: *PTEN*, *TP53*, microribonucleic acids (microRNAs), circulating tumor DNA, and DNA methylation. Protein biomarkers include *pRb2/p130, Ki 67, ARID1A*, cell adhesion molecules (CAMs), phosphohistone-H3 (*pHH3*), angiotensin factors, etc. The most commonly mutated genes detected in EC patients using Tao brush samples were *PTEN* and *TP53* [83].

One of the gene-based biomarkers, *PTEN* tumor suppressor, antagonizes the phosphoinositol-3-kinase/AKT signaling pathway, suppressing cell survival as well as cell proliferation [105]. A recent study suggests that *PTEN* expression in endometrial hyperplasia can be used as an early warning of heightened cancer risk [105,195]. Complete loss of *PTEN* protein expression is most commonly found in EC and endometrial hyperplasia with cytological atypia.

Another potentially useful molecular biomarker is *TP53*, which belongs to cell cycle proteins [105], and triggers cellular responses that can lead to cell-cycle arrest, senescence, differentiation, DNA repair, apoptosis, and inhibition of angiogenesis [196]. The role of *TP53* in EC and hyperplasia has been studied, showing that TP53 gene mutation is present in EC, but it is absent in endometrial hyperplasia [105,197].

The expression of the cell cycle regulator *pRb2/p130* was evaluated in EC and endometrial hyperplasia and was found to be highly expressed in the proliferative endometrium and in hyperplasia without atypia, but it was downregulated in secretory endometrium, atypical hyperplasia, and EC [105,197].

The most promising serum biomarker for EC is human epididymis protein 4 (HE4) [105]. A number of studies have looked at HE4 as a prognostic marker for EC [86,105,198,199]. Diagnostic levels range between 50 and 70 pmol/L, with a minimum 78% sensitivity and 100% specificity, even in early-stage disease [105,198]. Serum HE4 levels are found to be significantly higher in advanced stages of EC [105,199] and are predictive for disease recurrence [105].

There are many novel biomarkers under investigation. Introduction of them into clinical practice could improve timely EC diagnosis, treatment outcomes, and surveillance of EC patients.

6. Conclusions

Although diagnostic methods of endometriosis are well-developed in modern gynecology, the etiopathogenesis of the disease remains largely unknown. Lack of clear understanding of the pathologic process leads to inferable outcomes in patients suffering from endometriosis and may be linked to development of related female genital malignancy. Existing studies have reported inconclusive data for an association between endometriosis and risk of EC. Further large-scale investigations could help to answer this query. Molecular studies of endometrial tissue function and endometriosis might shed light on the real cause of the condition and the factors leading to EC development. As a result of a better understanding of the molecular basis of endometriosis and EC, patient management and outcomes could be improved.

Author Contributions: Conceptualization, M.T. and A.S.L.; methodology, M.T., A.S.L.; resources, M.T.; data curation, G.A., G.B., S.T.; writing—original draft preparation, G.A., J.K., B.A.; writing—review and editing, M.T., A.S.L.; supervision, G.B.; project administration, M.T.; funding acquisition, M.T. All authors have read and agreed to the published version of the manuscript.

Funding: This study was supported by the Nazarbayev University Grant Number 110119FD4540, 2019–2021.

Institutional Review Board Statement: Not applicable.

Informed Consent Statement: Not applicable.

Data Availability Statement: No raw data to share.

Conflicts of Interest: The authors declare no conflict of interest.

References

1. Garry, R.; Hart, R.; Karthigasu, K.A.; Burke, C. A re-appraisal of the morphological changes within the endometrium during menstruation: A hysteroscopic, histological and scanning electron microscopic study. *Hum. Reprod.* **2009**, *24*, 1393–1401. [CrossRef]
2. Emera, D.; Wagner, G. Transposable element recruitments in the mammalian placenta: Impacts and mechanisms. *Brief. Funct. Genom.* **2012**, *11*, 267–276. [CrossRef]
3. Amant, F.; Moerman, P.; Neven, P.; Timmerman, D.; Van Limbergen, E.; Vergote, I. Endometrial cancer. *Lancet* **2005**, *366*, 491–505. [CrossRef]
4. Yamaguchi, M.; Yoshihara, K.; Suda, K.; Nakaoka, H.; Yachida, N.; Ueda, H.; Sugino, K.; Mori, Y.; Yamawaki, K.; Tamura, R.; et al. Three-dimensional understanding of the morphological complexity of the human uterine endometrium. *iScience* **2021**, *24*, 102258. [CrossRef]
5. Cooke, P.S.; Spencer, T.; Bartol, F.F.; Hayashi, K. Uterine glands: Development, function and experimental model systems. *Mol. Hum. Reprod.* **2013**, *19*, 547–558. [CrossRef]
6. Gray, C.A.; Bartol, F.F.; Tarleton, B.J.; Wiley, A.A.; Johnson, G.A.; Bazer, F.W.; Spencer, T.E. Developmental Biology of Uterine Glands1. *Biol. Reprod.* **2001**, *65*, 1311–1323. [CrossRef] [PubMed]
7. Kyo, S.; Maida, Y.; Inoue, M. Stem cells in endometrium and endometrial cancer: Accumulating evidence and unresolved questions. *Cancer Lett.* **2011**, *308*, 123–133. [CrossRef]
8. Miyazaki, K.; Maruyama, T.; Masuda, H.; Yamasaki, A.; Uchida, S.; Oda, H.; Uchida, H.; Yoshimura, Y. Stem Cell-Like Differentiation Potentials of Endometrial Side Population Cells as Revealed by a Newly Developed In Vivo Endometrial Stem Cell Assay. *PLoS ONE* **2012**, *7*, e50749. [CrossRef]
9. Prianishnikov, V.A. A functional model of the structure of the epithelium of normal, hyperplastic, and malignant human endometrium: A review. *Gynecol. Oncol.* **1978**, *6*, 420–428. [CrossRef]
10. Garry, R.; Hart, R.; Karthigasu, K.; Burke, C. Structural changes in endometrial basal glands during menstruation. *BJOG Int. J. Obstet. Gynaecol.* **2010**, *117*, 1175–1185. [CrossRef]
11. Gellersen, B.; Brosens, J. Cyclic Decidualization of the Human Endometrium in Reproductive Health and Failure. *Endocr. Rev.* **2014**, *35*, 851–905. [CrossRef]

12. Santamaria, X.; Mas, A.; Cervelló, I.; Taylor, H.; Simón, C. Uterine stem cells: From basic research to advanced cell therapies. *Hum. Reprod. Updat.* **2018**, *24*, 673–693. [CrossRef]
13. E McLennan, C.; Rydell, A.H. Extent of endometrial shedding during normal menstruation. *Obstet. Gynecol.* **1965**, *26*, 605–621.
14. Filho, J.H.; Cedenho, A.P.; De Freitas, V. Correlation between endometrial dating of luteal phase days 6 and 10 of the same menstrual cycle. *Sao Paulo Med. J.* **1998**, *116*, 1734–1737. [CrossRef]
15. Johannisson, E.; Parker, R.A.; Landgren, B.-M.; Diczfalusy, E. Morphometric analysis of the human endometrium in relation to peripheral hormone levels. *Fertil. Steril.* **1982**, *38*, 564–571. [CrossRef]
16. García-Solares, J.; Donnez, J.; Donnez, O.; Dolmans, M.-M. Pathogenesis of uterine adenomyosis: Invagination or metaplasia? *Fertil. Steril.* **2018**, *109*, 371–379. [CrossRef] [PubMed]
17. Koninckx, P.R.; Ussia, A.; Adamyan, L.; Wattiez, A.; Gomel, V.; Martin, D.C. Pathogenesis of endometriosis: The genetic/epigenetic theory. *Fertil. Steril.* **2019**, *111*, 327–340. [CrossRef] [PubMed]
18. Morice, P.; Leary, A.; Creutzberg, C.; Abu-Rustum, N.; Darai, E. Endometrial cancer. *Lancet* **2016**, *387*, 1094–1108. [CrossRef]
19. Matalliotaki, C.; Matalliotakis, M.; Zervou, M.I.; Patelarou, A.; Koliarakis, I.; Spandidos, D.A.; Arici, A.; Matalliotakis, I.; Goulielmos, G.N. Epidemiological aspects of the outcomes from the treatment of endometriosis: Experience from two different geographical areas. *Exp. Ther. Med.* **2019**, *19*, 1079–1083. [CrossRef]
20. Johnatty, S.E.; Tan, Y.; Buchanan, D.D.; Bowman, M.; Walters, R.J.; Obermair, A.; Quinn, M.A.; Blomfield, P.B.; Brand, A.; Leung, Y.; et al. Family history of cancer predicts endometrial cancer risk independently of Lynch Syndrome: Implications for genetic counselling. *Gynecol. Oncol.* **2017**, *147*, 381–387. [CrossRef]
21. Laganà, A.S.; Vitale, S.G.; Salmeri, F.M.; Triolo, O.; Frangež, H.B.; Vrtačnik-Bokal, E.; Stojanovska, L.; Apostolopoulos, V.; Granese, R.; Sofo, V. Unus pro omnibus, omnes pro uno: A novel, evidence-based, unifying theory for the pathogenesis of endometriosis. *Med. Hypotheses* **2017**, *103*, 10–20. [CrossRef] [PubMed]
22. Raffaelli, R.; Garzon, S.; Baggio, S.; Genna, M.; Pomini, P.; Laganà, A.S.; Ghezzi, F.; Franchi, M. Mesenteric vascular and nerve sparing surgery in laparoscopic segmental intestinal resection for deep infiltrating endometriosis. *Eur. J. Obstet. Gynecol. Reprod. Biol.* **2018**, *231*, 214–219. [CrossRef]
23. Bulun, S.E. Endometriosis. *N. Engl. J. Med.* **2009**, *360*, 268–279. [CrossRef]
24. E Bulun, S.; Yilmaz, B.D.; Sison, C.; Miyazaki, K.; Bernardi, L.; Liu, S.; Kohlmeier, A.; Yin, P.; Milad, M.; Wei, J. Endometriosis. *Endocr. Rev.* **2019**, *40*, 1048–1079. [CrossRef] [PubMed]
25. Falcone, T.; Flyckt, R. Clinical Management of Endometriosis. *Obstet. Gynecol.* **2018**, *131*, 557–571. [CrossRef] [PubMed]
26. Terzic, M.; Aimagambetova, G.; Garzon, S.; Bapayeva, G.; Ukybassova, T.; Terzic, S.; Norton, M.; Laganà, A.S. Ovulation induction in infertile women with endometriotic ovarian cysts: Current evidence and potential pitfalls. *Minerva Med.* **2020**, *111*, 50–61. [CrossRef]
27. Hemmert, R.; Schliep, K.C.; Willis, S.; Peterson, C.M.; Louis, G.B.; Allen-Brady, K.; Simonsen, S.E.; Stanford, J.B.; Byun, J.; Smith, K.R. Modifiable life style factors and risk for incident endometriosis. *Paediatr. Périnat. Epidemiol.* **2019**, *33*, 19–25. [CrossRef] [PubMed]
28. Shafrir, A.; Farland, L.; Shah, D.; Harris, H.; Kvaskoff, M.; Zondervan, K.; Missmer, S. Risk for and consequences of endometriosis: A critical epidemiologic review. *Best Pr. Res. Clin. Obstet. Gynaecol.* **2018**, *51*, 1–15. [CrossRef] [PubMed]
29. Adam, A.M.; Altalhi, T.A.; El-Megharbel, S.M.; Saad, H.A.; Refat, M.S. Using a Modified Polyamidoamine Fluorescent Dendrimer for Capturing Environment Polluting Metal Ions Zn^{2+}, Cd^{2+}, and Hg^{2+}: Synthesis and Characterizations. *Crystals* **2021**, *11*, 92. [CrossRef]
30. Capezzuoli, T.; Clemenza, S.; Sorbi, F.; Campana, D.; Vannuccini, S.; Chapron, C.; Petraglia, F. Classification/staging systems for endometriosis: The state of the art. *Gynecol. Reprod. Endocrinol. Metab.* **2020**, *1*, 14–22.
31. Canis, M.; Donnez, J.G.; Guzick, D.S.; Halme, J.K.; Rock, J.A.; Schenken, R.S.; Vernon, M.W. Revised American Society for Reproductive Medicine classification of endometriosis: 1996. *Fertil. Steril.* **1997**, *67*, 817–821. [CrossRef]
32. Vercellini, P.; Viganò, P.; Somigliana, E.; Fedele, L. Endometriosis: Pathogenesis and treatment. *Nat. Rev. Endocrinol.* **2014**, *10*, 261–275. [CrossRef] [PubMed]
33. Laganà, A.S.; Vitale, S.G.; Trovato, M.A.; Palmara, V.I.; Rapisarda, A.M.C.; Granese, R.; Sturlese, E.; De Dominici, R.; Alecci, S.; Padula, F.; et al. Full-Thickness Excision versus Shaving by Laparoscopy for Intestinal Deep Infiltrating Endometriosis: Rationale and Potential Treatment Options. *BioMed Res. Int.* **2016**, *2016*, 3617179. [CrossRef] [PubMed]
34. Mehedintu, C.; Plotogea, M.N.; Ionescu, S.; Antonovici, M. Endometriosis still a challenge. *J. Med. Life* **2014**, *7*, 349–357. [PubMed]
35. Maruyama, S.; Imanaka, S.; Nagayasu, M.; Kimura, M.; Kobayashi, H. Relationship between adenomyosis and endometriosis; Different phenotypes of a single disease? *Eur. J. Obstet. Gynecol. Reprod. Biol.* **2020**, *253*, 191–197. [CrossRef]
36. Tosti, C.; Pinzauti, S.; Santulli, P.; Chapron, C.; Petraglia, F. Pathogenetic Mechanisms of Deep Infiltrating Endometriosis. *Reprod. Sci.* **2015**, *22*, 1053–1059. [CrossRef] [PubMed]
37. Guo, S.-W. The Pathogenesis of Adenomyosis vis-à-vis Endometriosis. *J. Clin. Med.* **2020**, *9*, 485. [CrossRef]
38. Chapron, C.; Tosti, C.; Marcellin, L.; Bourdon, M.; Lafay-Pillet, M.-C.; Millischer, A.-E.; Streuli, I.; Borghese, B.; Petraglia, F.; Santulli, P. Relationship between the magnetic resonance imaging appearance of adenomyosis and endometriosis phenotypes. *Hum. Reprod.* **2017**, *32*, 1393–1401. [CrossRef]
39. Rolla, E. Endometriosis: Advances and controversies in classification, pathogenesis, diagnosis, and treatment. *F1000Research* **2019**, *8*, 529. [CrossRef]

40. Vitale, S.G.; La Rosa, V.L.; Rapisarda, A.M.C.; Laganà, A.S. Impact of endometriosis on quality of life and psychological well-being. *J. Psychosom. Obstet. Gynecol.* **2016**, *38*, 317–319. [CrossRef]
41. Brasil, D.L.; Montagna, E.; Trevisan, C.M.; La Rosa, V.L.; Laganà, A.S.; Barbosa, C.P.; Bianco, B.; Zaia, V. Psychological stress levels in women with endometriosis: Systematic review and meta-analysis of observational studies. *Minerva Med.* **2020**, *111*, 90–102. [CrossRef]
42. Abrao, M.S.; Miller, C.E. An endometriosis classification, designed to be validated. *NewsScope* **2012**, *25*, 6.
43. Dai, Y.; Li, X.; Shi, J.; Leng, J. A review of the risk factors, genetics and treatment of endometriosis in Chinese women: A comparative update. *Reprod. Health* **2018**, *15*, 82. [CrossRef] [PubMed]
44. Baranov, V.S.; Ivaschenko, T.E.; Liehr, T.; Yarmolinskaya, M.I. Systems genetics view of endometriosis: A common complex disorder. *Eur. J. Obstet. Gynecol. Reprod. Biol.* **2015**, *185*, 59–65. [CrossRef] [PubMed]
45. Laganà, A.S.; Garzon, S.; Götte, M.; Viganò, P.; Franchi, M.; Ghezzi, F.; Martin, D.C. The Pathogenesis of Endometriosis: Molecular and Cell Biology Insights. *Int. J. Mol. Sci.* **2019**, *20*, 5615. [CrossRef]
46. Williams, C.; Long, A.J.; Noga, H.; Allaire, C.; Bedaiwy, M.A.; Lisonkova, S.; Yong, P.J. East and South East Asian Ethnicity and Moderate-to-Severe Endometriosis. *J. Minim. Invasive Gynecol.* **2018**, *26*, 507–515. [CrossRef] [PubMed]
47. Missmer, S.A.; Hankinson, S.E.; Spiegelman, D.; Barbieri, R.L.; Marshall, L.M.; Hunter, D.J. Incidence of Laparoscopically Confirmed Endometriosis by Demographic, Anthropometric, and Lifestyle Factors. *Am. J. Epidemiol.* **2004**, *160*, 784–796. [CrossRef] [PubMed]
48. McLeod, B.S.; Retzloff, M.G. Epidemiology of endometriosis: An assessment of risk factors. *Clin. Obstet. Gynecol.* **2010**, *53*, 389–396. [CrossRef] [PubMed]
49. Schliep, K.C.; Schisterman, E.; Mumford, S.; Pollack, A.; Zhang, C.; Ye, A.; Stanford, J.B.; O Hammoud, A.; Porucznik, C.; Wactawski-Wende, J. Caffeinated beverage intake and reproductive hormones among premenopausal women in the BioCycle Study. *Am. J. Clin. Nutr.* **2012**, *95*, 488–497. [CrossRef]
50. Fiuza-Luces, C.; Garatachea, N.; Berger, N.A.; Lucia, A. Exercise is the Real Polypill. *Physiology* **2013**, *28*, 330–358. [CrossRef]
51. Sofo, V.; Götte, M.; Laganà, A.S.; Salmeri, F.M.; Triolo, O.; Sturlese, E.; Retto, G.; Alfa, M.; Granese, R.; Abrão, M.S. Correlation between dioxin and endometriosis: An epigenetic route to unravel the pathogenesis of the disease. *Arch. Gynecol. Obstet.* **2015**, *292*, 973–986. [CrossRef] [PubMed]
52. Painter, J.N.; O'Mara, T.A.; Morris, A.P.; Cheng, T.H.T.; Gorman, M.; Martin, L.; Hodson, S.; Jones, A.; Martin, N.G.; Gordon, S.; et al. Genetic overlap between endometriosis and endometrial cancer: Evidence from cross-disease genetic correlation and GWAS meta-analyses. *Cancer Med.* **2018**, *7*, 1978–1987. [CrossRef] [PubMed]
53. Burney, R.O.; Giudice, L.C. Pathogenesis and pathophysiology of endometriosis. *Fertil. Steril.* **2012**, *98*, 511–519. [CrossRef]
54. Coxon, L.; Horne, A.W.; Vincent, K. Pathophysiology of endometriosis-associated pain: A review of pelvic and central nervous system mechanisms. *Best Pr. Res. Clin. Obstet. Gynaecol.* **2018**, *51*, 53–67. [CrossRef]
55. Sasson, I.E.; Taylor, H.S. Stem Cells and the Pathogenesis of Endometriosis. *Ann. N. Y. Acad. Sci.* **2008**, *1127*, 106–115. [CrossRef]
56. Poli-Neto, O.B.; Meola, J.; Rosa-E-Silva, J.C.; Tiezzi, D. Transcriptome meta-analysis reveals differences of immune profile between eutopic endometrium from stage I-II and III-IV endometriosis independently of hormonal milieu. *Sci. Rep.* **2020**, *10*, 313. [CrossRef] [PubMed]
57. Cousins, F.L.; Dorien, F.O.; Gargett, C.E. Endometrial stem/progenitor cells and their role in the pathogenesis of endometriosis. *Best Pract. Res. Clin. Obstet. Gynaecol.* **2018**, *50*, 27–38. [CrossRef] [PubMed]
58. Vetvicka, V.; Laganà, A.S.; Salmeri, F.M.; Triolo, O.; Palmara, V.I.; Vitale, S.G.; Sofo, V.; Kralickova, M. Regulation of apoptotic pathways during endometriosis: From the molecular basis to the future perspectives. *Arch. Gynecol. Obstet.* **2016**, *294*, 897–904. [CrossRef] [PubMed]
59. Salmeri, F.M.; Laganà, A.S.; Sofo, V.; Triolo, O.; Sturlese, E.; Retto, G.; Pizzo, A.; D'Ascola, A.; Campo, S. Behavior of Tumor Necrosis Factor-α and Tumor Necrosis Factor Receptor 1/Tumor Necrosis Factor Receptor 2 System in Mononuclear Cells Recovered From Peritoneal Fluid of Women With Endometriosis at Different Stages. *Reprod. Sci.* **2014**, *22*, 165–172. [CrossRef] [PubMed]
60. Sturlese, E.; Salmeri, F.M.; Retto, G.; Pizzo, A.; De Dominici, R.; Ardita, F.V.; Borrielli, I.; Licata, N.; Laganà, A.S.; Sofo, V. Dysregulation of the Fas/FasL system in mononuclear cells recovered from peritoneal fluid of women with endometriosis. *J. Reprod. Immunol.* **2011**, *92*, 74–81. [CrossRef]
61. Patel, B.G.; Lenk, E.E.; Lebovic, D.I.; Shu, Y.; Yu, J.; Taylor, R.N. Pathogenesis of endometriosis: Interaction between Endocrine and inflammatory pathways. *Best Pract. Res. Clin. Obstet. Gynaecol.* **2018**, *50*, 50–60. [CrossRef] [PubMed]
62. Chapron, C.; Marcellin, L.; Borghese, B.; Santulli, P. Rethinking mechanisms, diagnosis and management of endometriosis. *Nat. Rev. Endocrinol.* **2019**, *15*, 666–682. [CrossRef] [PubMed]
63. Terzic, M.; Aimagambetova, G.; Norton, M.; Della Corte, L.; Marín-Buck, A.; Lisón, J.F.; Amer-Cuenca, J.J.; Zito, G.; Garzon, S.; Caruso, S.; et al. Scoring systems for the evaluation of adnexal masses nature: Current knowledge and clinical applications. *J. Obstet. Gynaecol.* **2021**, *41*, 340–347. [CrossRef] [PubMed]
64. Terzic, M.; Rapisarda, A.M.C.; Della Corte, L.; Manchanda, R.; Aimagambetova, G.; Norton, M.; Garzon, S.; Riemma, G.; King, C.R.; Chiofalo, B.; et al. Diagnostic work-up in paediatric and adolescent patients with adnexal masses: An evidence-based approach. *J. Obstet. Gynaecol.* **2021**, *41*, 503–515. [CrossRef]
65. Giudice, L.C. Clinical practice. Endometriosis. *N. Engl. J. Med.* **2010**, *362*, 2389–2398. [CrossRef]

66. DiVasta, A.D.; Vitonis, A.F.; Laufer, M.R.; Missmer, S.A. Spectrum of symptoms in women diagnosed with endometriosis during adolescence vs adulthood. *Am. J. Obstet. Gynecol.* **2018**, *218*, 324.e1–324.e11. [CrossRef]
67. D'Alterio, M.N.; Saponara, S.; D'Ancona, G.; Russo, M.; Laganà, A.S.; Sorrentino, F.; Nappi, L.; Angioni, S. Role of surgical treatment in endometriosis. *Minerva Obstet. Gynecol.* **2021**, *73*, 317–332. [CrossRef]
68. Chapron, C.; Santulli, P.; De Ziegler, D.; Noel, J.-C.; Anaf, V.; Streuli, I.; Foulot, H.; Souza, C.; Borghese, B. Ovarian endometrioma: Severe pelvic pain is associated with deeply infiltrating endometriosis. *Hum. Reprod.* **2012**, *27*, 702–711. [CrossRef]
69. Tanbo, T.; Fedorcsak, P. Endometriosis-associated infertility: Aspects of pathophysiological mechanisms and treatment options. *Acta Obstet. Gynecol. Scand.* **2017**, *96*, 659–667. [CrossRef] [PubMed]
70. Terzic, M.; Dotlic, J.; Brndusic, N.; Likic, I.; Andrijasevic, S.; Arsenovic, N.; Ladjevic, N.; Maričić, S. Histopathological diagnoses of adnexal masses: Which parameters are relevant in preoperative assessment? *Ginekol. Polska* **2013**, *84*, 700–708. [CrossRef]
71. Terzic, M.; Dotlic, J.; Likic, I.; Nikolic, B.; Brndusic, N.; Pilic, I.; Bila, J.; Maricic, S.; Arsenovic, N. Diagnostic value of serum tumor markers evaluation for adnexal masses. *Open Med.* **2014**, *9*, 210–216. [CrossRef]
72. Bazot, M.; Daraï, E. Diagnosis of deep endometriosis: Clinical examination, ultrasonography, magnetic resonance imaging, and other techniques. *Fertil. Steril.* **2017**, *108*, 886–894. [CrossRef]
73. Scioscia, M.; Virgilio, B.A.; Laganà, A.S.; Bernardini, T.; Fattizzi, N.; Neri, M.; Guerriero, S. Differential Diagnosis of Endometriosis by Ultrasound: A Rising Challenge. *Diagnostics* **2020**, *10*, 848. [CrossRef]
74. Djokovic, D.; Pinto, A.P.; van Herendael, B.J.; Laganà, A.S.; Thomas, V.; Keckstein, J. Structured report for dynamic ultrasonography in patients with suspected or known endometriosis: Recommendations of the International Society for Gynecologic Endoscopy (ISGE). *Eur. J. Obstet. Gynecol. Reprod. Biol.* **2021**, *263*, 252–260. [CrossRef] [PubMed]
75. Barra, F.; Biscaldi, E.; Scala, C.; Laganà, A.S.; Vellone, V.G.; Stabilini, C.; Ghezzi, F.; Ferrero, S. A Prospective Study Comparing Three-Dimensional Rectal Water Contrast Transvaginal Ultrasonography and Computed Tomographic Colonography in the Diagnosis of Rectosigmoid Endometriosis. *Diagnostics* **2020**, *10*, 252. [CrossRef] [PubMed]
76. Noventa, M.; Scioscia, M.; Schincariol, M.; Cavallin, F.; Pontrelli, G.; Virgilio, B.; Vitale, S.G.; Laganà, A.S.; Dessole, F.; Cosmi, E.; et al. Imaging Modalities for Diagnosis of Deep Pelvic Endometriosis: Comparison between Trans-Vaginal Sonography, Rectal Endoscopy Sonography and Magnetic Resonance Imaging. A Head-to-Head Meta-Analysis. *Diagnostics* **2019**, *9*, 225. [CrossRef]
77. Nisenblat, V.; Bossuyt, P.M.M.; Farquhar, C.; Johnson, N.; Hull, M.L. Imaging modalities for the non-invasive diagnosis of endometriosis. *Cochrane Database Syst. Rev.* **2016**, *2*, CD009591. [CrossRef] [PubMed]
78. Raglan, O.; Kalliala, I.; Markozannes, G.; Cividini, S.; Gunter, M.J.; Nautiyal, J.; Gabra, H.; Paraskevaidis, E.; Martin-Hirsch, P.; Tsilidis, K.K.; et al. Risk factors for endometrial cancer: An umbrella review of the literature. *Int. J. Cancer* **2019**, *145*, 1719–1730. [CrossRef]
79. Terzic, M.; Norton, M.; Terzic, S.; Bapayeva, G.; Aimagambetova, G. Fertility preservation in endometrial cancer patients: Options, challenges and perspectives. *Ecancermedicalscience* **2020**, *14*, 1030. [CrossRef]
80. Lortet-Tieulent, J.; Ferlay, J.; Bray, F.; Jemal, A. International Patterns and Trends in Endometrial Cancer Incidence, 1978–2013. *J. Natl. Cancer Inst.* **2017**, *110*, 354–361. [CrossRef]
81. Moore, K.; Brewer, M.A. Endometrial Cancer: Is This a New Disease? *Am. Soc. Clin. Oncol. Educ. Book* **2017**, *37*, 435–442. [CrossRef]
82. American Cancer Society. *Facts & Figures 2021*; American Cancer Society: Atlanta, GA, USA, 2021; Available online: https://www.cancer.org/cancer/endometrial-cancer.html (accessed on 2 July 2021).
83. Urick, M.E.; Bell, D.W. Clinical actionability of molecular targets in endometrial cancer. *Nat. Rev. Cancer* **2019**, *19*, 510–521. [CrossRef]
84. Terzic, M.; Aimagambetova, G.; Terzic, S.; Norton, M.; Bapayeva, G.; Garzon, S. Current role of Pipelle endometrial sampling in early diagnosis of endometrial cancer. *Transl. Cancer Res.* **2020**, *9*, 7716–7724. [CrossRef]
85. Braun, M.M.; Overbeek-Wager, E.A.; Grumbo, R.J. Diagnosis and Management of Endometrial Cancer. *Am. Fam. Phys.* **2016**, *93*, 468–474.
86. Vitale, S.G.; Capriglione, S.; Zito, G.; Lopez, S.; Gulino, F.A.; Di Guardo, F.; Vitagliano, A.; Noventa, M.; La Rosa, V.L.; Sapia, F.; et al. Management of endometrial, ovarian and cervical cancer in the elderly: Current approach to a challenging condition. *Arch. Gynecol. Obstet.* **2018**, *299*, 299–315. [CrossRef]
87. Howlader, N.N.A.K.M.; Noone, A.M.; Krapcho, M.; Garshell, J.; Miller, D.; Altekruse, S.F.; Kosary, C.L.; Yu, M.; Ruhl, J.; Tatalovich, Z.; et al. *SEER Cancer Statistics Review, 1975–2015*; National Cancer Institute: Bethesda, MD, USA, 2015. Available online: https://seer.cancer.gov/csr/1975_2015/ (accessed on 2 July 2021).
88. Lu, K.H.; Broaddus, R.R. Endometrial Cancer. *New Engl. J. Med.* **2020**, *383*, 2053–2064. [CrossRef] [PubMed]
89. Benati, M.; Montagnana, M.; Danese, E.; Mazzon, M.; Paviati, E.; Garzon, S.; Laganà, A.S.; Casarin, J.; Giudici, S.; Raffaelli, R.; et al. Aberrant Telomere Length in Circulating Cell-Free DNA as Possible Blood Biomarker with High Diagnostic Performance in Endometrial Cancer. *Pathol. Oncol. Res.* **2020**, *26*, 2281–2289. [CrossRef]
90. Passarello, K.; Kurian, S.; Villanueva, V. Endometrial Cancer: An Overview of Pathophysiology, Management, and Care. *Semin. Oncol. Nurs.* **2019**, *35*, 157–165. [CrossRef]
91. Chiofalo, B.; Mazzon, I.; Antonio, S.D.A.; Amadore, D.; Vizza, E.; Laganà, A.S.; Vocaturo, G.; Calagna, G.; Favilli, A.; Palmara, V.; et al. Hysteroscopic Evaluation of Endometrial Changes in Breast Cancer Women with or without Hormone Therapies: Results from a Large Multicenter Cohort Study. *J. Minim. Invasive Gynecol.* **2020**, *27*, 832–839. [CrossRef] [PubMed]

92. Lindemann, K.; Vatten, L.J.; Ellstrøm-Engh, M.; Eskild, A. Body mass, diabetes and smoking, and endometrial cancer risk: A follow-up study. *Br. J. Cancer* **2008**, *98*, 1582–1585. [CrossRef] [PubMed]
93. Njoku, K.; Campbell, A.; Geary, B.; MacKintosh, M.; Derbyshire, A.; Kitson, S.; Sivalingam, V.; Pierce, A.; Whetton, A.; Crosbie, E. Metabolomic Biomarkers for the Detection of Obesity-Driven Endometrial Cancer. *Cancers* **2021**, *13*, 718. [CrossRef]
94. Renehan, A.G.; Tyson, M.; Egger, M.; Heller, R.F.; Zwahlen, M. Body-mass index and incidence of cancer: A systematic review and meta-analysis of prospective observational studies. *Lancet* **2008**, *371*, 569–578. [CrossRef]
95. Kalliala, I.; Markozannes, G.; Gunter, M.J.; Paraskevaidis, E.; Gabra, H.; Mitra, A.; Terzidou, V.; Bennett, P.; Martin-Hirsch, P.; Tsilidis, K.K.; et al. Obesity and gynaecological and obstetric conditions: Umbrella review of the literature. *BMJ* **2017**, *359*, j4511. [CrossRef] [PubMed]
96. Kyrgiou, M.; Kalliala, I.; Markozannes, G.; Gunter, M.J.; Paraskevaidis, E.; Gabra, H.; Martin-Hirsch, P.; Tsilidis, K.K. Adiposity and cancer at major anatomical sites: Umbrella review of the literature. *BMJ* **2017**, *356*, j477. [CrossRef]
97. Tsilidis, K.K.; Kasimis, J.C.; Lopez, D.S.; E Ntzani, E.; Ioannidis, J.P.A. Type 2 diabetes and cancer: Umbrella review of meta-analyses of observational studies. *BMJ* **2015**, *350*, g7607. [CrossRef] [PubMed]
98. Nead, K.T.; Sharp, S.J.; Thompson, D.J.; Painter, J.N.; Savage, D.B.; Semple, R.; Barker, A.; Perry, J.R.B.; Attia, J.; Dunning, A.M.; et al. Evidence of a Causal Association Between Insulinemia and Endometrial Cancer: A Mendelian Randomization Analysis. *J. Natl. Cancer Inst.* **2015**, *107*, 178. [CrossRef] [PubMed]
99. Collaborative Group on Epidemiological Studies on Endometrial Cancer. Endometrial cancer and oral contraceptives: An in-dividual participant meta-analysis of 27,276 women with endometrial cancer from 36 epidemiological studies. *Lancet Oncol.* **2015**, *16*, 1061–1070. [CrossRef]
100. Wang, A.; Wang, S.; Zhu, C.; Huang, H.; Wu, L.; Wan, X.; Yang, X.; Zhang, H.; Miao, R.; He, L.; et al. Coffee and cancer risk: A meta-analysis of prospective observational studies. *Sci. Rep.* **2016**, *6*, 33711. [CrossRef] [PubMed]
101. Zhou, Q.; Luo, M.-L.; Li, H.; Li, M.; Zhou, J.-G. Coffee consumption and risk of endometrial cancer: A dose-response meta-analysis of prospective cohort studies. *Sci. Rep.* **2015**, *5*, 13410. [CrossRef]
102. Al-Zoughool, M.; Dossus, L.; Kaaks, R.; Clavel-Chapelon, F.; Tjønneland, A.; Olsen, A.; Overvad, K.; Boutron-Ruault, M.-C.; Gauthier, E.; Linseisen, J.; et al. Risk of endometrial cancer in relationship to cigarette smoking: Results from the EPIC study. *Int. J. Cancer* **2007**, *121*, 2741–2747. [CrossRef] [PubMed]
103. Setiawan, V.W.; Pike, M.C.; Kolonel, L.N.; Nomura, A.M.; Goodman, M.T.; Henderson, B.E. Racial/Ethnic Differences in Endometrial Cancer Risk: The Multiethnic Cohort Study. *Am. J. Epidemiol.* **2006**, *165*, 262–270. [CrossRef]
104. Arend, R.C.; Jones, B.A.; Martinez, A.; Goodfellow, P. Endometrial cancer: Molecular markers and management of advanced stage disease. *Gynecol. Oncol.* **2018**, *150*, 569–580. [CrossRef] [PubMed]
105. Hutt, S.; Tailor, A.; Ellis, P.; Michael, A.; Butler-Manuel, S.; Chatterjee, J. The role of biomarkers in endometrial cancer and hyperplasia: A literature review. *Acta Oncol.* **2019**, *58*, 342–352. [CrossRef] [PubMed]
106. Aimagambetova, G.; Kaiyrlykyzy, A.; Bapayeva, G.; Ukybassova, T.; Kenbayeva, K.; Ibrayimov, B.; Lyasova, A.; Bonaldo, G.; Buzzaccarini, G.; Noventa, M.; et al. Validation of Pipelle endometrial biopsy in patients with abnormal uterine bleeding in Kazakhstani healthcare setting. *Clin. Exp. Obstet. Gynecol.* **2021**, *48*, 670–675. [CrossRef]
107. Terzic, M.M.; Aimagambetova, G.; Terzic, S.; Norton, M.; Bapayeva, G.; Garzon, S. Pipelle endometrial sampling success rates in Kazakhstani settings: Results from a prospective cohort analysis. *J. Obstet. Gyn.* **2021**. [CrossRef]
108. Scioscia, M.; Noventa, M.; Laganà, A.S. Abnormal uterine bleeding and the risk of endometrial cancer: Can subendometrial vascular ultrasound be of help to discriminate cancer from adenomyosis? *Am. J. Obstet. Gynecol.* **2020**, *223*, 605–606. [CrossRef]
109. Laganà, A.S.; Scioscia, M. Endometrial Cancer in Women with Adenomyosis: An Underestimated Risk? *Int. J. Fertil. Steril.* **2020**, *14*, 260–261.
110. Stachowicz, N.; Smoleń, A.; Ciebiera, M.; Łoziński, T.; Poziemski, P.; Borowski, D.; Czekierdowski, A. Risk Assessment of Endometrial Hyperplasia or Endometrial Cancer with Simplified Ultrasound-Based Scoring Systems. *Diagnostics* **2021**, *11*, 442. [CrossRef]
111. Will, A.J.; Sanchack, K.E. Endometrial Biopsy. In *StatPearls [Internet]*; StatPearls Publishing: Treasure Island, FL, USA, 2021.
112. Costas, T.; Belda, R.; Alcazar, J.L. Transvaginal three-dimensional ultrasound for preoperative assessment of myometrial invasion in patients with endometrial cancer: A systematic review and meta-analysis. *Med. Ultrason.* **2021**. [CrossRef]
113. Capozzi, V.A.; Rosati, A.; Rumolo, V.; Ferrari, F.; Gullo, G.; Karaman, E.; Karaaslan, O.; Hacioğlu, L. Novelties of ultrasound imaging for endometrial cancer preoperative workup. *Minerva Med.* **2021**, *112*, 3–11. [CrossRef] [PubMed]
114. Zondervan, K.T.; Becker, C.M.; Koga, K.; Missmer, S.A.; Taylor, R.N.; Viganò, P. Endometriosis. *Nat. Rev. Dis. Primers* **2018**, *4*, 9. [CrossRef] [PubMed]
115. Zondervan, K.T.; Becker, C.M.; Missmer, S.A. Endometriosis. *New Engl. J. Med.* **2020**, *382*, 1244–1256. [CrossRef] [PubMed]
116. Gardner, G.H.; Greene, R.R.; Ranney, B. The histogenesis of endometriosis; recent contributions. *Obstet. Gynecol.* **1953**, *1*, 615–637.
117. Simpson, J.L.; Elias, S.; Malinak, L.; Buttram, V.C. Heritable aspects of endometriosis. *Am. J. Obstet. Gynecol.* **1980**, *137*, 327–331. [CrossRef]
118. Parasar, P.; Ozcan, P.; Terry, K.L. Endometriosis: Epidemiology, Diagnosis and Clinical Management. *Curr. Obstet. Gynecol. Rep.* **2017**, *6*, 34–41. [CrossRef]
119. Frey, G. The Familial Occurrence of Endometriosis. *Am. J. Obstet. Gynecol.* **1957**, *73*, 418–421. [CrossRef]

120. Kennedy, S.; Hadfield, R.; Mardon, H.; Barlow, D. Age of onset of pain symptoms in non-twin sisters concordant for endometriosis. *Hum. Reprod.* **1996**, *11*, 403–405. [CrossRef] [PubMed]
121. A Treloar, S.; O'Connor, D.T.; O'Connor, V.M.; Martin, N. Genetic influences on endometriosis in an Australian twin sample. *Fertil. Steril.* **1999**, *71*, 701–710. [CrossRef]
122. Stefansson, H.; Geirsson, R.; Steinthorsdottir, V.; Jonsson, H.; Manolescu, A.; Kong, A.; Ingadottir, G.; Gulcher, J. Genetic factors contribute to the risk of developing endometriosis. *Hum. Reprod.* **2002**, *17*, 555–559. [CrossRef] [PubMed]
123. Treloar, S.A.; Wicks, J.; Nyholt, D.; Montgomery, G.; Bahlo, M.; Smith, V.; Dawson, G.; Mackay, I.J.; Weeks, D.; Bennett, S.T.; et al. Genomewide Linkage Study in 1,176 Affected Sister Pair Families Identifies a Significant Susceptibility Locus for Endometriosis on Chromosome 10q26. *Am. J. Hum. Genet.* **2005**, *77*, 365–376. [CrossRef] [PubMed]
124. Zondervan, K.T.; Treloar, S.A.; Lin, J.; Weeks, D.; Nyholt, D.; Mangion, J.; Mackay, I.J.; Cardon, L.R.; Martin, N.; Kennedy, S.H.; et al. Significant evidence of one or more susceptibility loci for endometriosis with near-Mendelian inheritance on chromosome 7p13–15. *Hum. Reprod.* **2007**, *22*, 717–728. [CrossRef]
125. Daftary, G.S.; Taylor, H.S. EMX2 Gene Expression in the Female Reproductive Tract and Aberrant Expression in the Endometrium of Patients with Endometriosis. *J. Clin. Endocrinol. Metab.* **2004**, *89*, 2390–2396. [CrossRef]
126. Du, H.; Taylor, H.S. Molecular Regulation of Müllerian Development by Hox Genes. *Ann. N. Y. Acad. Sci.* **2004**, *1034*, 152–165. [CrossRef] [PubMed]
127. Dinulescu, D.M.; A Ince, T.; Quade, B.J.; A Shafer, S.; Crowley, D.; Jacks, T. Role of K-ras and Pten in the development of mouse models of endometriosis and endometrioid ovarian cancer. *Nat. Med.* **2005**, *11*, 63–70. [CrossRef]
128. Mutter, G.L.; Lin, M.-C.; Fitzgerald, J.T.; Kum, J.B.; Baak, J.P.A.; Lees, J.A.; Weng, L.-P.; Eng, C. Altered PTEN Expression as a Diagnostic Marker for the Earliest Endometrial Precancers. *J. Natl. Cancer Inst.* **2000**, *92*, 924–930. [CrossRef] [PubMed]
129. Maxwell, G.L.; I Risinger, J.; Gumbs, C.; Shaw, H.; Bentley, R.C.; Barrett, J.C.; Berchuck, A.; A Futreal, P. Mutation of the PTEN tumor suppressor gene in endometrial hyperplasias. *Cancer Res.* **1998**, *58*, 2500–2503.
130. Martini, M.; Ciccarone, M.; Garganese, G.; Maggiore, C.; Evangelista, A.; Rahimi, S.; Zannoni, G.; Vittori, G.; Larocca, L.M. Possible involvement ofhMLH1, p16INK4a andPTEN in the malignant transformation of endometriosis. *Int. J. Cancer* **2002**, *102*, 398–406. [CrossRef]
131. Treloar, S.A.; Zhao, Z.Z.; Le, L.; Zondervan, K.; Martin, N.; Kennedy, S.; Nyholt, D.; Montgomery, G. Variants in EMX2 and PTEN do not contribute to risk of endometriosis. *Mol. Hum. Reprod.* **2007**, *13*, 587–594. [CrossRef] [PubMed]
132. Painter, J.N.; Nyholt, D.; Morris, A.; Zhao, Z.Z.; Henders, A.; Lambert, A.; Wallace, L.; Martin, N.; Kennedy, S.H.; Treloar, S.A.; et al. High-density fine-mapping of a chromosome 10q26 linkage peak suggests association between endometriosis and variants close to CYP2C19. *Fertil. Steril.* **2011**, *95*, 2236–2240. [CrossRef]
133. Painter, J.N.; Nyholt, D.R.; Krause, L.; Zhao, Z.Z.; Chapman, B.; Zhang, C.; Medland, S.; Martin, N.G.; Kennedy, S.; Treloar, S.; et al. Common variants in the CYP2C19 gene are associated with susceptibility to endometriosis. *Fertil. Steril.* **2014**, *102*, 496–502. [CrossRef]
134. Zanger, U.M.; Schwab, M. Cytochrome P450 enzymes in drug metabolism: Regulation of gene expression, enzyme activities, and impact of genetic variation. *Pharmacol. Ther.* **2013**, *138*, 103–141. [CrossRef]
135. Lee, A.J.; Cai, M.X.; Thomas, P.E.; Conney, A.H.; Zhu, B.T. Characterization of the Oxidative Metabolites of 17β-Estradiol and Estrone Formed by 15 Selectively Expressed Human Cytochrome P450 Isoforms. *Endocrinology* **2003**, *144*, 3382–3398. [CrossRef]
136. Painter, J.N.; Anderson, C.A.; Nyholt, D.; MacGregor, S.; Lin, J.; Lee, S.H.; Lambert, A.; Zhao, Z.Z.; Roseman, F.; Guo, Q.; et al. Genome-wide association study identifies a locus at 7p15.2 associated with endometriosis. *Nat. Genet.* **2010**, *43*, 51–54. [CrossRef] [PubMed]
137. Nyholt, D.R.; Low, S.-K.; Anderson, C.A.; Painter, J.N.; Uno, S.; Morris, A.P.; MacGregor, S.; Gordon, S.D.; Henders, A.; Martin, N.; et al. Genome-wide association meta-analysis identifies new endometriosis risk loci. *Nat. Genet.* **2012**, *44*, 1355–1359. [CrossRef] [PubMed]
138. Uno, S.; Zembutsu, H.; Hirasawa, A.; Takahashi, A.; Kubo, M.; Akahane, T.; Aoki, D.; Kamatani, N.; Hirata, K.; Nakamura, Y. A genome-wide association study identifies genetic variants in the CDKN2BAS locus associated with endometriosis in Japanese. *Nat. Genet.* **2010**, *42*, 707–710. [CrossRef] [PubMed]
139. Adachi, S.; Tajima, A.; Quan, J.; Haino, K.; Yoshihara, K.; Masuzaki, H.; Katabuchi, H.; Ikuma, K.; Suginami, H.; Nishida, N.; et al. Meta-analysis of genome-wide association scans for genetic susceptibility to endometriosis in Japanese population. *J. Hum. Genet.* **2010**, *55*, 816–821. [CrossRef] [PubMed]
140. Albertsen, H.M.; Chettier, R.; Farrington, P.; Ward, K. Genome-Wide Association Study Link Novel Loci to Endometriosis. *PLoS ONE* **2013**, *8*, e58257. [CrossRef]
141. Uimari, O.; Rahmioglu, N.; Nyholt, D.; Vincent, K.; Missmer, S.A.; Becker, C.; Morris, A.P.; Montgomery, G.; Zondervan, K.T. Genome-wide genetic analyses highlight mitogen-activated protein kinase (MAPK) signaling in the pathogenesis of endometriosis. *Hum. Reprod.* **2017**, *32*, 780–793. [CrossRef] [PubMed]
142. Sapkota, Y.; De Vivo, I.; Steinthorsdottir, V.; Fassbender, A.; Bowdler, L.; Buring, J.E.; Edwards, T.L.; Jones, S.; Dorien, O.; Peterse, D.; et al. Analysis of potential protein-modifying variants in 9000 endometriosis patients and 150,000 controls of European ancestry. *Sci. Rep.* **2017**, *7*, 11380. [CrossRef] [PubMed]
143. Sapkota, Y.; Fassbender, A.; Bowdler, L.; Fung, J.N.T.; Peterse, D.O.D.; Montgomery, G.; Nyholt, D.; D'Hooghe, T.M. Independent Replication and Meta-Analysis for Endometriosis Risk Loci. *Twin Res. Hum. Genet.* **2015**, *18*, 518–525. [CrossRef]

144. Sapkota, Y.; Steinthorsdottir, V.; Morris, A.P.; Fassbender, A.; Rahmioglu, N.; De Vivo, I.; Buring, J.E.; Zhang, F.; Edwards, T.L.; Jones, S.; et al. Meta-analysis identifies five novel loci associated with endometriosis highlighting key genes involved in hormone metabolism. *Nat. Commun.* **2017**, *8*, 15539. [CrossRef] [PubMed]
145. Rahmioglu, N.; Missmer, S.A.; Montgomery, G.W.; Zondervan, K.T. Insights into Assessing the Genetics of Endometriosis. *Curr. Obstet. Gynecol. Rep.* **2012**, *1*, 124–137. [CrossRef] [PubMed]
146. Rahmioglu, N.; Montgomery, G.; Zondervan, K. Genetics of Endometriosis. *Women's Health* **2015**, *11*, 577–586. [CrossRef] [PubMed]
147. Neto, J.S.; Kho, R.M.; Siufi, D.F.D.S.; Baracat, E.C.; Anderson, K.S.; Abrão, M.S. Cellular, Histologic, and Molecular Changes Associated with Endometriosis and Ovarian Cancer. *J. Minim. Invasive Gynecol.* **2014**, *21*, 55–63. [CrossRef]
148. Wiegand, K.C.; Shah, S.P.; Al-Agha, O.M.; Zhao, Y.; Tse, K.; Zeng, T.; Senz, J.; McConechy, M.K.; Anglesio, M.S.; Kalloger, S.E.; et al. ARID1AMutations in Endometriosis-Associated Ovarian Carcinomas. *N. Engl. J. Med.* **2010**, *363*, 1532–1543. [CrossRef]
149. Melin, A.; Sparén, P.; Persson, I.; Bergqvist, A. Endometriosis and the risk of cancer with special emphasis on ovarian cancer. *Hum. Reprod.* **2006**, *21*, 1237–1242. [CrossRef] [PubMed]
150. Anglesio, M.S.; Papadopoulos, N.; Ayhan, A.; Nazeran, T.M.; Noë, M.; Horlings, H.M.; Lum, A.; Jones, S.; Senz, J.; Seckin, T.; et al. Cancer-Associated Mutations in Endometriosis without Cancer. *N. Engl. J. Med.* **2017**, *376*, 1835–1848. [CrossRef]
151. Suda, K.; Nakaoka, H.; Yoshihara, K.; Ishiguro, T.; Tamura, R.; Mori, Y.; Yamawaki, K.; Adachi, S.; Takahashi, T.; Kase, H.; et al. Clonal Expansion and Diversification of Cancer-Associated Mutations in Endometriosis and Normal Endometrium. *Cell Rep.* **2018**, *24*, 1777–1789. [CrossRef] [PubMed]
152. Noë, M.; Ayhan, A.; Wang, T.-L.; Shih, I.-M. Independent development of endometrial epithelium and stroma within the same endometriosis. *J. Pathol.* **2018**, *245*, 265–269. [CrossRef]
153. Rathore, N.; Kriplani, A.; Yadav, R.K.; Jaiswal, U.; Netam, R. Distinct peritoneal fluid ghrelin and leptin in infertile women with endometriosis and their correlation with interleukin-6 and vascular endothelial growth factor. *Gynecol. Endocrinol.* **2014**, *30*, 671–675. [CrossRef]
154. Martincorena, I.; Campbell, P.J. Somatic mutation in cancer and normal cells. *Science* **2015**, *349*, 1483–1489. [CrossRef] [PubMed]
155. Moore, L.; Leongamornlert, D.; Coorens, T.H.H.; Sanders, M.A.; Ellis, P.; Dentro, S.C.; Dawson, K.J.; Butler, T.; Rahbari, R.; Mitchell, T.J.; et al. The mutational landscape of normal human endometrial epithelium. *Nat. Cell Biol.* **2020**, *580*, 640–646. [CrossRef] [PubMed]
156. Pon, J.R.; Marra, M.A. Driver and Passenger Mutations in Cancer. *Annu. Rev. Pathol. Mech. Dis.* **2015**, *10*, 25–50. [CrossRef] [PubMed]
157. Leyendecker, G.; Herbertz, M.; Kunz, G.; Mall, G. Endometriosis results from the dislocation of basal endometrium. *Hum. Reprod.* **2002**, *17*, 2725–2736. [CrossRef] [PubMed]
158. Králíčková, M.; Laganà, A.S.; Ghezzi, F.; Vetvicka, V. Endometriosis and risk of ovarian cancer: What do we know? *Arch. Gynecol. Obstet.* **2019**, *301*, 1–10. [CrossRef] [PubMed]
159. Alderman, M.H.; Yoder, N.; Taylor, H.S. The Systemic Effects of Endometriosis. *Semin. Reprod. Med.* **2017**, *35*, 263–270. [CrossRef]
160. Kajiyama, H.; Suzuki, S.; Yoshihara, M.; Tamauchi, S.; Yoshikawa, N.; Niimi, K.; Shibata, K.; Kikkawa, F. Endometriosis and cancer. *Free. Radic. Biol. Med.* **2019**, *133*, 186–192. [CrossRef]
161. Vargas-Hernández, V.M. La endometriosis como factor de riesgo para cáncer de ovario. *Cirugía Cirujanos* **2013**, *81*, 163–168. (in Spanish)
162. Saavalainen, L.; Lassus, H.; But, A.; Tiitinen, A.; Härkki, P.; Gissler, M.; Pukkala, E.; Heikinheimo, O. Risk of Gynecologic Cancer According to the Type of Endometriosis. *Obstet. Gynecol.* **2018**, *131*, 1095–1102. [CrossRef]
163. Poole, E.M.; Lin, W.T.; Kvaskoff, M.; De Vivo, I.; Terry, K.L.; Missmer, S.A. Endometriosis and risk of ovarian and endometrial cancers in a large prospective cohort of U.S. nurses. *Cancer Causes Control* **2017**, *28*, 437–445. [CrossRef]
164. Rowlands, I.J.; Nagle, C.M.; Spurdle, A.B.; Webb, P.M. Gynecological conditions and the risk of endometrial cancer. *Gynecol. Oncol.* **2011**, *123*, 537–541. [CrossRef]
165. Kalaitzopoulos, D.R.; Mitsopoulou, A.; Iliopoulou, S.M.; Daniilidis, A.; Samartzis, E.P.; Economopoulos, K.P. Association between endometriosis and gynecological cancers: A critical review of the literature. *Arch. Gynecol. Obstet.* **2020**, *301*, 355–367. [CrossRef]
166. Chen, J.-J.; Xiao, Z.-J.; Meng, X.; Wang, Y.; Yu, M.K.; Huang, W.Q.; Sun, X.; Chen, H.; Duan, Y.-G.; Jiang, C.; et al. MRP4 sustains Wnt/β-catenin signaling for pregnancy, endometriosis and endometrial cancer. *Theranostics* **2019**, *9*, 5049–5064. [CrossRef]
167. Johnatty, S.E.; Stewart, C.J.R.; Smith, D.; Nguyen, A.; Dwyer, J.O.; O'Mara, T.A.; Webb, P.M.; Spurdle, A.B. Co-existence of leiomyomas, adenomyosis and endometriosis in women with endometrial cancer. *Sci. Rep.* **2020**, *10*, 3621. [CrossRef] [PubMed]
168. Mogensen, J.B.; Kjaer, S.K.; Mellemkjaer, L.; Jensen, A. Endometriosis and risks for ovarian, endometrial and breast cancers: A nationwide cohort study. *Gynecol. Oncol.* **2016**, *143*, 87–92. [CrossRef] [PubMed]
169. Yu, H.-C.; Lin, C.-Y.; Chang, W.-C.; Shen, B.-J.; Chang, W.-P.; Chuang, C.-M. Increased association between endo-metriosis and endometrial cancer: A nationwide population-based retrospective cohort study. *Int. J. Gynecol. Cancer* **2015**, *25*, 447–452. [CrossRef]
170. Franchi, M.; Garzon, S.; Zorzato, P.C.; Laganà, A.S.; Casarin, J.; Locantore, L.; Raffaelli, R.; Ghezzi, F. PET-CT scan in the preoperative workup of early stage intermediate- and high-risk endometrial cancer. *Minim. Invasive Ther. Allied Technol.* **2019**, *29*, 232–239. [CrossRef] [PubMed]

171. Cignini, P.; Vitale, S.G.; Laganà, A.S.; Biondi, A.; La Rosa, V.L.; Cutillo, G. Preoperative work-up for definition of lymph node risk involvement in early stage endometrial cancer: 5-year follow-up. *Updates Surg.* **2017**, *69*, 75–82. [CrossRef]
172. Vitale, S.G.; Rossetti, D.; Tropea, A.; Biondi, A.; Laganà, A.S. Fertility sparing surgery for stage IA type I and G2 endometrial cancer in reproductive-aged patients: Evidence-based approach and future perspectives. *Updates Surg.* **2017**, *69*, 29–34. [CrossRef]
173. Casarin, J.; Bogani, G.; Piovano, E.; Falcone, F.; Ferrari, F.; Odicino, F.; Puppo, A.; Bonfiglio, F.; Donadello, N.; Pinelli, C.; et al. Survival implication of lymphadenectomy in patients surgically treated for apparent early-stage uterine serous carcinoma. *J. Gynecol. Oncol.* **2020**, *31*, e64. [CrossRef]
174. Freytag, D.; Pape, J.; Dhanawat, J.; Günther, V.; Maass, N.; Gitas, G.; Laganà, A.S.; Allahqoli, L.; Meinhold-Heerlein, I.; Moawad, G.N.; et al. Challenges Posed by Embryonic and Anatomical Factors in Systematic Lymphadenectomy for Endometrial Cancer. *J. Clin. Med.* **2020**, *9*, 4107. [CrossRef]
175. Lee, S.-Y. Tailored Therapy Based on Molecular Characteristics in Endometrial Cancer. *BioMed Res. Int.* **2021**, *2021*, 2068023. [CrossRef]
176. Casarin, J.; Bogani, G.; Serati, M.; Pinelli, C.; Laganà, A.S.; Garzon, S.; Raspagliesi, F.; Ghezzi, F. Presence of Glandular Cells at the Preoperative Cervical Cytology and Local Recurrence in Endometrial Cancer. *Int. J. Gynecol. Pathol.* **2020**, *39*, 522–528. [CrossRef] [PubMed]
177. Winterhoff, B.; Thomaier, L.; Mullany, S.; Powell, M.A. Molecular characterization of endometrial cancer and therapeutic implications. *Curr. Opin. Obstet. Gynecol.* **2020**, *32*, 76–83. [CrossRef]
178. Cancer Genome Atlas Research Network, Kandoth C, Schultz N, et al Integrated genomic characterization of endometrial carcinoma. *Nature* **2013**, *497*, 67–73. [CrossRef]
179. Huvila, J.; Pors, J.; Thompson, E.F.; Gilks, C.B. Endometrial carcinoma: Molecular subtypes, precursors and the role of pathology in early diagnosis. *J. Pathol.* **2021**, *253*, 355–365. [CrossRef] [PubMed]
180. León-Castillo, A.; De Boer, S.M.; Powell, M.E.; Mileshkin, L.R.; Mackay, H.J.; Leary, A.; Nijman, H.W.; Singh, N.; Pollock, P.M.; Bessette, P.; et al. Molecular Classification of the PORTEC-3 Trial for High-Risk Endometrial Cancer: Impact on Prognosis and Benefit from Adjuvant Therapy. *J. Clin. Oncol.* **2020**, *38*, 3388–3397. [CrossRef] [PubMed]
181. McAlpine, J.; Leon-Castillo, A.; Bosse, T. The rise of a novel classification system for endometrial carcinoma; integration of mo-lecular subclasses. *J. Pathol.* **2018**, *244*, 538–549. [CrossRef]
182. Carlson, J.; McCluggage, W.G. Reclassifying endometrial carcinomas with a combined morphological and molecular approach. *Curr. Opin. Oncol.* **2019**, *31*, 411–419. [CrossRef] [PubMed]
183. Nakamura, M.; Obata, T.; Daikoku, T.; Fujiwara, H. The Association and Significance of p53 in Gynecologic Cancers: The Potential of Targeted Therapy. *Int. J. Mol. Sci.* **2019**, *20*, 5482. [CrossRef] [PubMed]
184. Salvesen, H.B.; Haldorsen, I.S.; Trovik, J. Markers for individualised therapy in endometrial carcinoma. *Lancet Oncol.* **2012**, *13*, e353–e361. [CrossRef]
185. Alexa, M.; Hasenburg, A.; Battista, M. The TCGA Molecular Classification of Endometrial Cancer and Its Possible Impact on Adjuvant Treatment Decisions. *Cancers* **2021**, *13*, 1478. [CrossRef] [PubMed]
186. Menderes, G.; Lopez, S.; Han, C.; Altwerger, G.; Gysler, S.; Varughese, J.; E Schwartz, P.; Santin, A.D. Mechanisms of resistance to HER2-targeted therapies in HER2-amplified uterine serous carcinoma, and strategies to overcome it. *Discov. Med.* **2018**, *26*, 39–50. [PubMed]
187. Erickson, B.K.; Zeybek, B.; Santin, A.D.; Fader, A.N. Targeting human epidermal growth factor receptor 2 (HER2) in gynecologic malignancies. *Curr. Opin. Obstet. Gynecol.* **2020**, *32*, 57–64. [CrossRef]
188. Ferriss, J.S.; Erickson, B.K.; Shih, I.-M.; Fader, A.N. Uterine serous carcinoma: Key advances and novel treatment approaches. *Int. J. Gynecol. Cancer* **2021**, *31*, 1165–1174. [CrossRef] [PubMed]
189. Stelloo, E.; Nout, R.A.; Osse, E.M.; Juergenliemk-Schulz, I.J.; Jobsen, J.J.; Lutgens, L.C.; Van Der Steen-Banasik, E.M.; Nijman, H.W.; Putter, H.; Bosse, T.; et al. Improved Risk Assessment by Integrating Molecular and Clinicopathological Factors in Early-stage Endometrial Cancer—Combined Analysis of the PORTEC Cohorts. *Clin. Cancer Res.* **2016**, *22*, 4215–4224. [CrossRef] [PubMed]
190. Talhouk, A.; DeRocher, H.; Schmidt, P.; Leung, S.; Milne, K.; Gilks, C.B.; Anglesio, M.S.; Nelson, B.H.; McAlpine, J.N. Molecular Subtype Not Immune Response Drives Outcomes in Endometrial Carcinoma. *Clin. Cancer Res.* **2019**, *25*, 2537–2548. [CrossRef]
191. Reijnen, C.; Küsters-Vandevelde, H.V.; Prinsen, C.F.; Massuger, L.F.; Snijders, M.P.; Kommoss, S.; Brucker, S.Y.; Kwon, J.S.; McAlpine, J.N.; Pijnenborg, J.M. Mismatch repair deficiency as a predictive marker for response to adjuvant radiotherapy in endometrial cancer. *Gynecol. Oncol.* **2019**, *154*, 124–130. [CrossRef]
192. Mackay, H.J.; Freixinos, V.R.; Fleming, G.F. Therapeutic Targets and Opportunities in Endometrial Cancer: Update on Endocrine Therapy and Nonimmunotherapy Targeted Options. *Am. Soc. Clin. Oncol. Educ. Book* **2020**, *40*, 245–255. [CrossRef]
193. Gómez-Raposo, C.; Salvador, M.M.; Zamora, C.A.; de Santiago, B.G.; Sáenz, E.C. Immune checkpoint inhibitors in endometrial cancer. *Crit. Rev. Oncol.* **2021**, *161*, 103306. [CrossRef]
194. Jamieson, A.; Thompson, E.F.; Huvila, J.; Gilks, C.B.; McAlpine, J.N. p53abn Endometrial Cancer: Understanding the most aggressive endometrial cancers in the era of molecular classification. *Int. J. Gynecol. Cancer* **2021**, *31*, 907–913. [CrossRef] [PubMed]
195. Nm, A.E.M.; El-Gelany, S. Differential Expression Patterns of PTEN in Cyclic, Hyperplastic and Malignant Endome-trium: Its Relation with ER, PR and Clinicopathological Parameters. *J. Egypt. Natl. Cancer Inst.* **2009**, *21*, 323–331.
196. Giono, L.E.; Manfredi, J.J. The p53 tumor suppressor participates in multiple cell cycle checkpoints. *J. Cell. Physiol.* **2006**, *209*, 13–20. [CrossRef] [PubMed]

197. D'Andrilli, G.; Bovicelli, A.; Paggi, M.G.; Giordano, A. New insights in endometrial carcinogenesis. *J. Cell. Physiol.* **2012**, *227*, 2842–2846. [CrossRef]
198. Angioli, R.; Miranda, A.; Aloisi, A.; Montera, R.; Capriglione, S.; Nardone, C.D.C.; Terranova, C.; Plotti, F. A critical review on HE4 performance in endometrial cancer: Where are we now? *Tumor Biol.* **2014**, *35*, 881–887. [CrossRef] [PubMed]
199. Kemik, P.; Saatli, B.; Yıldırım, N.; Kemik, V.D.; Deveci, B.; Terek, M.C.; Koçtürk, S.; Koyuncuoğlu, M.; Saygılı, U. Diagnostic and prognostic values of preoperative serum levels ofYKL-40, HE-4 and DKK-3 in endometrial cancer. *Gynecol. Oncol.* **2016**, *140*, 64–69. [CrossRef]

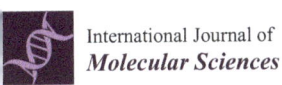

Review

The Role of Long Non-Coding RNAs in Endometriosis

Quanah J. Hudson †, Katharina Proestling †, Alexandra Perricos, Lorenz Kuessel, Heinrich Husslein, René Wenzl and Iveta Yotova *

Department of Obstetrics and Gynecology, Medical University of Vienna, Waehringer Guertel 18-20, A-1090 Vienna, Austria; quanah.hudson@univie.ac.at (Q.J.H.); katharina.proestling@meduniwien.ac.at (K.P.); alexandra.perricos@meduniwien.ac.at (A.P.); lorenz.kuessel@meduniwien.ac.at (L.K.); heinrich.husslein@meduniwien.ac.at (H.H.); rene.wenzl@meduniwien.ac.at (R.W.)
* Correspondence: iveta.yotova@meduniwien.ac.at
† These authors contributed equally to this work.

Abstract: Endometriosis is a chronic gynecological disorder affecting the quality of life and fertility of many women around the world. Heterogeneous and non-specific symptoms may lead to a delay in diagnosis, with treatment options limited to surgery and hormonal therapy. Hence, there is a need to better understand the pathogenesis of the disease to improve diagnosis and treatment. Long non-coding RNAs (lncRNAs) have been increasingly shown to be involved in gene regulation but remain relatively under investigated in endometriosis. Mutational and transcriptomic studies have implicated lncRNAs in the pathogenesis of endometriosis. Single-nucleotide polymorphisms (SNPs) in lncRNAs or their regulatory regions have been associated with endometriosis. Genome-wide transcriptomic studies have identified lncRNAs that show deregulated expression in endometriosis, some of which have been subjected to further experiments, which support a role in endometriosis. Mechanistic studies indicate that lncRNAs may regulate genes involved in endometriosis by acting as a molecular sponge for miRNAs, by directly targeting regulatory elements via interactions with chromatin or transcription factors or by affecting signaling pathways. Future studies should concentrate on determining the role of uncharacterized lncRNAs revealed by endometriosis transcriptome studies and the relevance of lncRNAs implicated in the disease by in vitro and animal model studies.

Keywords: endometriosis; long non-coding RNAs; lncRNAs; sponging; ceRNA; chromatin; chronic pain

1. Introduction

Endometriosis is a chronic inflammatory disorder defined by endometrial-like lesions growing ectopically outside of the uterus that affects many reproductive-age women worldwide. The disease has heterogeneous symptoms that may not be specific to the disease, such as different types of chronic gynecological pain and reduced fertility. The cause of the disease remains unclear, but lesions are thought to originate from endometrial cells that escape the uterus [1], although the presence of rare endometriosis-like lesions in males supports a trans-differentiation origin [2]. Endometriosis is thought to be an immunological disease, first because lesions must evade the immune system in order to establish and develop, and second because the inflammatory nature of the disease accounts for many of the symptoms [3]. Additionally, a meta-analysis has found that there is some association between endometriosis and a risk for developing an autoimmune disease [4]. Treatment options for the disease remain limited to laparoscopic surgery to remove lesions and hormone-based treatments that are not compatible with pregnancy [3]. Given that diagnosis is often delayed due to the non-specific symptoms and that there are limited treatment options, there is a need to better understand the molecular pathogenesis of the disease in order to identify key players that may be used as biomarkers for diagnosis or as targets for new treatments. One class of molecules that may play a role in the disease are long non-coding RNAs (lncRNAs).

LncRNAs are a class of genes that since the advent of high-throughput sequencing technology have been revealed to be much more numerous than was previously realized. Currently over 16,000 human lncRNAs are annotated by the GENCODE project, while some other studies have indicated that the total number may be over 100,000 [5]. Although most of these lncRNAs remain uncharacterized, an increasing number have been shown to have a biological function, often involved in gene regulation [6]. LncRNAs remain relatively under investigated in endometriosis, but given their roles in development and disease in other contexts [7], it is reasonable to assume that there may be lncRNAs that also play a role in endometriosis.

LncRNAs may exert their function in either the nucleus or the cytoplasm via a variety of mechanisms. In the nucleus, lncRNAs may act as epigenetic gene regulators by recruiting chromatin remodeling or modification complexes to target gene promoters either in *cis* (Figure 1a) [8] and/or in *trans* to activate or suppress their transcription (Figure 1b) [9]. LncRNAs can act as decoys of specific chromatin modifiers by sequestering them from the promoters of target genes (Figure 1c) [10]. In other contexts, lncRNAs may act as transcriptional regulators by competing with a transcription factor for binding DNA and/or by binding its DNA binding domain (Figure 1d) [11]. LncRNAs have also been associated with the regulation of pre-mRNA alternative splicing in the nucleus, thereby affecting which isoforms predominate (Figure 1e) [12]. In the cytoplasm, lncRNAs are involved in post-transcriptional regulation processes that can affect the stability of transcripts (Figure 1f) [13] or whether a transcript is translated into a protein or not (Figure 1g) [14]. LncRNAs can also be involved in the modulation of cell signaling pathways by binding to signaling proteins and affecting their activation state (Figure 1h) [15]. Finally, a common mechanism whereby lncRNAs are thought to affect mRNA abundance is by acting as so-called "sponges" of miRNAs to reduce miRNA-mediated degradation. Here, lncRNAs may share miRNA target sequences with mRNAs, thereby reducing miRNA availability to target mRNAs (Figure 1i) [16,17].

These studies show that lncRNAs can act at multiple subcellular sites to affect various aspects of cell biology, although in most cases they affect either transcription or processing of mRNAs and their steady state levels in the cell. That is, in a broad sense, they regulate other genes. An increasing body of literature implicates abnormal expression of specific lncRNAs in disease, particularly in different types of cancer [18], but also in a variety of other diseases including neural disorders [19], cardiovascular disease [20], and diabetes [21]. Evidence for the involvement of individual lncRNAs in the pathogenesis of these diseases ranges from a correlation with dysregulated lncRNA expression to detailed mechanistic studies that indicate a functional role in the disease. The implication from these studies and others is that lncRNAs are important players in the pathogenesis of many diseases, suggesting that there may be lncRNAs that play a role in endometriosis. Furthermore, a number of studies in have shown that lncRNAs can either be regulated by estrogen-dependent enhancers [22] or that lncRNAs can regulate estrogen receptor expression [23]. As endometriosis is an estrogen-dependent disease [3], these studies give further impetus to investigate the role of lncRNAs in the disease. Given this evidence for the role of lncRNAs in other contexts, in this review, we aim to provide a comprehensive picture of the current state of knowledge over the role of lncRNAs in endometriosis.

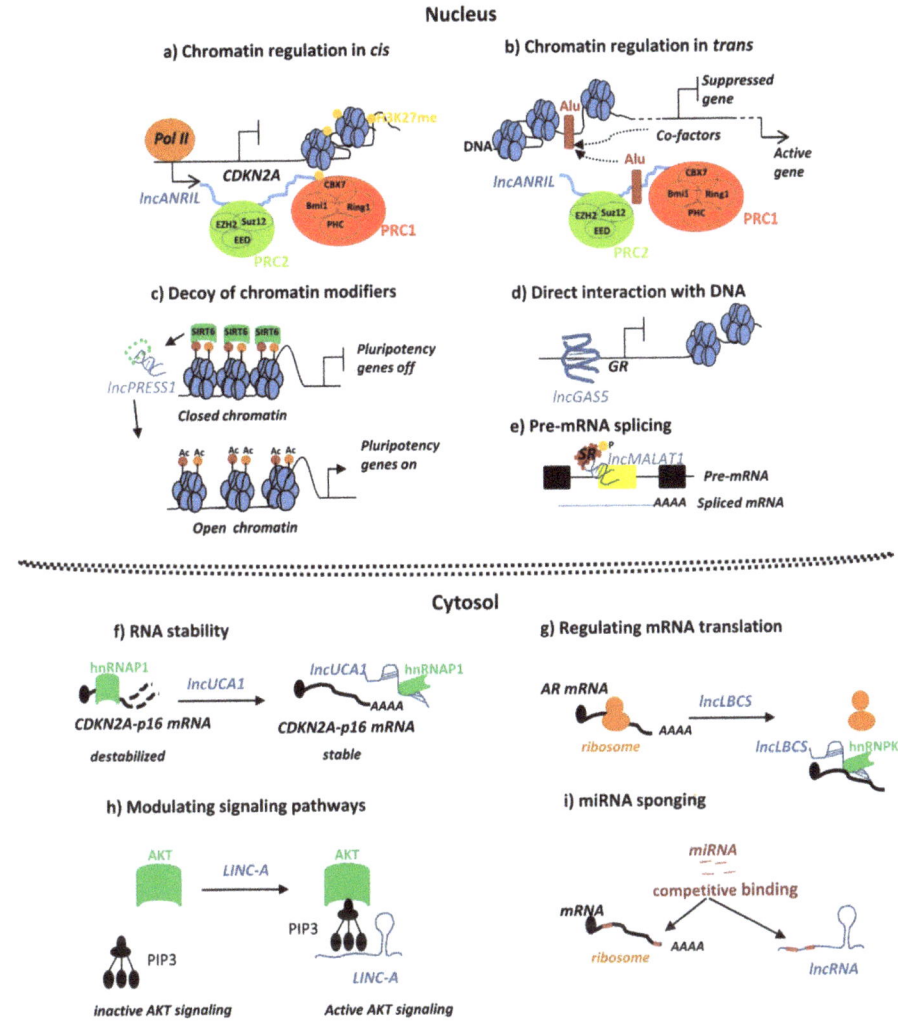

Figure 1. Description of the general mechanisms of the lncRNA actions in the nucleus (**a**–**e**) or in the cytosol (**f**–**i**). (**a**) Regulation in *cis* by lncRNA *ANRIL*, which mediates polycomb repressive complex (PRC) 1 and 2 recruitment to the promoter of the neighboring *CDKN2A* and *CDKN2B* genes, thereby controlling their expression [8]. (**b**) Regulation in *trans* by *ANRIL*, which acts through Alu sequences to recruit PRC1 and PRC2 complexes to distant targets [9]. (**c**) The embryonic stem cell–specific lncRNA *lncPRESS1* sequesters the histone deacetylase Sirtuin 6 (SIRT6) from the promoters of numerous pluripotency genes. *LncPRESS1* keeps histone H3 acetylated, thereby activating the transcription of pluripotency genes. During differentiation or following depletion of *lncPRESS1*, SIRT6 localizes to the chromatin, blocking the transcription of pluripotency genes [10]. (**d**) The lncRNA *GAS5* folds into a DNA-like structure and binds to the glucocorticoid receptor (GR), thereby inhibiting its transcriptional activity [11]. (**e**) The nuclear-retained lncRNA *MALAT1* can regulate alternative splicing by modulating the phosphorylation of the SR splicing factor [12]. (**f**) In the cytosol, the lncRNA *urothelial carcinoma associated 1* (*UCA1*) stabilizes *CDKN2A-p16* mRNA by sequestering the heterogeneous nuclear ribonucleoprotein A1 (hnRNPA1) [13]. (**g**) LncRNA *LBCS* suppresses the androgen receptor (AR) translation efficiency by forming a complex with hnRNPK and *AR* mRNA [14]. (**h**) The *lncRNA for kinase activation* (*LINK-A*) directly interacts with the AKT pleckstrin homology domain and PIP3 facilitating AKT–PIP3 interaction and consequent enzymatic activation [15]. (**i**) The lncRNA *PVT1* sponges *miR-503* to upregulate *ARL2* expression in cervical cancer [17].

2. Aims and Methodology of This Review

In this review, we aim to provide a comprehensive picture of the current knowledge of the role of lncRNAs in the pathogenesis of endometriosis and the mechanisms by which they affect the disease. We included patient studies to detect lncRNAs that have been associated with endometriosis, along with in vitro studies and in vivo animal studies to analyze the mechanism of action and function of lncRNAs in the disease. To gather studies for this review, we searched both the PubMed and Google Scholar databases for endometriosis and lncRNA combined with the following keywords: mechanism of action, sponging, ceRNA networks, chromatin, biomarkers, genome-wide, microenvironment, and infertility. We concentrated on original research papers, excluding literature reviews, pre-prints, meeting abstracts, and articles that were not in English and then assessed the remaining publications for this review.

3. Evidence for the Role of lncRNAs in Endometriosis

The evidence for the role of lncRNAs in the pathogenesis of endometriosis has been largely uncovered by using high-throughput screening technologies to detect differences between control and disease cohorts from either patient samples or animal models. Selected lncRNAs identified using these approaches were then subjected to further validation experiments to confirm their role. Below, we discuss the current evidence, most of which is derived from genome-wide genomic or transcriptomic studies.

3.1. Genetic Evidence for lncRNA Involvement in Endometriosis

Genome-wide association studies (GWAS) have been conducted for many diseases including endometriosis [24,25]. This powerful approach surveys single-nucleotide polymorphisms (SNPs) throughout the genome in a large cohort of individuals to identify variants and genomic regions associated with an increased chance of developing the disease. SNPs identified in GWAS studies often occur in intergenic regions, and therefore, it has been speculated that they may affect the regulation of nearby genes [26]. One mechanism by which this could work is via changing the sequence of an lncRNA and, thereby, affecting its regulatory function [27].

Genome-wide DNA sequencing technology has identified genetic variations in lncRNA loci that may affect the pathogenesis of endometriosis. The rs10965235 SNP located on chromosome 9p21.3 is associated with severe endometriosis in a Korean patient cohort and lies within the *CDKN2B-AS* gene locus [28]. This indicates that disruption of lncRNA function by the SNP is a possible mechanism through which this variant may predispose patients to endometriosis. The rs3820282 SNP located within a *WNT4* intron on chromosome 1p36.12 is associated with endometriosis and appears to affect an enhancer–promoter interaction resulting in the downregulation of *LINC00339* and upregulation of *CDC42* [29]. This indicates another possible mechanism for lncRNA regulation, whereby dysregulation of *CDC42* due to the risk of an SNP affecting enhancer competition with the *LINC00339* promoter leads to predisposition to endometriosis. Recently, genetic variations at the rs1838169 and rs17720428 SNPs sites on chromosome 12q13.3 in *HOTAIR* have been shown to be frequently detected in patients with endometriosis [30]. These variants appear to increase the stability of the lncRNA, resulting in reduced levels of *HOXD10* and *HOXA5* transcripts regulated by *HOTAIR*. A variant of the rs591291 SNP located on chromosome 11q13.1 in the promoter region of *MALAT1* was associated with an increase in endometriosis risk in a Chinese population, indicating that a change in the *MALAT1* expression level may affect endometriosis risk, although this was not examined in this study [31]. Finally, the rs710886 SNP in *PCAT1* has been associated with increased risk of developing endometriosis [32]. This SNP appears to disrupt sponging by *PCAT1* of *miR-145*, affecting the expression of *FASCIN1*, *SOX2*, *MSI2*, *SERPINE1*, and *JAM-A*, and the proliferative and invasive ability of endometriosis stem cells. Together, these studies indicate that genetic variants associated with endometriosis may predispose patients to the disease by disrupting the lncRNA gene regulatory function via diverse mechanisms.

3.2. Transcriptional Evidence for lncRNA Involvement in Endometriosis

To date, there have been around 14 genome-wide profiling transcriptome studies of human patient samples and animal models for endometriosis (Table 1). These studies are mainly descriptive in nature, with experimental validation limited to a few selected candidates. These studies often include in silico analysis examining the relationship between differentially expressed protein coding and lncRNA transcripts. Further bioinformatic approaches, such as gene ontology analysis, are then often used to predict the relevance of the identified targets to biological pathways involved in the pathogenesis of endometriosis. Initial studies were mostly conducted using microarray platforms to assess the expression of lncRNAs and mRNAs. Using a human lncRNA expression microarray, Sun et al. [33] were the first to assess genome-wide the relationship between lncRNA and mRNA expression in ovarian endometriosis lesions compared to paired autologous eutopic endometrial samples. They identified 948 lncRNAs and 4088 mRNAs as differentially expressed in the study cohort and validated the differential expression of the top 10 lncRNA candidates using qRT-PCR. Based on co-expression with mRNAs, lncRNAs in this study were predicted to take part in tissue adhesion, angiogenesis, estrogen production, and immune response, all processes known to be associated with the pathogenesis of endometriosis. Co-expression and genomic proximity were then used to predict 49 *cis*-regulating lncRNAs and their protein coding targets, while *trans*-regulating lncRNAs were predicted by co-expression with transcription factors and network analysis. This indicated that the top candidates were in a network with MYC, CTCF, and E2F4. Another study from Cai et al. (2019) used microarrays to profile lncRNA and mRNA expression in an endometriosis rat model, resulting in the identification of 115 upregulated and 51 downregulated lncRNAs together with 182 differentially expressed protein coding mRNA transcripts [34]. Co-expression analysis revealed five lncRNAs (*LOC102551276, NONRTT006252, LOC103691820, LOC102546604,* and *NONRATT003997*) that show a similar expression pattern to four protein coding mRNAs (*Adamts7, P2ry6, Dlx3,* and *TP53*), indicating a possible functional relationship in endometriosis.

Using a transcriptome array, Wang et al. [35] investigated the expression profile of lncRNAs in serum and tissue samples from patients with and without endometriosis. Following qRT-PCR validation of differentially expressed lncRNAs, they identified a combination of five circulating lncRNAs (*NR_038395, NR_038452, ENST00000482343, ENST00000544649,* and *ENST00000393610*) that they proposed could act as non-invasive biomarkers for the disease.

In the last few years, high-throughput RNA sequencing technology has surpassed microarrays as the preferred genome-wide technology for the identification of differentially expressed lncRNAs in endometriosis. Unlike microarrays, RNA sequencing is not biased by prior knowledge, enabling the discovery and characterization of lncRNAs that may play a role in the disease. A number of RNA sequencing studies have now been conducted comparing tissues from either patients or endometriosis animal models (Table 1). For example, using RNA sequencing, Cui et al. identified 86 differentially expressed lncRNAs and 1228 differentially expressed mRNAs in patients with ovarian endometriosis lesions compared to eutopic endometrial controls [36]. Pathway and gene ontology analysis showed that differentially expressed lncRNAs were involved in the regulation of cell proliferation, adhesion, migration, steroidogenesis, and angiogenesis, all processes implicated in endometriosis lesion formation and survival at ectopic sites of implantation.

Table 1. Genome-wide studies that identified differentially expressed lncRNAs in endometriosis.

Method (Reference)	Cohort (Tissue Type)	Validation (Type; Cohort; lncRNAs)	Predicted Function in Endometriosis	Limitations
Expression Microarray [33]	$n = 8$ (paired ovarian: 4 eutopic and 4 ectopic tissues)	RT-qPCR $n = 42$ (paired ovarian: 21 eutopic and 21 ectopic tissues) CHL1-AS2, MGC24103, XLOC_007433, HOXA11-AS, KLF1, LOC100505776, XLOC_012981, LIMS3-LOC4408, LOC389906	*Cis* and *trans* regulation of protein coding genes	1, 6

Table 1. Cont.

Method (Reference)	Cohort (Tissue Type)	Validation (Type; Cohort; lncRNAs)	Predicted Function in Endometriosis	Limitations
Expression Microarray [37]	$n = 6$ (3 eutopic tissues of women with EM of undefined entity and 3 eutopic tissues of women without EM)	RT-qPCR $n = 68$ (40 eutopic tissues of women with EM of undefined entity and 28 eutopic tissues of women without EM) RP11-369C8.1, RP11-432J24.5, AC068282.3, GBP1P1, SNHG1, AC002454.1, AC007246.3, FTX	Cell cycle regulation and immune response	1, 2, 4, 6
Expression Microarray [35]	Serum: $n = 20$ (10 women with peritoneal and/or ovarian EM and 10 women without EM) Tissue: $n = 15$ (paired peritoneal and/or ovarian: 5 eutopic and 5 ectopic EM patients and 5 eutopic tissues of women without EM	RT-qPCR Serum: $n = 110$ (59 women with peritoneal and/or ovarian EM and 51 women without EM) Tissue: qPCR $n = 24$ (paired peritoneal and/or ovarian: 9 eutopic and 9 ectopic tissues of EM patients and 6 eutopic tissues of women without EM) DE lncRNAs 16	Combination of NR_038395, NR_038452, ENST00000482343, ENST00000544649, and ENST00000393610 suggested as a non-invasive diagnosis marker	1, 2 (because of pooling)
Expression microarray [38]	$n = 8$ (paired ovarian: 4 eutopic and 4 ectopic tissues of EM patients)	RT-qPCR $n = 87$ (paired ovarian: 30 eutopic and 30 ectopic tissues of EM patients and 27 eutopic tissues of women without EM)) CHL1-AS2	CCDC144NL-AS1 expression was upregulated in ectopic tissues compared to eutopic and control endometrial tissues	1
Re-analysis of existing microarray data [39]	$n = 18$ GSE120103 (eutopic tissue from 9 fertile and 9 infertile women with ovarian EM)	Validation of 14 hub mRNAs using GSE26787 (5 fertile and 5 infertile women with unknown EM status)	Identification of putative infertility-associated lncRNAs LOC390705 and LOC100505854	1, 3, 6
Re-analysis of existing microarray data [40]	GSE7305 (paired ovarian: 10 eutopic and 10 ectopic tissues of EM patients and 10 eutopic tissues of women without EM) GSE7846 (HEECs of eutopic tissues of 5 EM patients with ovarian EM and HEECs of eutopic tissues of 5 women without EM), GSE29981 (LMD epithelial cells of 20 women without EM) E-MTAB-694 (paired peritoneal: 18 eutopic and 18 ectopic tissues of EM patients and 17 eutopic tissues of women without EM)	No validation	Proposed cell cycle regulatory functions for LINC01279	2, 3, 4, 5
RNA-Seq [41]	$n = 16$ (8 eutopic tissues of women with EM of undefined entity and 8 eutopic tissues of women without EM)	No validation	Predicted oxidative stress and endometrial receptivity regulatory functions	1, 2, 3, 4, 6
RNA-Seq [36]	$n = 10$ (5 eutopic tissues of patients with ovarian EM and 5 eutopic tissues of women without EM)	RT-qPCR $n = 24$ (12 eutopic tissues of patients with ovarian EM and 12 eutopic tissues of women without EM) USP46-AS1, RP11-1143G9.4, RP11-217B1.2, AC004951.6, RP11-182J1.12	Predicted proliferation, adhesion, migration, invasion, and angiogenesis regulatory functions	1, 4, 6

Table 1. Cont.

Method (Reference)	Cohort (Tissue Type)	Validation (Type; Cohort; lncRNAs)	Predicted Function in Endometriosis	Limitations
RNA-Seq [42]	n = 9 (paired ovarian: 3 eutopic and 3 ectopic tissues of EM patients and 3 eutopic tissues of women without EM)	RT-qPCR n = 45 (paired:15 eutopic and 15 ectopic tissues of EM patients with undefined entity and 15 eutopic tissues of women without EM) PRKAR2B, CLEC2D	Predicted angiogenesis, cell adhesion, cell migration, immune response, inflammatory response, NF-κB signaling, regulatory functions	1, 2, 4
Re-analysis of existing RNA-Seq and expression array datasets [43]	GSE105764 (paired ovarian: 8 eutopic and 8 ectopic tissues of EM patients) GSE121406 (paired ovarian: FACS sorted stromal cells of 4 eutopic and 4 ectopic tissues of EM patients) GSE105765 (same as GSE105764)	in silico validation by microarray GSE124010 (3 ectopic tissues of patients with EM of undefined entity and 3 eutopic tissues of women without EM) GSE86534 (paired ovarian: 4 eutopic and 4 ectopic tissues of patients with EM)	Predicted function in regulation of inflammation and prediction of sponging LINC01018 and SMIM25 functions for hsa-miR-182-5p in the regulation of CHL1 protein coding gene to promote endometriosis	1, 4 (validation study), 5, 6
Re-analysis of existing RNA-Seq datasets [44]	n = 28 (paired ovarian: 14 eutopic and 14 ectopic tissues of infertile EM patients) GSE105764 (paired ovarian: 8 eutopic and 8 ectopic tissues of EM patients) GSE105765 (same patients as in GSE105764) GSE25628 (unpaired DIE: 8 eutopic and 8 ectopic tissues of EM patients and 6 eutopic tissues of women without EM)	No validation	Construction of a competitive endogenous (ce) RNA network promoting growth and death of endometrial stroma cells. CDK1 and PCNA proposed as treatment targets for endometriosis-associated infertility	1, 3, 5
RNA-Seq [45]	n = 12 (paired ovarian: 6 eutopic and 6 ectopic tissues of EM patients)	RT-qPCR n = 60 (paired ovarian: 30 eutopic and 30 ectopic tissues of EM patients) MIR202HG, LINC00261, UCA1, GAGA2-AS1	Immunity, inflammation	1, 6
Re-analysis of existing RNA-Seq data [46]	GSE105764 and GSE105765 include same patients n = 16 (paired ovarian: 8 eutopic and 8 ectopic tissues of EM patients)	No validation	LncRNAs:H19, GS1-358P8.4, and RP11-96D1.10 strongly associated with ovarian endometriosis	1, 3, 6
Animal Studies				
Expression microarray [34]	Rat n = 35 (EM uterine tissue EM = 13, adipose tissue control = 8, blank = 14)	RT-qPCR; NONRATT003997; gi|672033904|ref|, XR_589853.1|; NONRATT006252; gi|672027621|ref|; XR_592747.1|; gi|672045999|ref|; XR_591544.1|	Regulation of endometrial receptivity	

EM, endometriosis; HEECs, human endometrial endothelial cells; LMD, laser microdissection; DIE, deep infiltrating endometriosis. 1, small sample size (less than 30 per group); 2, no comprehensive clinical information (i.e., American Fertility Society (rAFS) disease stage, lesion entities, menstrual cycle phase); 3, no validation in an adequate independent cohort; 4, EM-free controls are not appropriate (i.e., CIN patients, no laparoscopic proof); 5, combining heterogeneous datasets (i.e., different lesion entities, cycle phases, stages, cell types); 6, not all relevant tissues analyzed (i.e., eutopic tissues of EM-free controls, eutopic and ectopic tissues of EM patients).

In spite of the advantages listed above, RNA sequencing studies have some limitations. Due to their high cost, they are often limited to a small number of samples and lack extensive validation. However, they can form the basis for further studies that perform functional validation of candidate genes and investigate their value as diagnostic and prognostic markers in endometriosis. These validation studies usually have cohorts with a larger sample size and may include functional experiments that attempt to uncover the molecular mechanism of lncRNA action (Table S1). For example, AFAP1-AS1 was identified as one of the most differentially expressed lncRNAs in the microarray study of Sun et al. [33]. In a new study, Lin et al. [47] could confirm and extend these findings in a cohort of $n = 36$ patients. They show that *AFAP1-AS1* is overexpressed in ectopic endometrium of women with endometriosis ($n = 18$), compared to paired eutopic endometriosis tissue ($n = 18$) and normal endometrium of women without the disease ($n = 10$). In vitro gene targeting assays in primary human endometriotic stroma cells (ESCs) indicated that this lncRNA regulates epithelial–mesenchymal transition (EMT) in endometriosis by regulating transcription of the EMT-related transcription factor ZEB1. Furthermore, experiments in a xenograft mouse model indicated that AFAP1-AS1 was required for the growth of ectopic tissue. In this case, a shRNA knockdown of AFAP1-AS1 in the Ishikawa endometrial cancer cell line led to reduction of the subcutaneous tumor size, compared to animals injected with a non-targeting shRNA-transfected cell line [47].

Liu et al. analyzed the value of lncRNA H19 expression as an endometriosis biomarker [48]. They found that H19 expression in the both the ectopic and eutopic endometrium of endometriosis patients was significantly higher than in the normal endometrium. Overexpression of H19 lncRNA in endometriosis lesions was associated with infertility, recurrence of disease, bilateral ovarian lesions, an increased CA125 level and with progression in the revised American Fertility Society (rAFS) disease stage. Further multivariate logistic regression analysis showed that H19 overexpression in endometriosis lesions is a prognostic factor for endometriosis recurrence.

In summary, recently there has been an effort by a number of studies using genome-wide high-throughput technologies to identify differentially expressed lncRNAs in endometriosis not only for their potential clinical application as diagnostic or prognostic biomarkers of the disease, but also in order to gain insights into the pathogenesis of the disease (Table 1). The lncRNAs where further work has been done to validate a role in endometriosis are listed in Table S1 and summarized in Figure 2.

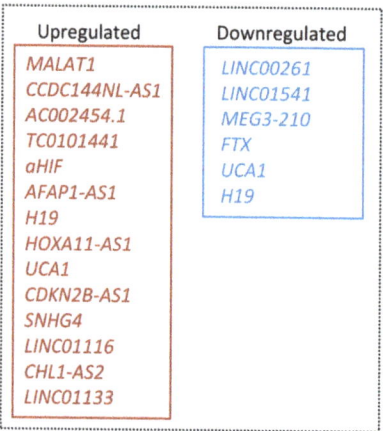
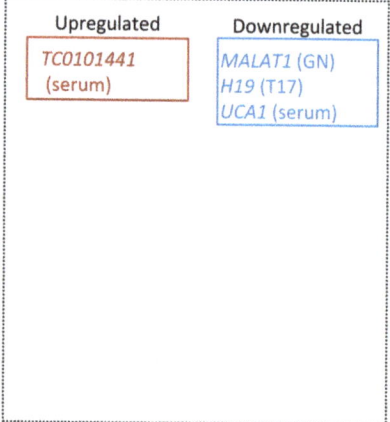

Figure 2. Differentially expressed (DE) lncRNAs in endometriosis based on validation studies: (**a**) Up- and downregulated lncRNAs in endometriosis tissues and/or cells (**b**) in body fluids or lesion microenvironment.

3.3. Critical Assessment of the Evidence for the Role of lncRNAs in Endometriosis

In the previous sections, and in Table 1 and Table S1, we summarized the evidence for a role for lncRNAs candidates in endometriosis derived from genomic and transcriptomic studies. However, the strengths and weaknesses of these studies should be taken into account when assessing the role of individual lncRNAs in the pathology of the disease.

We have assessed the studies listed in Table 1 and Table S1 and noted common limitations, namely small sample size, incomplete clinical information, no validation in an independent cohort, inappropriate controls, or failure to examine all relevant tissues. A limitation that can apply in particular to re-analysis of published datasets is that differences in the type of tissue collected, such as lesion type, menstrual cycle stage, or the type of controls, used may limit the validity of comparisons between studies. Following assessment of all the studies in Table 1 and Table S1, we found that 38.5% (5/13) of the transcriptome studies had no validation in an adequate independent cohort and that 23.1% (3/13) compared heterogeneous datasets that containing either different lesion types, cell types, or disease stages, and/or samples from different menstrual cycle phases. In total, 81.1% (30/37) of all studies analyzing lncRNA expression in human tissues had a small sample size (defined as less than 30 per group), and 45.9% (17/37) did not provide comprehensive clinical information regarding the lesion type, rAFS stage, or menstrual cycle phase. Around half of the studies (19/37) had inappropriate endometriosis-free controls, in that they included cervical intraepithelial neoplasia (CIN) patients or had no laparoscopic proof that the controls were endometriosis free. Finally, 45.9% (17/37) of the studies did not evaluate all the relevant tissue types, which are eutopic tissues of endometriosis-free controls and eutopic and ectopic tissues from endometriosis patients. Therefore, while these genome-wide studies can be valuable in detecting lncRNAs that may be novel players in endometriosis pathogenesis, careful validation studies are required, as well as mechanistic studies to understand how they may function.

4. Functional Evidence for the Mechanism of lncRNA Action in Endometriosis

The diverse range of mechanisms for lncRNA action described above show what is possible, but so far, only a subset of these mechanisms have been described in the context of endometriosis. Based on the current knowledge, the mechanism of lncRNA action in endometriosis can be divided into the following groups: (i) lncRNAs that recruit and target chromatin remodeling or transcriptional regulatory factors, (ii) lncRNAs with miRNA sponging functions, and (iii) lncRNAs that modulate cellular signaling pathways.

4.1. Chromatin Remodeling and Transcriptional Control by lncRNAs in Endometriosis

The HOTAIR lncRNA is known as a critical regulator of HOX gene expression. Maintaining appropriate expression of genes within the HOX-gene network has been shown to be critical for endometrial homeostasis during embryonic implantation, and alterations in HOXA10 and HOXA11 expression have been associated with endometriosis-associated infertility [49,50]. Mechanistically, *HOTAIR* interacts with the PRC2 or REST/CoREST chromatin remodeling complex to guide the recruitment of H3K27 tri-methylation or H3K4-demethylation at target gene loci resulting in target gene silencing [51]. As described above, it has been shown that genetic variations at SNPs sites in *HOTAIR* are relatively frequently detected in patients with endometriosis [30]. These genetic changes alter the thermostability of mature *HOTAIR* leading to epigenetic silencing of *HOXD10* and *HOXA5* genes and are associated with more advanced endometriosis [30].

Overexpression of the lncRNA *AFAP1-AS1* has been shown to be associated with ovarian endometriosis [33]. In another example of direct transcriptional regulation by an lncRNA in endometriosis, *AFAP1-AS1* directly activates expression of EMT-related transcription factor ZEB1 in vitro [47]. ZEB1 has been previously shown to be involved in 17β-estradiol-induced EMT in endometriosis [52], indicating a possible mechanism by which *AFAP1-AS1* could affect endometriosis.

4.2. MiRNA Sponging by LncRNAs in Endometriosis

A growing body of evidence indicates that lncRNAs can act as miRNA sponges in endometriosis (summarized in Table 2). In these cases, a binding site for the miRNA is present in both the lncRNA and the targeted protein-coding gene, and there is a correlation between expression of the lncRNA and the protein-coding gene. In the first reported example of sponging in endometriosis, decreased levels of the H19 lncRNA was shown to be associated with an increase in *let-7* miRNA activity, which inhibits *IGF1R* expression resulting in the reduced proliferation of endometrial stroma cells [53]. These results suggested that the *H19/let7/IGF1R* pathway may contribute to impaired endometrial receptivity in women suffering from the disease. *H19* was also shown to regulate cell proliferation and invasion of ectopic endometrial cells by increasing ITGB3 expression via sponging of *miR-124-3p* [54]. *H19* has also been implicated in the impaired immune responses of women with the disease, by acting as a sponge for *miR-342-3p*, which regulates the IER3 pathway. This pathway has been implicated in Th-17 cell differentiation and endometrial stroma cell proliferation in ectopic sites in women with the disease [55]. Another lncRNA that has been shown to act as a sponge in endometriosis is *CDKN2B-AS1*, which acts as a regulator of AKT3 expression by sponging *miR-424-5p* in an in vitro model of ovarian endometriosis [56]. In another example, *LINC01116* promoted the proliferation and migration of endometrial stroma cells by targeting FOXP1 via sponging of *miR-9-5p*, thereby promoting endometriosis lesion formation and growth [57]. *MALAT1* was identified as a sponge of *miR-200c* involved in the regulation of endometriosis stoma cell proliferation and migration by promoting ZEB1 and ZEB2 expression in women with the disease [58]. This regulation is not restricted to *miR-200c* and may include the entire *miR-200* family, consisting of *miR-200a, miR-200b, miR-200c, miR-141*, and *miR-429* [59]. In addition to these examples, other lncRNAs have also been implicated in endometriosis via their role as sponges for miRNAs, as summarized in Table 2.

Table 2. LncRNAs involved in endometriosis as molecular sponges of miRNAs.

lncRNA (Reference)	Sponged miRNA	Target mRNA (Pathway) in Endometriosis
H19 [53]	Let-7; miR-125-3p; miR-342-3p; miR-216a-5p	IGF1R; ITGB3; IER3; ACTA2
CDKN2B-AS1 [56]	miR-424-5p	AKT3
LINC01541 [60]	miR-506-3p	WIF1 (Wnt/β-catenin)
LINC01116 [57]	miR-9-5p	FOXP1
SNHG4 [61]	miR-148a-3p	c-Met
LINC01018 [43]	miR-182-5p	CHLI (inflammatory)
SMIM25 [43]	miR-182-5p	CHLI (inflammatory)
MALAT1 [62]	miR-126-5p; miR200s; miR200c	CREB1 (PI3K/AKT); ZEB1, ZEB2, VIM (EMT); ZEB1, ZEB2, CDH2 (EMT)
LINC00261 [63]	miR-132-3p	BCL2L11
PCAT1 [32]	miR-145	FASCIN1, SOX2, MSI2, SERPIN

4.3. LncRNAs Modulating Cellular Signaling Pathways in Endometriosis

Cell signaling pathways have a pivotal role in the regulation of a variety of cellular processes in response to intracellular or extracellular stimuli. The regulation of components of a signaling pathway by lncRNAs can be direct or indirect and result in functional changes in the signaling cascades. Direct regulation can be achieved by direct binding of the lncRNA to signaling proteins leading to changes in either their free cellular levels or their activity. We define indirect regulation as cases where no direct lncRNA binding to signaling molecules has been shown and where the lncRNA is thought to alter the transcription of genes associated with the signaling pathway resulting in an altered cellular response. In Table 3, we summarize currently known cases where a lncRNA directly or indirectly affects a signaling pathway in endometriosis.

Table 3. Mechanisms of cell signaling regulation via lncRNAs in endometriosis.

lncRNA (Reference)	Model System	Signaling Molecules	Signaling Pathways	Type of Regulation	Function in Endometriosis
MEG3-210 [64]	Primary HESC, HEEC, EM mouse model	Galectin-1	P38 MAPK, PKA/SERCA2	direct	Regulation of migration, invasion and apoptosis, lesion growth and vascularization
MALAT1 [65]	EMs cells	Caspase-3, MMP-9	NFkB/iNOS	Indirect	Regulation of apoptosis, migration, invasion
MALAT1 [66]	Granulosa cells (KGN cell line)	p21, p53, CDK1	ERK/MAPK	Indirect	Regulation of cell proliferation, ovarian follicle count, infertility
MALAT1 [67]	HESC	HIF-1α, LC3-II, beclin1	-	Indirect	Regulation of hypoxia-induced pro-survival and autophagy
LINC01541 [68]	HESC	β-Catenin, VEGFA, BCL2, caspase-3	WNT/β-Catenin	Indirect	Regulates EMT, migration, invasion, survival, and angiogenesis
LINC01541 [69]	12Z epithelial endometriosis cell line	p21, cyclin A	TESK1/Cofilin	Indirect	Regulation of cell proliferation and invasion
FTX [70]	EESC (ectopic endometrial stromal cells), HESC (normal)	E-Cadherin, N-cadherin, ZEB1, vimentin	PI3K/AKT	Indirect	Regulates EMT and cell cycle
BANCR [71]	Rat model of EM, ectopic tissue, and serum	VEGF, MMP-9, MMP-2	MAPK/ERK	Indirect	Regulation of angiogenesis
UCA1 [72]	HESC	IC3, VMP1	-	Indirect	Regulation of autophagy and apoptosis
AC002454.1 [73]	EESC	CDK6	-	Indirect	Regulation of cell migration and invasion
CCDC144NL-AS1 [74]	HESC	Vimentin, MMP-9	-	Indirect	Regulation of cell migration and invasion
TC0101441 [75]	ECSC	N-Cadherin, SNAIL, SLUG, TCF8/ZEB1	-	Indirect	Promotes endometriosis cyst stromal cell (ECSC) migration and invasion

In an example of direct regulation of a signaling pathway in endometriosis, the lncRNA *MEG3-210* has been shown to regulate endometriosis stromal cell migration, invasion, and apoptosis through the p38 MAPK and PKA/SERCA2 signaling pathways. In this case, *MEG3-210* directly interacts with Galectin-1 in vitro and affects the growth of endometriotic lesions in vivo in a murine model of the disease [64]. Mechanistically, *MEG3-210* titrates away the cellular levels of Galectin-1, preventing its action on the p38 MAPK and PKA/SERCA2 signaling cascades in endometrial stromal cells. In endometriosis, the levels of *MEG3-210* are downregulated and the levels of free Galectin-1 are upregulated, which is associated with the subsequent activation of p38 MAPK signaling–mediated phosphorylation of ATF2. Activated ATF2 increases the expression of BCL-2 and MMP contributing to the anti-apoptotic, pro-migratory, and invasive phenotype of endometriosis cells. Simultaneously, *MEG3-210* downregulation leads to suppression of the PKA/SERCA2 signaling cascade [64].

In an example of indirect regulation of signaling pathway, knockdown of *MALAT1* lncRNA in endometriosis cells leads to enhanced cell death, reduced migration and invasion associated with activation of Caspase-3, and downregulation of MMP-9 and the NFkB/iNOS signaling pathway (Figure 3a) [65]. In contrast to endometriosis tissue where *MALAT1* is overexpressed, in the granulosa cells of women with endometriosis *MALAT1* expression is reduced [66]. This is associated with a reduced follicle count, due to impaired cell proliferation resulting from ERK/MAPK-dependent p21/p53 cell cycle arrest. This implicates altered expression of *MALAT1* in endometriosis-related infertility. In cultured primary endometrial stromal cells, depletion of *MALAT1* by siRNA knockdown results in the suppression of hypoxia-induced autophagy, as indicated by a reduction in the expression of autophagy markers Beclin-1 and LC3-II [67]. In this signaling cascade, expression of *MALAT1* is regulated by the HIF1α transcription factor, known to be overexpressed in endometriosis lesions and to regulate multiple gene targets in response to hypoxia (Figure 3a) (reviewed in [76]).

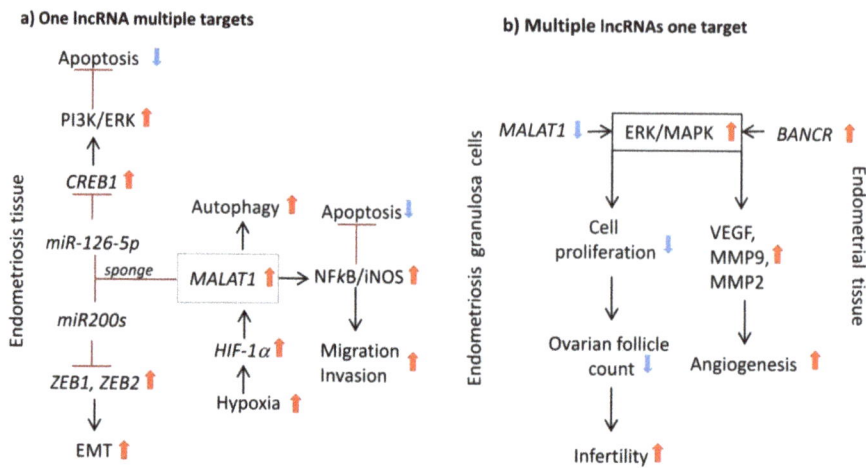

Figure 3. (a) *MALAT1* was identified as a sponge of *miR-200c*. This regulation is not restricted to *miR-200c* and might include the entire *miR-200* family (*miR-200s*), consisting of *miR-200a*, *miR-200b*, *miR-200c*, *miR-141*, and *miR-429*. Upregulation of *MALAT1* in women with endometriosis leads to enhanced sponging of *miR200s* and promotes zinc finger E-box binding homeobox transcription factor 1 (ZEB1) and ZEB2 expression leading to higher EMT. In HESCs, the lncRNA *MALAT1* directly interacts with *miR-126-5p*, which regulates cAMP responsive element-binding protein (CREB1) expression. Upregulation of *MALAT1* inhibits apoptosis probably via activation of the PI3K–AKT pathway through the *miR-126-5p*–CREB1 axis. *MALAT1* lncRNA can also lead to reduced apoptosis in HESCs through the upregulation of the NFkB/iNOS signaling pathway activity, which also enhances migration and invasion of cells. In cultured primary endometrial stromal cells, *MALAT1* leads to upregulation of hypoxia-induced autophagy. In this signaling cascade, regulation of *MALAT1* expression is under the control of the HIF1α transcription factor. (b) In granulosa cells (GCs) of women with endometriosis, significant downregulation of *MALAT1* expression was reported. *MALAT1* knockdown induced an increase in phosphorylated ERK1/2 (p-ERK1/2) that was associated with altered follicle count, due to impaired cell proliferation resulting from ERK/MAPK-dependent activation of p21/p53 cell cycle arrest. In an autograft transplantation rat model of endometriosis, inhibition of the lncRNA *BANCR* led to a decrease in ectopic tissue volume associated with a significant reduction in serum levels of *VEGF*, *MMP-2*, and *MMP-9*, *ERK*, and *MAPK* mRNA and in phosphorylated ERK and MAPK protein levels in tissues. HESCs: human endometrial stromal cells.

In another example, the most downregulated lncRNA in ectopic tissue of women with ovarian endometriosis was *LINC01541* [33], which has been shown respond to levels of estradiol [68]. A gene-targeting in vitro study in human endometrial stromal cells showed that the cellular levels of *LINC01541* affect the activity of WNT/β-catenin, pro- and anti-apoptotic signaling regulators Caspase-3 and BCL2 and the levels of VEGFA production [68].

The presence of extracellular lncRNA in exosomes or microvesicles raises the possibility that these lncRNAs may be able to serve as extracellular signals for cell signaling regulation in endometriosis. This was supported by reports that exosomal lncRNAs promote angiogenesis in endometriosis [77]. Based on an in vitro co-culture model and patient serum analysis, the authors developed a novel mechanistic model explaining how endometriosis stromal cells of the lesion induce angiogenesis. They suggested that these cells in an ectopic environment can produce exosomes that are enriched in *aHIF* lncRNA, a pro-angiogenic lncRNA, highly expressed in ectopic endometrial stromal tissue. These *aHIF*-rich exosomes are then taken up by recipient macrovascular cells, where they cause upregulation of the angiogenesis-related genes VEGF-A, VEGF-D, and bFGF.

Endometriosis is an estrogen-dependent disease, and therefore, lncRNAs involved in the estrogen pathway or those targeted by estrogen signaling could play a role in the disease. The lncRNA *H19* is positively regulated by estrogen, and its expression in the endometrium increases during the proliferative stage of the menstrual cycle [78,79]. *H19* has been shown regulate several pathways that are relevant in endometriosis including IGF1R, ITGB3, IER3, and ACTA2 [53–55,80]. Another lncRNA, *steroid receptor RNA activator 1 (SRA1)* lncRNA, has been reported to act in concert with SRA1 to regulate the expression of estrogen receptors by affecting alternative splicing, and thereby the growth of stromal cells in ovarian endometriosis [81]. These examples illustrate how lncRNAs could play a role in endometriosis via the estrogen pathway or as targets of estrogen regulation.

Conceptually, the mechanism of lncRNAs' action in endometriosis may involve influencing cellular pathways, where one lncRNA may regulate several targets using different molecular strategies (Figure 3a) or one targeted signaling pathway may be affected by multiple lncRNAs (Figure 3b). To better understand this complexity, integrative in silico and experimental analyses interrogating the molecular networks in endometriosis cells need to be applied. This approach should help to dissect the relationship between lncRNA, mRNA, miRNA expression, genetic- and epigenetic-driven chromatin remodeling, and signal transduction activity and to enable lncRNA target identification. The use of such in silico bioinformatics algorithms for cellular network construction in endometriosis has already been attempted by several studies [41,43,46]. For example, Wang et al. [41] constructed an lncRNA–miRNA–mRNA network, revealing lncRNAs that act as competing endogenous RNAs (ceRNA), the miRNAs they sponge, and the target genes that were involved in regulating endometrial receptivity in endometriosis. Moreover, Jiang et al. [43] identified the lncRNAs (*SMIM25*, *LINC01018*), miRNA (*miR-182-5p*), and mRNA (*CHLI*) as part of a ceRNA network implicated in the regulation of immune responses in endometriosis. These in silico studies may be valuable to predict how lncRNAs may function in endometriosis, but experimental validation is required in order for these predictions to be confirmed.

5. Summary and Perspectives

In recent years, a growing number of studies have implicated the abnormal expression of specific lncRNAs with various aspects of endometriosis pathogenesis. This altered expression may be due to genetic predisposition or an unknown environmental trigger and affect pathogenetic processes including EMT, endometriosis cell stemness, angiogenesis, lesion establishment and growth, endometriosis cell survival, proliferation and invasion, oxidative stress, autophagy, and endometrial receptivity (summarized in Figure 4). Evidence for the role of lncRNAs has mainly come from large-scale transcriptome studies comparing normal and diseased tissue, followed by validation studies of a small number of candidate lncRNAs. These studies can be valuable for uncovering potential novel players in endometriosis but often have weaknesses that should be considered including small sample size, incomplete clinical information on patient samples, and inappropriate controls (Table 1, Table S1). A general weakness of these studies is that they do not assess the complexity of the disease to take into account different lesion types, the stage or severity of the disease, or the effect of hormone status or age of the patient. The vast majority of lncRNAs revealed in these studies remain unvalidated by an independent method or by functional studies. One challenge for future work is to prioritize lncRNAs identified in these studies for validation and then conduct further functional studies to determine their role in endometriosis and their possible use as biomarkers or targets for treatment.

One avenue of endometriosis research that should be pursued in the future is the connection between genetic variants and abnormal lncRNA expression that affects aspects of endometriosis pathogenesis. The majority of disease-associated SNPs in GWAS studies, including those investigating endometriosis, are in non-coding regions. The hypothesis that these SNPs may affect lncRNA function is supported by a number of studies in endometriosis, with SNPs in or near lncRNAs including *HOTAIR*, *MALAT1*, *CDKN2B-AS*, *PCAT1*, and *LINC00339* affecting their expression and regulation of genes and the endometriosis phenotype [28–32]. The possibility that other non-coding SNPs associated with endometriosis may also affect the disease via lncRNAs should be investigated.

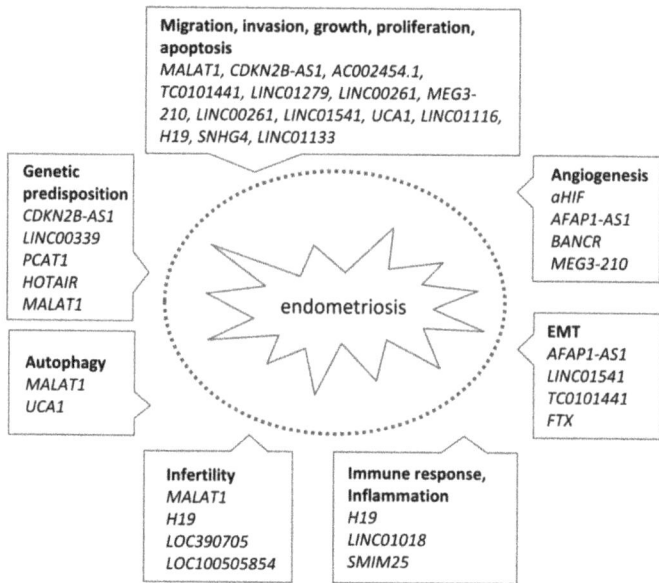

Figure 4. Phenotypical changes caused by altered expression of lncRNAs in endometriosis. Altered expression of lncRNAs in endometriosis is involved in the regulation of numerous processes known to be associated with the pathogenesis of the disease. These processes include EMT, endometriosis cell stemness, angiogenesis, lesion establishment and growth, endometriosis cell survival, proliferation and invasion, oxidative stress, autophagy, and endometrial receptivity.

In vitro cell culture models and in vivo animal models are valuable systems that enable the mechanism of action and function of individual lncRNAs to be investigated experimentally. However, a weakness of some studies investigating endometriosis, including those investigating the role of lncRNAs, is that the available in vitro and in vivo models may not always represent all aspects of the disease accurately. Therefore, it should be a priority for the field to continue to strive for improved models to investigate the disease.

To conclude, genome-wide genomic and transcriptomic studies have implicated numerous lncRNAs in a wide range of diseases, including in endometriosis. The challenge remains to distinguish the lncRNAs that play a relevant role in the disease from those that are merely associated with the transcriptional changes in the disease and to functionally show their role.

Supplementary Materials: The following are available online at https://www.mdpi.com/article/10.3390/ijms222111425/s1.

Author Contributions: Conceptualization, Q.J.H., K.P. and I.Y.; methodology, Q.J.H., K.P. and I.Y.; data curation, Q.J.H., K.P. and I.Y.; writing—original draft preparation, Q.J.H., K.P. and I.Y.; writing—review and editing, A.P., L.K., H.H. and R.W.; visualization, Q.J.H., K.P. and I.Y.; supervision, I.Y.; funding acquisition, H.H. All authors have read and agreed to the published version of the manuscript.

Funding: This work was co-funded by the Ingrid Flick Foundation (grant no. FA751C0801), which played no role in the review design and analysis, decision to publish, or preparation of the manuscript.

Data Availability Statement: Not applicable.

Conflicts of Interest: The authors declare no conflict of interest.

References

1. Sampson, J.A. Peritoneal Endometriosis Due to the Menstrual Dissemination of Endometrial Tissue into the Peritoneal Cavity. *Am. J. Obstet. Gynecol.* **1927**, *14*, 442–469. [CrossRef]
2. Rei, C.; Williams, T.; Feloney, M. Endometriosis in a Man as a Rare Source of Abdominal Pain: A Case Report and Review of the Literature. *Case Rep. Obstet. Gynecol.* **2018**, *2018*, 2083121. [CrossRef] [PubMed]
3. Zondervan, K.T.; Becker, C.M.; Missmer, S.A. Endometriosis. *N. Engl. J. Med.* **2020**, *382*, 1244–1256. [CrossRef] [PubMed]
4. Shigesi, N.; Kvaskoff, M.; Kirtley, S.; Feng, Q.; Fang, H.; Knight, J.C.; Missmer, S.A.; Rahmioglu, N.; Zondervan, K.T.; Becker, C.M. The association between endometriosis and autoimmune diseases: A systematic review and meta-analysis. *Hum. Reprod. Update* **2019**, *25*, 486–503. [CrossRef] [PubMed]
5. Statello, L.; Guo, C.-J.; Chen, L.-L.; Huarte, M. Gene regulation by long non-coding RNAs and its biological functions. *Nat. Rev. Mol. Cell Biol.* **2021**, *22*, 96–118. [CrossRef] [PubMed]
6. Gil, N.; Ulitsky, I. Regulation of gene expression by cis-acting long non-coding RNAs. *Nat. Rev. Genet.* **2020**, *21*, 102–117. [CrossRef] [PubMed]
7. Delás, M.J.; Hannon, G.J. lncRNAs in development and disease: From functions to mechanisms. *Open Biol.* **2017**, *7*, 170121. [CrossRef] [PubMed]
8. Yap, K.L.; Li, S.; Munoz-Cabello, A.M.; Raguz, S.; Zeng, L.; Mujtaba, S.; Gil, J.; Walsh, M.J.; Zhou, M.M. Molecular interplay of the noncoding RNA ANRIL and methylated histone H3 lysine 27 by polycomb CBX7 in transcriptional silencing of INK4a. *Mol. Cell* **2010**, *38*, 662–674. [CrossRef] [PubMed]
9. Holdt, L.M.; Hoffmann, S.; Sass, K.; Langenberger, D.; Scholz, M.; Krohn, K.; Finstermeier, K.; Stahringer, A.; Wilfert, W.; Beutner, F.; et al. Alu elements in ANRIL non-coding RNA at chromosome 9p21 modulate atherogenic cell functions through trans-regulation of gene networks. *PLoS Genet.* **2013**, *9*, e1003588. [CrossRef] [PubMed]
10. Jain, A.K.; Xi, Y.; McCarthy, R.; Allton, K.; Akdemir, K.C.; Patel, L.R.; Aronow, B.; Lin, C.; Li, W.; Yang, L.; et al. LncPRESS1 Is a p53-Regulated LncRNA that Safeguards Pluripotency by Disrupting SIRT6-Mediated De-acetylation of Histone H3K56. *Mol. Cell* **2016**, *64*, 967–981. [CrossRef] [PubMed]
11. Kino, T.; Hurt, D.E.; Ichijo, T.; Nader, N.; Chrousos, G.P. Noncoding RNA Gas5 Is a Growth Arrest– and Starvation-Associated Repressor of the Glucocorticoid Receptor. *Sci. Signal.* **2010**, *3*, ra8. [CrossRef] [PubMed]
12. Tripathi, V.; Ellis, J.D.; Shen, Z.; Song, D.Y.; Pan, Q.; Watt, A.T.; Freier, S.M.; Bennett, C.F.; Sharma, A.; Bubulya, P.A.; et al. The nuclear-retained noncoding RNA MALAT1 regulates alternative splicing by modulating SR splicing factor phosphorylation. *Mol. Cell* **2010**, *39*, 925–938. [CrossRef] [PubMed]
13. Kumar, P.P.; Emechebe, U.; Smith, R.; Franklin, S.; Moore, B.; Yandell, M.; Lessnick, S.L.; Moon, A.M. Coordinated control of senescence by lncRNA and a novel T-box3 co-repressor complex. *Elife* **2014**, *3*, e02805. [CrossRef] [PubMed]
14. Gu, P.; Chen, X.; Xie, R.; Xie, W.; Huang, L.; Dong, W.; Han, J.; Liu, X.; Shen, J.; Huang, J.; et al. A novel AR translational regulator lncRNA LBCS inhibits castration resistance of prostate cancer. *Mol. Cancer* **2019**, *18*, 109. [CrossRef] [PubMed]
15. Lin, A.; Hu, Q.; Li, C.; Xing, Z.; Ma, G.; Wang, C.; Li, J.; Ye, Y.; Yao, J.; Liang, K.; et al. The LINK-A lncRNA interacts with PtdIns(3,4,5)P3 to hyperactivate AKT and confer resistance to AKT inhibitors. *Nat. Cell Biol.* **2017**, *19*, 238–251. [CrossRef] [PubMed]
16. Gong, C.; Maquat, L.E. lncRNAs transactivate STAU1-mediated mRNA decay by duplexing with 3′ UTRs via Alu elements. *Nature* **2011**, *470*, 284–288. [CrossRef] [PubMed]
17. Liu, W.; Yao, D.; Huang, B. LncRNA PVT1 promotes cervical cancer progression by sponging miR-503 to upregulate ARL2 expression. *Open Life Sci.* **2021**, *16*, 1–13. [CrossRef] [PubMed]
18. Jiang, M.C.; Ni, J.J.; Cui, W.Y.; Wang, B.Y.; Zhuo, W. Emerging roles of lncRNA in cancer and therapeutic opportunities. *Am. J. Cancer Res.* **2019**, *9*, 1354–1366. [PubMed]
19. Policarpo, R.; Sierksma, A.; De Strooper, B.; d'Ydewalle, C. From Junk to Function: LncRNAs in CNS Health and Disease. *Front. Mol. Neurosci.* **2021**, *14*, 151. [CrossRef] [PubMed]
20. Yu, B.; Wang, S. Angio-LncRs: LncRNAs that regulate angiogenesis and vascular disease. *Theranostics* **2018**, *8*, 3654–3675. [CrossRef] [PubMed]
21. He, X.; Ou, C.; Xiao, Y.; Han, Q.; Li, H.; Zhou, S. LncRNAs: Key players and novel insights into diabetes mellitus. *Oncotarget* **2017**, *8*, 71325–71341. [CrossRef] [PubMed]
22. Sedano, M.J.; Harrison, A.L.; Zilaie, M.; Das, C.; Choudhari, R.; Ramos, E.; Gadad, S.S. Emerging Roles of Estrogen-Regulated Enhancer and Long Non-Coding RNAs. *Int. J. Mol. Sci.* **2020**, *21*, 3711. [CrossRef] [PubMed]
23. Basak, P.; Chatterjee, S.; Bhat, V.; Su, A.; Jin, H.; Lee-Wing, V.; Liu, Q.; Hu, P.; Murphy, L.C.; Raouf, A. Long Non-Coding RNA H19 Acts as an Estrogen Receptor Modulator that is Required for Endocrine Therapy Resistance in ER+ Breast Cancer Cells. *Cell. Physiol. Biochem.* **2018**, *51*, 1518–1532. [CrossRef] [PubMed]
24. Sapkota, Y.; Steinthorsdottir, V.; Morris, A.P.; Fassbender, A.; Rahmioglu, N.; De Vivo, I.; Buring, J.E.; Zhang, F.; Edwards, T.L.; Jones, S.; et al. Meta-analysis identifies five novel loci associated with endometriosis highlighting key genes involved in hormone metabolism. *Nat. Commun.* **2017**, *8*, 15539. [CrossRef] [PubMed]
25. Gallagher, C.S.; Mäkinen, N.; Harris, H.R.; Rahmioglu, N.; Uimari, O.; Cook, J.P.; Shigesi, N.; Ferreira, T.; Velez-Edwards, D.R.; Edwards, T.L.; et al. Genome-wide association and epidemiological analyses reveal common genetic origins between uterine leiomyomata and endometriosis. *Nat. Commun.* **2019**, *10*, 4857. [CrossRef] [PubMed]

26. Giral, H.; Landmesser, U.; Kratzer, A. Into the Wild: GWAS Exploration of Non-coding RNAs. *Front. Cardiovasc. Med.* **2018**, *5*, 181. [CrossRef] [PubMed]
27. Mirza, A.H.; Kaur, S.; Brorsson, C.A.; Pociot, F. Effects of GWAS-associated genetic variants on lncRNAs within IBD and T1D candidate loci. *PLoS ONE* **2014**, *9*, e105723. [CrossRef] [PubMed]
28. Lee, G.H.; Choi, Y.M.; Hong, M.A.; Yoon, S.H.; Kim, J.J.; Hwang, K.; Chae, S.J. Association of CDKN2B-AS and WNT4 genetic polymorphisms in Korean patients with endometriosis. *Fertil. Steril.* **2014**, *102*, 1393–1397. [CrossRef] [PubMed]
29. Powell, J.E.; Fung, J.N.; Shakhbazov, K.; Sapkota, Y.; Cloonan, N.; Hemani, G.; Hillman, K.M.; Kaufmann, S.; Luong, H.T.; Bowdler, L.; et al. Endometriosis risk alleles at 1p36.12 act through inverse regulation of CDC42 and LINC00339. *Hum. Mol. Genet.* **2016**, *25*, 5046–5058. [PubMed]
30. Chang, C.Y.; Tseng, C.C.; Lai, M.T.; Chiang, A.J.; Lo, L.C.; Chen, C.M.; Yen, M.J.; Sun, L.; Yang, L.; Hwang, T.; et al. Genetic impacts on thermostability of onco-lncRNA HOTAIR during the development and progression of endometriosis. *PLoS ONE* **2021**, *16*, e0248168. [CrossRef] [PubMed]
31. Chen, G.; Zhang, M.; Liang, Z.; Chen, S.; Chen, F.; Zhu, J.; Zhao, M.; Xu, C.; He, J.; Hua, W.; et al. Association of polymorphisms in MALAT1 with the risk of endometriosis in Southern Chinese women. *Biol. Reprod.* **2019**, *102*, 943–949. [CrossRef] [PubMed]
32. Wang, L.; Xing, Q.; Feng, T.; He, M.; Yu, W.; Chen, H. SNP rs710886 A>G in long noncoding RNA PCAT1 is associated with the risk of endometriosis by modulating expression of multiple stemness-related genes via microRNA-145 signaling pathway. *J. Cell Biochem.* **2020**, *121*, 1703–1715. [PubMed]
33. Sun, P.R.; Jia, S.Z.; Lin, H.; Leng, J.H.; Lang, J.H. Genome-wide profiling of long noncoding ribonucleic acid expression patterns in ovarian endometriosis by microarray. *Fertil. Steril.* **2014**, *101*, 1038–1346. [CrossRef] [PubMed]
34. Cai, H.; Zhu, X.; Li, Z.; Zhu, Y.; Lang, J. lncRNA/mRNA profiling of endometriosis rat uterine tissues during the implantation window. *Int. J. Mol. Med.* **2019**, *44*, 2145–2160. [CrossRef] [PubMed]
35. Wang, W.T.; Sun, Y.M.; Huang, W.; He, B.; Zhao, Y.N.; Chen, Y.Q. Genome-wide Long Non-coding RNA Analysis Identified Circulating LncRNAs as Novel Non-invasive Diagnostic Biomarkers for Gynecological Disease. *Sci. Rep.* **2016**, *6*, 23343. [CrossRef] [PubMed]
36. Cui, D.; Ma, J.; Liu, Y.; Lin, K.; Jiang, X.; Qu, Y.; Lin, J.; Xu, K. Analysis of long non-coding RNA expression profiles using RNA sequencing in ovarian endometriosis. *Gene* **2018**, *673*, 140–148. [CrossRef] [PubMed]
37. Wang, Y.; Li, Y.; Yang, Z.; Liu, K.; Wang, D. Genome-Wide Microarray Analysis of Long Non-Coding RNAs in Eutopic Secretory Endometrium with Endometriosis. *Cell Physiol. Biochem.* **2015**, *37*, 2231–2245. [CrossRef] [PubMed]
38. Zhang, C.; Wu, W.; Ye, X.; Ma, R.; Luo, J.; Zhu, H.; Chang, X. Aberrant expression of CHL1 gene and long non-coding RNA CHL1-AS1, CHL1-AS2 in ovarian endometriosis. *Eur. J. Obstet. Gynecol. Reprod. Biol.* **2019**, *236*, 177–182. [CrossRef] [PubMed]
39. Wu, J.; Xia, X.; Hu, Y.; Fang, X.; Orsulic, S. Identification of Infertility-Associated Topologically Important Genes Using Weighted Co-expression Network Analysis. *Front. Genet.* **2021**, *12*, 580190. [CrossRef] [PubMed]
40. Liu, J.; Wang, Q.; Zhang, R.; Zhang, C.; Lin, J.; Huang, X. Identification of LINC01279 as a cell cycle-associated long non-coding RNA in endometriosis with GBA analysis. *Mol. Med. Rep.* **2018**, *18*, 3850–3858. [CrossRef] [PubMed]
41. Wang, X.; Yu, Q. Endometriosis-related ceRNA network to identify predictive biomarkers of endometrial receptivity. *Epigenomics* **2019**, *11*, 147–167. [CrossRef] [PubMed]
42. Liu, S.-P.; Tian, X.; Cui, H.-Y.; Zhang, Q.; Hua, K.-Q. The messenger RNA and long non-coding RNA expression profiles in ectopic and eutopic endometrium provide novel insights into endometriosis. *Reprod. Dev. Med.* **2019**, *3*, 11.
43. Jiang, L.; Zhang, M.; Wang, S.; Xiao, Y.; Wu, J.; Zhou, Y.; Fang, X. LINC01018 and SMIM25 sponged miR-182-5p in endometriosis revealed by the ceRNA network construction. *Int. J. Immunopathol. Pharmacol.* **2020**, *34*, 2058738420976309. [CrossRef] [PubMed]
44. Zhang, M.; Li, J.; Duan, S.; Fang, Z.; Tian, J.; Yin, H.; Zhai, Q.; Wang, X.; Zhang, L. Comprehensive characterization of endometrial competing endogenous RNA network in infertile women of childbearing age. *Aging* **2020**, *12*, 4204–4221. [CrossRef] [PubMed]
45. Bi, J.; Wang, D.; Cui, L.; Yang, Q. RNA sequencing-based long non-coding RNA analysis and immunoassay in ovarian endometriosis. *Am. J. Reprod. Immunol.* **2021**, *85*, e13359. [CrossRef] [PubMed]
46. Bai, J.; Wang, B.; Wang, T.; Ren, W. Identification of Functional lncRNAs Associated With Ovarian Endometriosis Based on a ceRNA Network. *Front. Genet.* **2021**, *12*, 534054. [CrossRef] [PubMed]
47. Lin, D.; Huang, Q.; Wu, R.; Dai, S.; Huang, Z.; Ren, L.; Huang, S.; Chen, Q. Long non-coding RNA AFAP1-AS1 promoting epithelial-mesenchymal transition of endometriosis is correlated with transcription factor ZEB1. *Am. J. Reprod. Immunol.* **2019**, *81*, e13074. [CrossRef] [PubMed]
48. Liu, S.; Xin, W.; Tang, X.; Qiu, J.; Zhang, Y.; Hua, K. LncRNA H19 Overexpression in Endometriosis and its Utility as a Novel Biomarker for Predicting Recurrence. *Reprod. Sci.* **2020**, *27*, 1687–1697. [CrossRef] [PubMed]
49. Du, H.; Taylor, H.S. The Role of Hox Genes in Female Reproductive Tract Development, Adult Function, and Fertility. *Cold Spring Harb. Perspect. Med.* **2015**, *6*, a023002. [CrossRef] [PubMed]
50. Liu, X.H.; Liu, Z.L.; Sun, M.; Liu, J.; Wang, Z.X.; De, W. The long non-coding RNA HOTAIR indicates a poor prognosis and promotes metastasis in non-small cell lung cancer. *BMC Cancer* **2013**, *13*, 464. [CrossRef] [PubMed]
51. Tsai, M.C.; Manor, O.; Wan, Y.; Mosammaparast, N.; Wang, J.K.; Lan, F.; Shi, Y.; Segal, E.; Chang, H.Y. Long noncoding RNA as modular scaffold of histone modification complexes. *Science* **2010**, *329*, 689–693. [CrossRef] [PubMed]

52. Wu, R.F.; Chen, Z.X.; Zhou, W.D.; Li, Y.Z.; Huang, Z.X.; Lin, D.C.; Ren, L.L.; Chen, Q.X.; Chen, Q.H. High expression of ZEB1 in endometriosis and its role in 17beta-estradiol-induced epithelial-mesenchymal transition. *Int. J. Clin. Exp. Pathol.* **2018**, *11*, 4744–4758. [PubMed]
53. Ghazal, S.; McKinnon, B.; Zhou, J.; Mueller, M.; Men, Y.; Yang, L.; Mueller, M.; Flannery, C.; Huang, Y.; Taylor, H.S. H19 lncRNA alters stromal cell growth via IGF signaling in the endometrium of women with endometriosis. *EMBO Mol. Med.* **2015**, *7*, 996–1003. [CrossRef] [PubMed]
54. Liu, S.; Qiu, J.; Tang, X.; Cui, H.; Zhang, Q.; Yang, Q. LncRNA-H19 regulates cell proliferation and invasion of ectopic endometrium by targeting ITGB3 via modulating miR-124-3p. *Exp. Cell Res.* **2019**, *381*, 215–222. [CrossRef] [PubMed]
55. Liu, Z.; Liu, L.; Zhong, Y.; Cai, M.; Gao, J.; Tan, C.; Han, X.; Guo, R.; Han, L. LncRNA H19 over-expression inhibited Th17 cell differentiation to relieve endometriosis through miR-342-3p/IER3 pathway. *Cell Biosci.* **2019**, *9*, 84. [CrossRef] [PubMed]
56. Wang, S.; Yi, M.; Zhang, X.; Zhang, T.; Jiang, L.; Cao, L.; Zhou, Y.; Fang, X. Effects of CDKN2B-AS1 on cellular proliferation, invasion and AKT3 expression are attenuated by miR-424-5p in a model of ovarian endometriosis. *Reprod. Biomed. Online* **2021**, *42*, 1057–1066. [CrossRef] [PubMed]
57. Cui, L.; Chen, S.; Wang, D.; Yang, Q. LINC01116 promotes proliferation and migration of endometrial stromal cells by targeting FOXP1 via sponging miR-9-5p in endometriosis. *J. Cell Mol. Med.* **2021**, *25*, 2000–2012. [CrossRef] [PubMed]
58. Liang, Z.; Chen, Y.; Zhao, Y.; Xu, C.; Zhang, A.; Zhang, Q.; Wang, D.; He, J.; Hua, W.; Duan, P. miR-200c suppresses endometriosis by targeting MALAT1 in vitro and in vivo. *Stem Cell Res. Ther.* **2017**, *8*, 251. [CrossRef] [PubMed]
59. Du, Y.; Zhang, Z.; Xiong, W.; Li, N.; Liu, H.; He, H.; Li, Q.; Liu, Y.; Zhang, L. Estradiol promotes EMT in endometriosis via MALAT1/miR200s sponge function. *Reproduction* **2019**, *157*, 179–188. [CrossRef] [PubMed]
60. Xu, Z.; Zhang, L.; Yu, Q.; Zhang, Y.; Yan, L.; Chen, Z.J. The estrogen-regulated lncRNA H19/miR-216a-5p axis alters stromal cell invasion and migration via ACTA2 in endometriosis. *Mol. Hum. Reprod.* **2019**, *25*, 550–561. [CrossRef] [PubMed]
61. Mai, H.; Xu, H.; Lin, H.; Wei, Y.; Yin, Y.; Huang, Y.; Huang, S.; Liao, Y. LINC01541 Functions as a ceRNA to Modulate the Wnt/beta-Catenin Pathway by Decoying miR-506-5p in Endometriosis. *Reprod. Sci.* **2021**, *28*, 665–674. [CrossRef] [PubMed]
62. Liu, Y.; Huang, X.; Lu, D.; Feng, Y.; Xu, R.; Li, X.; Yin, C.; Xue, B.; Zhao, H.; Wang, S.; et al. LncRNA SNHG4 promotes the increased growth of endometrial tissue outside the uterine cavity via regulating c-Met mediated by miR-148a-3p. *Mol. Cell Endocrinol.* **2020**, *514*, 110887. [CrossRef] [PubMed]
63. Feng, Y.; Tan, B.Z. LncRNA MALAT1 inhibits apoptosis of endometrial stromal cells through miR-126-5p-CREB1 axis by activating PI3K-AKT pathway. *Mol. Cell Biochem.* **2020**, *475*, 185–194. [CrossRef] [PubMed]
64. Wang, H.; Sha, L.; Huang, L.; Yang, S.; Zhou, Q.; Luo, X.; Shi, B. LINC00261 functions as a competing endogenous RNA to regulate BCL2L11 expression by sponging miR-132-3p in endometriosis. *Am. J. Transl. Res.* **2019**, *11*, 2269–2279. [PubMed]
65. Liu, Y.; Ma, J.; Cui, D.; Fei, X.; Lv, Y.; Lin, J. LncRNA MEG3-210 regulates endometrial stromal cells migration, invasion and apoptosis through p38 MAPK and PKA/SERCA2 signalling via interaction with Galectin-1 in endometriosis. *Mol. Cell Endocrinol.* **2020**, *513*, 110870. [CrossRef] [PubMed]
66. Yu, J.; Chen, L.H.; Zhang, B.; Zheng, Q.M. The modulation of endometriosis by lncRNA MALAT1 via NF-kappaB/iNOS. *Eur. Rev. Med. Pharmacol. Sci.* **2019**, *23*, 4073–4080. [PubMed]
67. Li, Y.; Liu, Y.D.; Chen, S.L.; Chen, X.; Ye, D.S.; Zhou, X.Y.; Zhe, J.; Zhang, J. Down-regulation of long non-coding RNA MALAT1 inhibits granulosa cell proliferation in endometriosis by up-regulating P21 via activation of the ERK/MAPK pathway. *Mol. Hum. Reprod.* **2019**, *25*, 17–29. [CrossRef] [PubMed]
68. Liu, H.; Zhang, Z.; Xiong, W.; Zhang, L.; Du, Y.; Liu, Y.; Xiong, X. Long non-coding RNA MALAT1 mediates hypoxia-induced pro-survival autophagy of endometrial stromal cells in endometriosis. *J. Cell Mol. Med.* **2019**, *23*, 439–452. [CrossRef] [PubMed]
69. Zhan, L.; Wang, W.; Zhang, Y.; Song, E.; Fan, Y.; Wei, B. Hypoxia-inducible factor-1alpha: A promising therapeutic target in endometriosis. *Biochimie* **2016**, *123*, 130–137. [CrossRef] [PubMed]
70. Mai, H.; Wei, Y.; Yin, Y.; Huang, S.; Lin, H.; Liao, Y.; Liu, X.; Chen, X.; Shi, H.; Liu, C.; et al. LINC01541 overexpression attenuates the 17beta-Estradiol-induced migration and invasion capabilities of endometrial stromal cells. *Syst. Biol. Reprod. Med.* **2019**, *65*, 214–222. [CrossRef] [PubMed]
71. Qiu, J.J.; Lin, X.J.; Zheng, T.T.; Tang, X.Y.; Zhang, Y.; Hua, K.Q. The Exosomal Long Noncoding RNA aHIF is Upregulated in Serum From Patients With Endometriosis and Promotes Angiogenesis in Endometriosis. *Reprod. Sci.* **2019**, *26*, 1590–1602. [CrossRef] [PubMed]
72. Yotova, I.; Hudson, Q.J.; Pauler, F.M.; Proestling, K.; Haslinger, I.; Kuessel, L.; Perricos, A.; Husslein, H.; Wenzl, R. LINC01133 Inhibits Invasion and Promotes Proliferation in an Endometriosis Epithelial Cell Line. *Int. J. Mol. Sci.* **2021**, *22*, 8385. [CrossRef] [PubMed]
73. Wang, H.; Ni, C.; Xiao, W.; Wang, S. Role of lncRNA FTX in invasion, metastasis, and epithelial-mesenchymal transition of endometrial stromal cells caused by endometriosis by regulating the PI3K/Akt signaling pathway. *Ann. Transl. Med.* **2020**, *8*, 1504. [CrossRef] [PubMed]
74. Zhu, M.B.; Chen, L.P.; Hu, M.; Shi, Z.; Liu, Y.N. Effects of lncRNA BANCR on endometriosis through ERK/MAPK pathway. *Eur. Rev. Med. Pharmacol. Sci.* **2019**, *23*, 6806–6812. [PubMed]
75. Jiang, L.; Wan, Y.; Feng, Z.; Liu, D.; Ouyang, L.; Li, Y.; Liu, K. Long Noncoding RNA UCA1 Is Related to Autophagy and Apoptosis in Endometrial Stromal Cells. *Front. Oncol.* **2020**, *10*, 618472. [CrossRef] [PubMed]

76. Liu, J.; Wang, Y.; Chen, P.; Ma, Y.; Wang, S.; Tian, Y.; Wang, A.; Wang, D. AC002454.1 and CDK6 synergistically promote endometrial cell migration and invasion in endometriosis. *Reproduction* **2019**, *157*, 535–543. [CrossRef] [PubMed]
77. Zhang, C.; Wu, W.; Zhu, H.; Yu, X.; Zhang, Y.; Ye, X.; Cheng, H.; Ma, R.; Cui, H.; Luo, J.; et al. Knockdown of long noncoding RNA CCDC144NL-AS1 attenuates migration and invasion phenotypes in endometrial stromal cells from endometriosis†. *Biol. Reprod.* **2019**, *100*, 939–949. [CrossRef] [PubMed]
78. Qiu, J.J.; Lin, Y.Y.; Tang, X.Y.; Ding, Y.; Yi, X.F.; Hua, K.Q. Extracellular vesicle-mediated transfer of the lncRNA-TC0101441 promotes endometriosis migration/invasion. *Exp. Cell Res.* **2020**, *388*, 111815. [CrossRef] [PubMed]
79. Korucuoglu, U.; Biri, A.A.; Konac, E.; Alp, E.; Onen, I.H.; Ilhan, M.N.; Turkyilmaz, E.; Erdem, A.; Erdem, M.; Menevse, S. Expression of the imprinted IGF2 and H19 genes in the endometrium of cases with unexplained infertility. *Eur. J. Obstet. Gynecol. Reprod. Biol.* **2010**, *149*, 77–81. [CrossRef] [PubMed]
80. Adriaenssens, E.; Lottin, S.; Dugimont, T.; Fauquette, W.; Coll, J.; Dupouy, J.P.; Boilly, B.; Curgy, J.J. Steroid hormones modulate H19 gene expression in both mammary gland and uterus. *Oncogene* **1999**, *18*, 4460–4473. [CrossRef] [PubMed]
81. Lin, K.; Zhan, H.; Ma, J.; Xu, K.; Wu, R.; Zhou, C.; Lin, J. Silencing of SRA1 Regulates ER Expression and Attenuates the Growth of Stromal Cells in Ovarian Endometriosis. *Reprod. Sci.* **2017**, *24*, 836–843. [CrossRef] [PubMed]

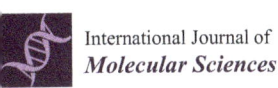

Review

Translational Applications of Linear and Circular Long Noncoding RNAs in Endometriosis

Xiyin Wang [1,2], Luca Parodi [3] and Shannon M. Hawkins [1,*]

1. Department of Obstetrics and Gynecology, Indiana University School of Medicine, Indianapolis, IN 46202, USA; wang.xiyin@mayo.edu
2. Mayo Clinic Graduate School of Biomedical Sciences, Rochester, MN 55905, USA
3. Obstetrics and Gynecology Department, Istituto Clinico Sant'Anna, 25127 Brescia, Italy; luca.parodi@grupposandonato.it
* Correspondence: shhawkin@iu.edu

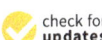

Citation: Wang, X.; Parodi, L.; Hawkins, S.M. Translational Applications of Linear and Circular Long Noncoding RNAs in Endometriosis. *Int. J. Mol. Sci.* **2021**, *22*, 10626. https://doi.org/10.3390/ijms221910626

Academic Editor: Antonio Simone Laganà

Received: 1 September 2021
Accepted: 28 September 2021
Published: 30 September 2021

Publisher's Note: MDPI stays neutral with regard to jurisdictional claims in published maps and institutional affiliations.

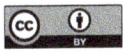

Copyright: © 2021 by the authors. Licensee MDPI, Basel, Switzerland. This article is an open access article distributed under the terms and conditions of the Creative Commons Attribution (CC BY) license (https://creativecommons.org/licenses/by/4.0/).

Abstract: Endometriosis is a chronic gynecologic disease that negatively affects the quality of life of many women. Unfortunately, endometriosis does not have a cure. The current medical treatments involve hormonal manipulation with unwanted side effects and high recurrence rates after stopping the medication. Sadly, a definitive diagnosis for endometriosis requires invasive surgical procedures, with the risk of complications, additional surgeries in the future, and a high rate of recurrence. Both improved therapies and noninvasive diagnostic tests are needed. The unique molecular features of endometriosis have been studied at the coding gene level. While the molecular components of endometriosis at the small RNA level have been studied extensively, other noncoding RNAs, such as long intergenic noncoding RNAs and the more recently discovered subset of long noncoding RNAs called circular RNAs, have been studied more limitedly. This review describes the molecular formation of long noncoding and the unique circumstances of the formation of circular long noncoding RNAs, their expression and function in endometriosis, and promising preclinical studies. Continued translational research on long noncoding RNAs, including the more stable circular long noncoding RNAs, may lead to improved therapeutic and diagnostic opportunities.

Keywords: endometriosis; human disease; noncoding RNA (ncRNA); long noncoding RNA (lncRNA); circular lncRNA (circRNA)

1. Introduction

Endometriosis is a progressive and debilitating gynecologic disease whereby endometrial-like tissue grows outside the uterine cavity, invading adjacent organs, such as the ovaries, bladder, colon, or pelvic peritoneum [1–3]. Endometriosis is often accompanied by chronic pelvic pain, dysmenorrhea, dyspareunia, dysuria, and dyschezia and can cause infertility [4,5]. The prevalence of endometriosis ranges from 5 to 15% of reproductive age women depending on the method of disease confirmation [3,6], affecting approximately 190 million women worldwide and 5 million women and adolescent girls in the United States [2].

Diagnosing endometriosis is exceptionally challenging since it shares non-specific symptoms, such as pelvic pain, with other conditions. The first-line imaging modality is typically pelvic ultrasound as it can allow for the diagnosis of other conditions that cause pelvic pain. However, the sensitivity and specificity of ultrasound are dependent on endometriosis lesion type and location. For example, transvaginal ultrasonography has high sensitivity and high specificity for ovarian endometriomas [7]. However, the diagnosis of deep infiltrating endometriosis lesions by ultrasound is related to operator expertise [7,8]. Surgical visual inspection by laparoscopy with histologic confirmation is currently the only way to diagnose pathology-proven endometriosis [5]. Surgery involves the risk of surgical complications, adhesion formation, and the need for future surgeries [9]. Because there is no gold standard for noninvasive diagnosis, there is often a significant delay in diagnosis [5]. The median time is seven years from the onset of symptoms with pain or infertility to endometriosis diagnosis [10]. Better diagnostic strategies must be developed.

Unfortunately, there is no cure for endometriosis. Non-steroidal anti-inflammatory medications are routinely used, but they are not more effective than a placebo [11]. Hormonal therapies, including gonadotropin-releasing hormone agonists and newer antagonists, can be prescribed only for a short time because of undesirable side effects, including irregular menstrual bleeding, the development of menopausal symptoms, and the detrimental impact on bone density [7,9,12]. Moreover, both medical and surgical therapies fail to prevent recurrence [2] as 20–50% of endometriosis recurs within five years of treatment [13]. The economic burden of endometriosis in the United States is estimated at $78 billion per year, including direct healthcare costs and indirect costs to patients [14]. Better treatment options are warranted.

Noncoding RNAs (ncRNAs), including microRNAs (miRNAs), long noncoding RNAs (lncRNAs), and circular RNAs (circRNAs), encompass large segments of the transcriptome that do not have apparent protein-coding roles [15]. ncRNAs are divided into two subclasses based on size: short ncRNAs and long ncRNAs. LncRNAs are commonly defined as transcripts longer than 200 nucleotides. Short ncRNAs, including the ~22 nucleotide long miRNAs, have emerged as critical post-transcriptional regulators of gene expression that are fundamental for many disease processes [16]. Although numerous studies have investigated the potential roles of miRNAs as diagnostic biomarkers, no particular miRNA has been translated from bench to clinic for diagnostic purposes [17]. The role of miRNAs in endometriosis has been recently reviewed [18] and will not be included again here.

Similar to messenger RNAs, most lncRNAs are transcribed by RNA polymerase II, and then they undergo post-transcription processes, leading to a 5′ cap, alternative splicing, and 3′ poly(A) tail [19]. Some lncRNAs have been re-defined as protein-encoding genes by closer inspection of the transcriptome and proteome with next-generation sequencing and mass spectrometry [20]. lncRNAs represent the largest class of ncRNAs as over 60,000 lncRNAs have been identified [21]. Many lncRNAs have substantial roles in several biological processes, including endometriosis [22]. As a unique subset of lncRNAs, circRNAs contain a circular secondary structure, characterized by a covalently closed continuous loop structure without 5′-3′ polarity or a poly(A) tail [23]. CircRNAs are involved in the pathogenesis of many diseases [24]. This review will discuss the fundamental roles of both linear and circular long noncoding RNAs in the molecular features of endometriosis and their relevance to current clinical practice. We will also discuss how these preclinical insights into ncRNA biology could develop into diagnostics and therapies in endometriosis.

2. Biogenesis, Structure, and Function of Linear and Circular lncRNAs

While more than 90% of the genome is transcribed into RNA, only about 2–5% of that genome contains protein-coding potential [25,26]. The remaining transcriptome comprises ncRNAs transcripts, consisting of small ncRNAs and lncRNAs and both linear and circular lncRNAs. To date, the GENCODE project has conservatively annotated the human genome and believes that it contains 19,954 protein-coding genes and 40,293 noncoding RNA genes [27]. Some 45% (17,957) of the noncoding RNA species are considered lncRNAs that give rise to more than 48,000 distinct transcripts [27]. CircRNAs are different from other long noncoding RNAs due to their single-stranded, circular secondary structure derived from the back splicing of exons from mRNAs and antisense RNAs [28]. In total, there are more than two million circRNAs present in all of the databases [29].

2.1. Biogenesis, Structure, and Function of Linear lncRNAs

The biogenesis of lncRNAs is like mRNA biogenesis since this process is mediated by RNA polymerase II. Similar to mRNA molecules, lncRNAs are characterized by alternative splicing, a 5′ 7-methylguanosine cap, and a 3′ poly (A) tail, although there is evidence that certain lncRNAs lack the 5′-cap or 3′poly (A) tail [30]. A comparison of the global features of lncRNAs and mRNAs shows that lncRNAs are less abundantly expressed, have less stability, are less evolutionarily conserved, and contain fewer numbers but longer exons [31]. The expression of lncRNAs is considered more cell- or tissue-specific than mRNA expression [32].

lncRNAs can be transcribed from the intergenic, exonic, or distal protein-coding regions of the genome. Based on genomic locations and orientation, lncRNAs can be classified into intergenic, intronic, sense, and antisense lncRNAs [33]. Intergenic lncRNAs (long intergenic noncoding RNAs or lincRNAs) are located between two protein-coding genes and transcribed in the same direction as those genes. Intronic lncRNAs are located entirely within the intronic region of a protein-coding gene and do not overlap with any exon. Sense lncRNAs are transcribed from the same strand and in the same direction as the protein-coding gene, possibly being exonic and/or intronic. Antisense lncRNAs are transcribed from the opposite strand of the protein-coding gene and can also be exonic and/or intronic. Pseudogene-derived RNAs are key components of lncRNAs with important functions in multiple biological processes [34].

Functionally, lncRNAs are classified under the mechanisms of action into these categories: signals (gene activators), decoys or sponges (gene repressors), guides (gene expression regulators), scaffolds (chromatin modifiers), and enhancer RNAs (eRNAs) [31,35]. As signals, lncRNAs function alone or combined with transcription factors or signaling pathways to activate transcriptional activity in time and space. As decoys, lncRNAs bind to functional sites to titrate the transcription factors away from chromatin or titrate miRNAs away from their targets to modulate transcription. As guides, lncRNAs recruit regulatory proteins to form ribonucleoprotein (RNP) complexes and direct them to their target sites to regulate the expression of target genes, either in cis or in trans. As scaffolds, lncRNAs provide platforms to bring different proteins together to form RNP complexes to activate or repress transcription. eRNAs are regulatory sequences from enhancer regions that in cis regulate the expression of target genes. LncRNAs can be nuclear, cytoplasmic, or both, and the subcellular localization determines its function [31,35].

2.2. CircRNA Biogenesis and Structure

CircRNAs are a unique subtype of lncRNAs that are covalently closed, single-stranded circular transcripts without 5′ caps or 3′ poly(A) tails. Although circRNAs were first described in the late 1970s, research in the past decade has dramatically improved our understanding of the expression and various biological functions due to the application of new technologies, mainly deep RNA sequencing [36]. The single-stranded, closed RNA molecules originate from precursor mRNAs (pre-mRNAs) and are usually from splicing within a protein-coding gene. CircRNAs have several biological functions in normal cells, including acting as sponges to efficiently subtract microRNAs and proteins [36].

CircRNAs can be classified into intronic circRNAs, exonic circRNAs, and exon-intron circRNAs (EIcirRNAs) (Figure 1). Multiple mechanisms have been used to describe the biogenesis of exonic circRNAs, including lariat-driven circularization, RNA binding protein (RBP) mediated circularization, and intron pairing-driven circularization [36]. During splicing, an exon skips, resulting in the back-splicing of RNA folding regions. EIciRNA is formed when the spliced intron lariat, or loop-like structure, remains. The loop-like structure can be mediated by an RBP or be intron-pairing-driven. The final structure is an exonic circRNA when the intron sequence is removed. The intronic circRNAs are formed both upstream and downstream of introns and are mainly accumulated in the nucleus. By contrast, exonic circRNAs without introns are most wielded in the cytoplasm to regulate past-transcriptional gene regulation [37].

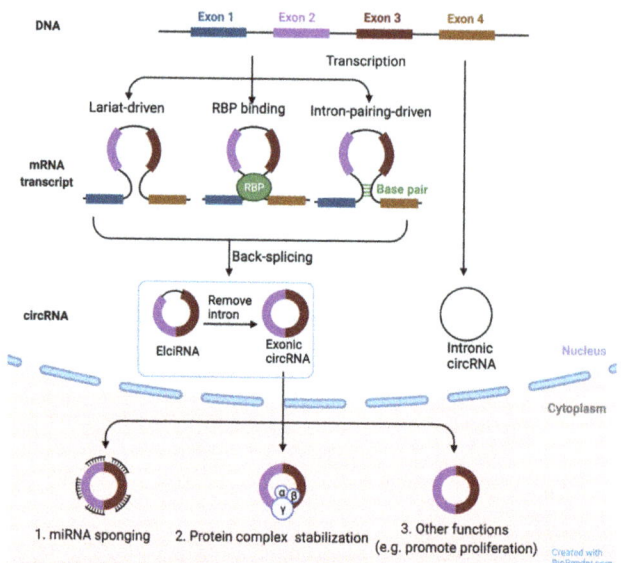

Figure 1. Biogenesis of circRNAs. Three types of circRNAs: exonic-intronic circRNA (EIciRNA), exonic circRNA, and intronic circRNA. EIcirRNAs and intronic circRNAs are abundant in the nucleus. Exonic circRNAs are exported from the nucleus to the cytoplasm and play functional roles in gene transcription and post-transcription. Adapted from [36].

3. Approaches for Discovering lncRNAs

Most lncRNAs and circRNAs are challenging to discover due to their low expression levels [38]. With the development of innovative technologies, an increasing number of novel linear lncRNAs and circRNAs have been identified by computational analysis of the transcriptomic datasets, high throughput sequencing, and experimental validation. Table 1 lists the techniques readily available for studying linear lncRNA and circRNA expression and function.

Table 1. Key experimental approaches for identifying and validating lncRNA expression and function.

Technique	Description	Ref
Microarray	Identify lncRNAs	[39]
RNA-sequencing	Identify lncRNAs	[40,41]
Tiling arrays	Identify and characterize lncRNAs	[42]
CAGE (Cap analysis of gene expression)	Identify lncRNAs	[43]
ChIRP-seq (chromatin isolation by RNA purification sequencing)	Identify lncRNA-chromatin interactions	[44,45]
CHART-seq (capture hybridization analysis of RNA targets)	Identify lncRNA-chromatin interactions	[46]
3C (chromosome confirmation capture)	Characterize lncRNA-genome binding site	[47]
RAP (RNA antisense purification)	Characterize lncRNA-genome binding site	[48]
RIP-seq (RNA immunoprecipitation)	Identify lncRNA-protein interactions	[49,50]
PAR-CLIP (Photoactivatable-ribonucleoside-enhanced cross-linking and immunoprecipitation)	Identify lncRNA-protein interactions	[51]
RNA pull-downs	Identify lncRNA-protein interactions	[52]
EMSA (Electrophoretic mobility shift assay)	Characterize lncRNA-protein complexes	[53]
RT-qPCR (real-time quantitative polymerase chain reactions)	Cellular localization and expression	[54]
RNA-FISH (RNA-fluorescent in situ hybridization)	Cellular localization	[55]
RNA-ISH (RNA- in situ hybridization)	Cellular localization	[54]
RNAi (RNA interference)	Knockdown lncRNAs	[56,57]
CRISPR-Cas9	Knockdown lncRNAs	[58–61]
ASO (Antisense oligonucleotides)	Knockdown lncRNAs	[62]

3.1. ncRNAs Databases

Public databases are one of the most important resources for ncRNAs research. More than 200 public databases are providing comprehensive associations between ncRNAs and their biological functions, including 25 for linear lncRNAs (i.e., TANRIC, CGS, GermlncRNA, LNCat, LncSNP, Lnc2Cancer, lnCeDB, LNCMap, Lnc2Meth, lncATLAS, lncPedia, lncRNAdisease, lncRNome, EVLnRNAs, GreeNC, LNCediting, and lncRNAdb for humans), and 13 for circRNAs (i.e., Circbase, Circnet, CirclncRNAnet, CircRNADb, CIRCpedia v2, DeepBase v2.0, CSCD, Circ2Traits, CircR2Disease, and MiOncoCirc) [36,38,63]. These databases are supported by high throughput sequencing or experimental validation.

3.2. High Throughput Identification

Multiple methods provide the systematic expression profiling of lncRNAs (Table 1). Although microarrays by predefined probes are not sensitive enough to identify low expression lncRNAs, microarrays have been used to discover novel ncRNAs at the whole-genome level [64]. The lncRNAs' sequence may match the previously built microarrays probe sequences and reannotate the initially protein-coding genes to lncRNAs [65]. A microarray, which hybridizes a selected panel of circRNAs explicitly, can be used to detect the annotated circRNAs expression [66]. For example, Shen et al. used a circRNA microarray and identified 262 upregulated and 291 downregulated circRNAs in ovarian endometriomas [67]. RNA-seq is currently the most widespread approach to discover linear lncRNAs and circRNAs. For example, Bi et al. performed RNA-seq experiments on six pairs of ectopic and eutopic endometria samples with endometriosis and identified 952 differentially expressed lncRNAs [68]. The limitations for RNA-seq data include the limited ability to discern linear and circular lncRNAs of similar sequence and the depth of sequencing required for low read count molecules, such as circRNAs [66,69,70]. Many deep sequencing studies on endometriosis have listed lncRNAs, including circRNAs, within the differentially expressed transcripts, but most of the manuscripts focus on protein-coding genes. Wu et al. identified 8660 upregulated and 651 downregulated lncRNAs [71], and Wang et al. detected 146 upregulated and 148 downregulated circRNAs in ovarian endometriosis by high throughput RNA-seq [72].

3.3. Experimental Validation

After discovering linear lncRNAs and circRNAs by databases or high throughput methods, experimental approaches can be used to study their expression and function (Table 1). RNA interference (RNAi), antisense oligonucleotides (AOs), and CRISPR systems have successfully been used to knock down lncRNAs [56–62,73]. However, RNAi and AOs may have non-specific and off-target effects. Further, Goyal et al. found only 38% of lncRNAs were safe to be targeted without deregulating neighboring genes by CRISPR applications [61]. It might be necessary to use multiple strategies to select the best gene silencing approach. Real-time quantitative reverse transcription-polymerase chain reaction (QPCR) is employed to validate the expression of linear lncRNAs and circRNAs [54]. The limitations of QPCR include the need for highly sensitive assays to detect low expression molecules and selecting appropriate endogenous control genes of similar low expression and transcript size. RNA in situ hybridization (ISH) is used to visualize and localize lncRNAs [54]. Holdsworth-Carson et al. performed RNA-seq, RT-PCR, and ISH in endometriosis samples. They found that the long intergenic non-protein coding RNA 339 (LINC00339) is localized in the nucleus of ectopic endometriotic lesions [74]. While ISH allows for the localization of lncRNA, it is generally not quantifiable. Newer technologies, including single-cell RNA-sequencing and spatial transcriptomics, are being used to quantify the expression and localization of protein-coding genes [31,75]. For example, spatial transcriptomics allows both the quantification of expression and localization, but the limited depth of sequencing at this time precludes the identification of low expression molecules [31]. Several groups have used approaches based on protein precipitation to detect key interactions of binding proteins with lncRNAs. Wang et al. used RNA immunoprecipitation to define the LINC00261/miR-132–3p/BCL2L11 regulatory networks [76]. In addition to functional studies, studies correlating expression, localization, and endometriosis phenotype (i.e., pain or infertility, anatomic location of disease, number of adhesions) may significantly impact the field.

4. The Importance of Noninvasive Biomarkers in Endometriosis

Laparoscopy remains the gold standard for pathology-confirmed endometriosis diagnosis [77]. While definitive diagnosis and anatomic characterization are critical for appropriate research studies, laparoscopy may not be ideal for all women with suspected endometriosis. Even as a minimally invasive surgical procedure, laparoscopy is associated with high costs, surgical complications, and time away from work and/or family obligations. The accurate diagnosis of visualized endometriosis lesions is surgeon-expertise-dependent [78,79]. Unfortunately, the lesions may not be visible. Biopsies of uterosacral ligaments without visible lesions in women undergoing laparoscopy for pelvic pain revealed 7% with histologically proven endometriosis [80]. Moreover, endometriosis is characterized by a broad panel of different symptoms depending on the localization of the lesions and the characteristics of the patient. Patients often present with intermenstrual bleeding, dysmenorrhea, dyspareunia, dyschezia, dysuria, or chronic pelvic pain. Non-painful endometriosis can be discovered during the surgical evaluation of infertility [81]. Ultrasonography has been proposed as a very good, cost-efficient noninvasive diagnostic tool. Still, this technique is strongly operator-dependent and, even in expert hands, can miss some lesions, particularly superficial lesions [8,82]. Unfortunately, the median time from the onset of symptoms to a diagnosis is seven years, leading to confusion, frustration, and other problems in terms of quality of life. Another aspect that must be considered is that it may be more successfully treated when endometriosis is diagnosed in the earlier stages [10]. Hence, a noninvasive, reliable test is needed to avoid the risks of surgery and shorten the time to diagnosis. Many studies in endometriosis have profiled linear lncRNAs and circRNAs in endometriotic lesions as a means of biomarker discovery, followed by a more focused examination of expression in circulation as a means of minimally invasive diagnosis (Table 2).

Table 2. Summary of the ncRNAs as biomarkers in endometriosis.

Clinical Application	ncRNA	Methods	Number of Patients	Tissue Types	Cycle Phase	Diagnostic Value	Study Type	Ref.
Noninvasive diagnostic biomarkers	NR_038395, NR_038452, ENST00000482343, ENST00000544649, ENST00000393610	Genome-wide transcriptome array	59 endometriosis 51 controls	Case: Endometriosis tissue (eutopic and ectopic endometrium) and blood samples Control: Eutopic endometrium, blood sample	Follicular, 50; luteal, 9 of 59 endometriosis patients Follicular, 44; luteal, 7 of 51 control patients	ENST0000048234 alone: 72.41% sensitivity and 71.74% specificity Panel of NR_038395, NR_038452, ENST00000482343, ENST00000544649 ENST00000393610: 89.66% sensitivity and 73.17% specificity	Case-Control	[83]
Biomarker discovery	86 total differently expressed SNORD3A TCONS_00006582 ABO TCONS_08347373	RNA Sequencing	17 endometriosis 17 controls	Case: Ectopic endometrium Control: eutopic endometrium	Proliferative	Not evaluated	Case-control	[84]
Noninvasive diagnostic biomarkers	UCA1	qRT PCR	98 endometriosis 28 controls	Case: Serum, eutopic-ectopic endometrium Controls: serum	Not evaluated	Stage I: specificity of 80.1% and sensitivity of 76.7% Stage II: specificity of 85.6% and sensitivity of 81.1% Stage III: specificity of 89.1% and sensitivity of 88.1 Stage IV: specificity of 90.5 % and sensitivity of 89.0%	Case-control	[85]
Biomarker discovery	circ_0004712 circ_0002198	CircRNA array	41 endometriosis 22 controls	Case: Ectopic, eutopic endometrium Control: Eutopic endometrium	Proliferative, 28; secretive, 13 of 41 endometriosis patients Proliferative, 16; secretive, 6 of 22 control patients	Not evaluated	Case-control	[86]
Biomarker discovery Therapeutic target discovery	circ_0004712, circ_0002198, circ_0003570, circ_0008951, circ_0017248	CircRNA array	41 endometriosis	Case: Ectopic, eutopic endometrium Control: Eutopic endometrium	Proliferative, 30; secretory, 11 of 41 endometriosis patients	Not evaluated	Discovery	[87]

Table 2. Cont.

Clinical Application	ncRNA	Methods	Number of Patients	Tissue Types	Cycle Phase	Diagnostic Value	Study Type	Ref.
Noninvasive diagnostic biomarkers	MEG8, SNHG25, LINC00293, LINC00929, RP5-898J17.1, NEAT1, H19	Small RNA sequencing	6 endometriosis Controls none	Case Eutopic ectopic endometrium, plasma, peritoneal fluid (PF)	Not evaluated	Not evaluated	Discovery	[88]
Noninvasive diagnostic biomarkers	TCO101441	FISH qRT-PCR	10 endometriosis 10 control	Case: Ectopic, eutopic endometrium, serum Controls: Eutopic endometrium, serum	Not evaluated	Not evaluated	Discovery	[89]
Noninvasive diagnostic biomarkers	TCO101441	qRT-PCR	29 endometriosis 16 controls	Case: Serum Controls: Serum	Not evaluated	Not evaluated	Discovery	[89]
Noninvasive diagnostic biomarker Recurrence	H19	qRT-PCR	104 endometriosis 50 controls	Case: Ectopic, eutopic endometrium Controls: Eutopic endometrium	Proliferative	sensitivity 90.9% and specificity 61.0%, for predicting recurrence	Case-control	[90]

The mechanism by which lncRNAs get from endometriotic tissues to circulation may be extracellular vesicles. Extracellular vesicles (EVs) are small membrane-bound vesicles that have emerged as mediators of cell-cell communication by transferring their contents, including lncRNAs [91]. Evidence has highlighted that miRNA, linear lncRNAs, and circRNAs can enter circulation and serve as noninvasive serum biomarkers for diagnosis or prognosis in other diseases, such as lung, colorectal, or prostate cancer [92]. For example, Qiu et al. found that serum extracellular vesicular TC0101441 levels are increased in patients at stage III/IV endometriosis in comparison with stage I/II endometriosis and non-endometriosis control patients. They further showed that this lncRNA played a role in the migration and invasion in cell lines through interaction with metastasis-related proteins, suggesting a possible role in endometriosis pathogenesis [89]. Beyond a functional role for lncRNAs, a potential diagnostic role of EVs lncRNAs has been proposed. Khalaj and collaborators showed a role for nuclear paraspeckle assembly transcript 1 (NEAT1) and H19 imprinted maternally expressed transcript (H19) in the context of a broad interaction with the miR-375, miR–30d-5p, and miR–27a-3p networks [88]. In this study, after the isolation of EVs, an analysis of the contents of the vesicles was performed. The EVs obtained from endometriotic lesions carried a unique miRNA signature compared with the EVs derived from matched patient eutopic endometrium and normal healthy endometrium. Moreover, endometriosis patient plasma-derived EVs carried unique ncRNAs compared with EVs from healthy control eutopic endometrium [88].

ncRNAs promise great results as biomarkers for noninvasive diagnosis purposes because they are resistant to RNase degradation and remain stable in biologic fluids, such as blood (i.e., serum or plasma), saliva, and urine [93]. Recently, circulating linear lncRNAs and circRNAs have been studied in gynecological diseases, gastric cancer, and hepatocellular carcinoma [83,94,95]. Specific to endometriosis, genome-wide profiling determined that a signature-based lncRNA profile, including the lncRNAs NR_038395, NR_038452, ENST00000482343, ENST00000544649, and ENST00000393610, can differentiate patients with and without endometriosis [83]. Notably, this group performed a genome-wide lncRNA analysis with the Glu Grant Transcriptome array in serum samples and eutopic and ectopic endometrium in endometriosis patients and a control group. While the control group had pelvic pain, the control group that had laparoscopy confirmed no evidence of endometriosis. This analysis identified 1682 lncRNAs with dysregulated expression in the sera of patients with endometriosis compared with controls and 1435 lncRNAs in the ectopic endometrium compared with the eutopic endometrium of negative controls. Of these differentially expressed lncRNAs in endometriosis tissues or serum, only 125 were differentially expressed in serum and tissue. After selecting for a similar change in gene expression direction (i.e., down or upregulated), they had a shortlist of 16 lncRNAs. The receiver operating characteristic (ROC) curve analysis used for cross-validation in the study population showed the highest area under the curve (AUC) of a circulating lncRNA was for ENST00000482343. Combining the expression of multiple lncRNAs into a signature-based profile revealed the highest AUC for a panel of NR_038395, NR_038452, ENST00000482343, ENST00000544649, and ENST00000393610. Significantly, the authors correlated the expression of this panel of lncRNAs with clinically relevant laparoscopic features (i.e., pelvic adhesions, ovarian involvement) [83]. A limitation of this study was the lack of external validation of results. The possibility of predicting a challenging surgery with a simple circulating biomarker during the preoperative workup would offer great help to make the right choices in terms of surgeons, surgical team, and surgical equipment. Additionally, women with endometriosis in remote areas without surgeons with expertise in endometriosis surgery could be referred appropriately.

The lncRNA urothelial cancer-associated 1 (UCA1) is another possible diagnostic biomarker for endometriosis. UCA1 was downregulated in the ectopic endometrium of a cohort of 98 endometriosis patients compared to 28 healthy controls. Endometriosis patients were classified with the American Fertility Society (AFS) staging: 19 patients in stage I, 21 patients in stage II, 33 patients in stage III, and 25 patients in stage IV. The relative expression of UCA1 in the serum was lower in women with increased AFS stage. A ROC curve analysis was performed among the study population to evaluate the diagnostic value of serum UCA1. The AUC for Stage I was 0.7509 [95% CI (0.6109 to 0.8910), $p = 0.003820$]; AUC for stage II was 0.9175 [95% CI (0.8308 to 1.004), $p < 0.0001$]; AUC for stage III was 0.9605 [95% CI (0.8982 to 1.023), $p < 0.0001$]; AUC for stage IV was 0.9921 [95% CI (0.9747 to 1.010), $p < 0.0001$]. To evaluate further, circulating UCA1 was examined immediately after surgery and periodically during follow-up. Interestingly, the serum levels of UCA1 were upregulated after treatment and downregulated in cases of relapse. These results suggest that UCA1 is a useful tool for diagnosis and monitoring recurrence [85]. A limitation of this study was the lack of external validation of the results. Similar studies should be performed for other treatment modalities, including medical management.

Up to 50% of women who experience infertility have endometriosis. Studies showed that women with endometriosis have endometrial dysfunction, including progesterone resistance, which may play a role in the timing of endometrial receptivity [96]. Understanding the appropriate timing for embryo transfer may improve pregnancy rates. Studies have examined miRNAs in the eutopic endometrium and peritoneal fluid for infertility evaluation [97–99]. Further, an association between endometriosis and some specific ovarian cancer histotypes, particularly endometrioid and clear cell carcinomas, have been shown epidemiologically [100]. Hence, a possible application of peritoneal fluid analysis could help in the early prediction of endometriosis-associated ovarian cancer, as already has been demonstrated for miRNAs [101,102]. Future work in lncRNAs is needed in these areas.

5. Therapeutic Opportunities for lncRNAs

As lncRNAs function to regulate gene expression, lncRNAs represent novel therapeutic molecules. Therapeutic noncoding RNAs as targeting molecules, including small interfering RNAs (siRNAs), short hairpin RNAs (shRNAs), miRNA mimics, miRNA sponges, and CRISPR–Cas9-based gene-editing technologies, have been experimentally developed to regulate gene expression and potentially treat disease, but therapeutic targeting using noncoding RNAs is in its infancy [103]. To date, 11 RNA-based therapeutics are approved by the United States Food and Drug Administration (US FDA) and/or the European Medicines Agency (EMA) [104]. While no RNA-based therapeutics are indicated for endometriosis, therapeutic linear lncRNAs and circRNAs may act to inhibit downstream genes and subsequent cellular function and offer significant promise for non-hormonal therapy. Understanding the precise mechanisms of lncRNAs and their antagonists is the first step towards translational applications, as indicated by several preclinical studies highlighted below.

First, the lncRNA H19 imprinted maternally expressed transcript (H19) regulates insulin grown factor receptor (IGF1R) expression by acting as a molecular sponge to let-7 [105]. An in vitro knockdown of H19 with siRNA led to the higher expression of let-7 by real-time quantitative polymerase chain reaction (qPCR) and subsequent inhibition of IGF1R transcript and protein. Functionally, the H19 knockdown resulted in the reduced proliferation of primary endometrial stromal cells isolated from the eutopic endometrium of subjects with endometriosis [105]. Secondly, the molecular sponge mechanism in a preclinical in vitro model can also be found for long intergenic non-protein coding RNA 261 (LINC00261), which binds miR-132-3p and subsequently acts as a regulator of BCL-2-like 11 (BCL2L11) expression. The overexpression of LINC00261 inhibited the proliferation and invasion of the endometriosis cell line CRL-7566 through the BCL2L11 network. Further, the overexpression of LINC00261 revealed a decrease in miR-132-3p expression and increased BCL2L11 expression [76]. The role of BCL2L11 in endometriosis was investigated by siRNA knockdown. BCL2L11 knockdown reduced epithelial-mesenchymal transition (EMT) markers and reduced invasion [76]. While clinically promising, the scientific reproducibility of this effect has not been tested due to the original study being performed in a single cell line, CRL-7566. The CRL-7566 cell line is derived from an ovarian endometrioma. While it was commercially available from American Type Tissue Culture Collection (ATCC), it is no longer available due to its slow growth rate. Further, while the CRL-7566 line was authenticated with short tandem repeat (STR) profiling, it was not well characterized in terms of molecular markers for endometrial epithelium and endometrial stroma [106,107]. Thus, these promising effects need to be replicated.

The in vitro studies on lncRNAs in endometriosis above led to preclinical mouse model studies. First, the lncRNA AFAP1 antisense RNA1 (AFAP1-AS1) mediates the signal transducer and activator of the transcription-transforming growth factor beta-SMAD (STAT3/TGF-β/SMAD) signaling pathway through miR-424-5p to influence endometriosis progression. Huan et al. reported that AFAP1-AS1 knockdown inhibited proliferation and migration and promoted apoptosis in an SV40-transformed, endometriosis eutopic endometrium stromal cell line, hEM15a [108]. Additionally, AFAP1-AS1 regulates EMT. Specifically, AFAP1-AS1 is thought to act in concert with steroid hormones, such as estradiol, to induce the expression of the transcription factor zinc finger E-box binding homeobox 1 (ZEB1). Interestingly, the shRNA knockdown of AFAP1-AS1 reduced the expression of ZEB1 in the spontaneously transformed endometrial cancer cell line Ishikawa. Further, Ishikawa cells with a knockdown of AFAP1-AS2 showed reduced tumor dimensions in a nude mouse model compared to non-targeted Ishikawa cells [109]. These studies highlight the impact of AFAP1-AS1 on proliferation and growth. While promising, the studies in an endometrial cancer cell line highlight the potential lack of clinical applicability to endometriosis. Finally, endometriosis is a disease of significant immunologic features. The use of nude mice, which are immunocompromised, may not be biologically applicable to endometriosis. Improved in vivo and in vitro models are needed to improve the translatability of studies.

Second, Liu and colleagues studied the lncRNA small nucleolar host gene 4 (SNHG4) in a heterologous mouse model of endometriosis. In this model, nude mice were injected subcutaneously with primary endometrial stromal cells (ESCs) isolated from ectopic endometrium and transfected with either NC-si, SNHG4-si1, or SNHG4-si1 combined with anti-miR-148-3p. After silencing SNHG4, the volume of endometriotic lesions was considerably reduced compared to the non-targeting control. Further, the expression of MET proto-oncogene receptor tyrosine kinase (MET) was inhibited, while miR-148a-3p was upregulated. The inhibitor of miR-148a-3p combined with SNHG4 knockdown rescued endometriotic lesions growth and upregulated the MET expression. The authors postulated that SNHG4 might upregulate proto-oncogene expression, in particular MET, via the suppression of miR-148a-3p, to promote the increased growth of endometrial tissue outside the uterine cavity and endometriosis lesions [110]. The impact of oncogenes and the manipulation of oncogenes in therapy for endometriosis deserves future study, particularly as non-hormonal therapies.

Third, studies showed that lncRNA maternally expressed 3 (MEG3-210) has a regulatory mechanism in endometriosis. MEG3-210 was downregulated in the eutopic endometrium of endometriosis patients and the primary cultures of endometrial stromal cells from women with endometriosis. The overexpression of MEG3-210 in the primary cultures of endometrial stromal cells from women with endometriosis revealed reduced invasion and migration. Further, flow cytometry detected a reduction in apoptosis. They examined two molecular pathways, including p38 signaling for its role in the endometriosis inflammatory response and PKA/SERCA2 signaling for its effects on cell motility and apoptosis. Western blotting showed that the protein levels of phosphorylated mitogen-activated protein kinase 14 (better known as p38) and phosphorylated activating transcription factor 2 (ATF2) were significantly increased after the downregulation of MEG3-210. Furthermore, the protein levels of protein kinase cAMP-activated catalytic subunit alpha (PRKACA, better known as PKA) and ATPase sarcoplasmic/endoplasmic reticulum Ca2+ transporting 2 (SERCA2) were decreased after MEG3-210 downregulation [111]. Previously, p38 activity was found to be higher in the eutopic and ectopic endometria in endometriosis patients. Increased p38 MAPK activity in endometriotic cells correlated with the activation of inflammatory cytokines, such as interleukin one beta (IL1b) and tumor necrosis factor-alpha

(TNFα) [112]. Finally, they found that p38/MAPK and PKA/SERCA2 signaling pathways act through Galectin1. Galectin-1 is a member of the sub-family of galectins that play a role in intracellular signal processing, molecular modification, cell motility, and malignant biological behavior [111,113]. Recently, MEG3 has regulated transforming growth factor-beta (TGFβ) signaling [114]. Previous work has shown the role of TGFβ signaling in ovarian endometriomas through small RNA signaling [115]. Further studies should examine the connection of lncRNA MEG3 in TGFβ signaling in endometriomas.

Like lncRNA, circular RNAs share the sponge mechanism of action. For example, the circular RNA circ_0007331 targets miR-200c-3p and, consequently, targets hypoxia-inducible factor 1 subunit alpha (HIF1A), a key transcription factor for angiogenesis and hypoxia mechanisms. Through this mechanistic axis, circ_0007331 knockdown, with the cooperation of HIF1A downstream, reduced the proliferation and invasion of primary endometrial cell cultures from women with endometriosis. With the overexpression of miR-200c-3p, proliferation and invasion increased, as did HIF1A. The inhibition of miR-200c-3p, conversely, reduced the proliferation and invasion caused by circ_0007331 knockdown, confirming that the circ_0007331/miR-200c-3p/HIF-1α axis has an important role in cell proliferation and invasion in endometriosis [116]. Using a homologous endometriosis mouse model, treatment with circ_0007331 shRNA, shRNA NC, or anti-miR-200c-3p showed that circ_0007331 knockdown reduced the lesion sizes. Further, treatment with anti-miR-200c-3p did not. Using immunohistochemistry, endometriosis lesions from mice treated with circ_0007331 shRNA were negative for HIF1A, but mice treated with anti-miR-200c-3p treatment maintained HIF1A expression [116]. These results show the importance of the circ_0007331/miR-200c-3p/HIF-1α axis in the endometrium of endometriosis patients.

Finally, the sponge mechanism of action has been proposed for the circular RNA circ_0004712, and miR-148a-3p. Notably, this axis plays an important role in estradiol (E2)-induced EMT processes in the development of endometriosis, potentially through the β-catenin pathway. The E2 treatment of either the endometrial cancer cell line Ishikawa or the human papillomavirus (HPV)-16 E6/E7 transformed endometriosis endocervical cell line End1/E6E7 showed the overexpression of circ_0004712. Further, E2 treatment increased migration in transwell assays and the induction of EMT through the b-catenin pathway. The E2- treatment effect was suppressed with the knockdown of circ_0004712 [117]. Interest in circRNA application in endometriosis is a relatively new area of research. However, the exciting data to date support additional preclinical studies.

While lncRNAs offer opportunities for targeting cellular function, lncRNAs themselves offer options as therapeutic targets. The dysregulation of lncRNA expression has been linked to diseases and complex biological processes [118]. Recently, lncRNA HOX transcript antisense RNA (HOTAIR) has been associated with a genetic susceptibility to endometriosis. Functional single nucleotide polymorphisms, including rs1838169 and rs17720428, were frequently found in endometriosis patients [119]. Moreover, endometriosis pathogenesis may revolve around a functional axis of HOTAIR/homeobox D10 and HOTAIR/homeobox A5. Homeobox proteins (HOXs) are critical in maintaining endometrium homeostasis during embryo implantation and menstrual cycles, highlighting their importance in endometriosis [120]. HOTAIR knockdown reduced cell proliferation and migration and increased HOXD10 and HOXA5 expression in two ovarian clear cell cancer cell lines, ES-2 and TOV-21G [119]. The overexpression of HOTAIR in epithelial ovarian cancer cells increases cancer invasiveness and metastasis. Moreover, the involvement of HOTAIR in cancer progression and response to standard chemotherapy, possibly promoting mesenchymal stem cell formation, has been highlighted [121,122]. Since endometriosis shares features with cancer, these results make HOTAIR a possible target for future endometriosis or ovarian cancer therapies. Secondly, Zhang et al. discovered that another potential target, CCDC144NL antisense RNA1 (CCDC144NL-AS1), was found to be upregulated in ectopic endometriosis and eutopic endometrium from women with endometriosis. The in vitro knockdown of CCDC144NL-AS1 in the SV40-transformed, endometriosis eutopic endometrium stromal cell line hEM15a was associated with decreased migration and invasion. Assuming that alterations in motility and invasion were related to cytoskeleton alteration, the authors found an altered distribution of cytoskeletal F-actin stress fibers compared to lower protein levels of vimentin filaments and matrix metallopeptidase 9 (MMP9) after CCDC144NL-AS1 knockdown [123]. Although there are yet no clinical studies, preclinical studies reveal a potential application of lncRNAs.

In the last few years, a growing interest in diet and nutrition as complementary therapeutic support for endometriosis was established even if randomized clinical trials do not show benefits [124]. Moreover, a connection between nutrition and ncRNA epigenetics has been found with sulforaphane, epigallocatechin gallate (EGCG), genistein, resveratrol, and curcumin in female reproductive tract cancers. A possible therapeutic role of these compounds combined with traditional therapies has been highlighted. As we know, endometriosis shares some pathways with neoplastic disease. Phytochemicals and nutraceuticals have been shown to influence pathways involving the miR-200 family, let-7 family, or miR-34a that can interact with inflammatory and oxidation mechanisms that play an important role in endometriosis [125].

6. Challenges to Clinical Application and Future Directions

Linear lncRNAs and circRNAs promise great results as biomarkers for the early detection and disease recurrence of endometriosis. ncRNAs are resistant to RNase degradation and remain stable in biologic fluids, allowing for transport stability to specialized clinical laboratories that may not be local for all women. Studies show promising results but with little consistency among them, especially if considering single lncRNAs as biomarkers. Signature panels of miRNAs, such as the miR-20 or miR-200 families, have been widely investigated but partially have the same problem [126]. A possible solution could be to combine different molecules to obtain a more powerful signature of lncRNAs and miRNAs or other circulating markers (such as CA125) to create a more accurate diagnostic tool.

The main contemporary challenge is the heterogeneity of endometriosis cases and controls. The World Endometriosis Research Foundation (WERF) Endometriosis Phenome and Biobanking Harmonisation Project (EPHect) has provided guidelines [127]. The detailed characterization of women with endometriosis in terms of pain symptoms, lesion location, and molecular profiles is critical to homing in on useful diagnostic tools. While most of the studies interrogate the use of medications, most do not consider nutritional factors, over-the-counter supplements, or drugs. For example, the dietary intake of omega-6 fatty acids, omega-3 fatty acids, vitamin D, and N-acetylcysteine may affect endometriosis development. Further, supplements containing quercetin and L-carnitine may be involved in the progression of endometriosis [128]. Nutraceuticals, nutritional products that are also used as medicines [129], are emerging within the realm of endometriosis therapy [130]. As studies within other gynecologic diseases have shown an effect of nutraceuticals on noncoding RNA expression [125], the role of these natural products, nutrients, and supplements on lncRNAs requires additional study in endometriosis.

Each woman with endometriosis is a unique individual, and small studies are insufficient to evaluate a large number of clinical features. The collaborative, detailed characterization of the phenotype of women with endometriosis is critical. Unfortunately, an optimal non-endometriosis control population is challenging without putting healthy women through laparoscopic surgery for research purposes. While detailed guidelines are helpful for translational studies, additional guidelines are needed to report endometriosis mouse models and in vitro model systems, including multicellular aggregates, spheroids, and organoids. Preclinical studies on lncRNAs and circRNAs show promise for the translation to well-characterized human studies.

Author Contributions: Conceptualization, X.W., L.P. and S.M.H. literature review, X.W., L.P. and S.M.H.; data curation, X.W., L.P. and S.M.H.; writing—original draft preparation, X.W., L.P. and S.M.H.; writing—review and editing, X.W., L.P. and S.M.H.; visualization, X.W., L.P. and S.M.H.; supervision, S.M.H.; project administration, S.M.H.; funding acquisition, S.M.H. All authors have read and agreed to the published version of the manuscript. All authors contributed substantially to the work reported.

Funding: This research was funded by R21HD102653-01A1 (to S.M.H.).

Institutional Review Board Statement: This review study did not involve human subjects directly. This review study did not involve animals directly.

Conflicts of Interest: The authors declare no conflict of interest.

References

1. Bulun, S.E. Endometriosis. *N. Engl. J. Med.* **2009**, *360*, 268–279. [CrossRef] [PubMed]
2. Zondervan, K.T.; Becker, C.M.; Missmer, S.A. Endometriosis. *N. Engl. J. Med.* **2020**, *382*, 1244–1256. [CrossRef]
3. Giudice, L.C.; Kao, L.C. Endometriosis. *Lancet* **2004**, *364*, 1789–1799. [CrossRef]
4. Holoch, K.J.; Lessey, B.A. Endometriosis and infertility. *Clin. Obs. Gynecol.* **2010**, *53*, 429–438. [CrossRef] [PubMed]
5. Hsu, A.L.; Khachikyan, I.; Stratton, P. Invasive and noninvasive methods for the diagnosis of endometriosis. *Clin. Obs. Gynecol.* **2010**, *53*, 413–419. [CrossRef] [PubMed]
6. Taylor, H.S.; Kotlyar, A.M.; Flores, V.A. Endometriosis is a chronic systemic disease: Clinical challenges and novel innovations. *Lancet* **2021**, *397*, 839–852. [CrossRef]
7. Falcone, T.; Flyckt, R. Clinical Management of Endometriosis. *Obs. Gynecol.* **2018**, *131*, 557–571. [CrossRef]
8. Somigliana, E.; Vercellini, P.; Vigano, P.; Benaglia, L.; Crosignani, P.G.; Fedele, L. Non-invasive diagnosis of endometriosis: The goal or own goal? *Hum. Reprod.* **2010**, *25*, 1863–1868. [CrossRef]
9. Practice bulletin, no. 114: Management of endometriosis. *Obs. Gynecol.* **2010**, *116*, 223–236.
10. Arruda, M.S.; Petta, C.A.; Abrao, M.S.; Benetti-Pinto, C.L. Time elapsed from onset of symptoms to diagnosis of endometriosis in a cohort study of Brazilian women. *Hum. Reprod.* **2003**, *18*, 756–759. [CrossRef]
11. Brown, J.; Crawford, T.J.; Allen, C.; Hopewell, S.; Prentice, A. Nonsteroidal anti-inflammatory drugs for pain in women with endometriosis. *Cochrane Database Syst Rev.* **2017**, *1*, CD004753. [CrossRef]
12. Taylor, H.S.; Giudice, L.C.; Lessey, B.A.; Abrao, M.S.; Kotarski, J.; Archer, D.F.; Diamond, M.P.; Surrey, E.; Johnson, N.P.; Watts, N.B.; et al. Treatment of Endometriosis-Associated Pain with Elagolix, an Oral GnRH Antagonist. *N. Engl. J. Med.* **2017**, *377*, 28–40. [CrossRef] [PubMed]
13. Farquhar, C. Endometriosis. *BMJ* **2007**, *334*, 249–253. [CrossRef] [PubMed]
14. Soliman, A.M.; Yang, H.; Du, E.X.; Kelley, C.; Winkel, C. The direct and indirect costs associated with endometriosis: A systematic literature review. *Hum. Reprod.* **2016**, *31*, 712–722. [CrossRef]
15. Zhang, P.; Wu, W.; Chen, Q.; Chen, M. Non-Coding RNAs and their Integrated Networks. *J. Integr. Bioinform.* **2019**, *16*, 20190027. [CrossRef] [PubMed]
16. Wendel, J.R.H.; Wang, X.; Hawkins, S.M. The Endometriotic Tumor Microenvironment in Ovarian Cancer. *Cancers* **2018**, *10*, 261. [CrossRef]
17. Saliminejad, K.; Khorram Khorshid, H.R.; Ghaffari, S.H. Why have microRNA biomarkers not been translated from bench to clinic? *Future Oncol.* **2019**, *15*, 801–803. [CrossRef] [PubMed]
18. Bjorkman, S.; Taylor, H.S. MicroRNAs in endometriosis: Biological function and emerging biomarker candidatesdagger. *Biol. Reprod.* **2019**, *100*, 1135–1146. [CrossRef]
19. Mercer, T.R.; Dinger, M.E.; Mattick, J.S. Long non-coding RNAs: Insights into functions. *Nat. Rev. Genet.* **2009**, *10*, 155–159. [CrossRef]
20. Quinn, J.J.; Chang, H.Y. Unique features of long non-coding RNA biogenesis and function. *Nat. Rev. Genet.* **2016**, *17*, 47–62. [CrossRef]
21. Charles Richard, J.L.; Eichhorn, P.J.A. Platforms for Investigating LncRNA Functions. *SLAS Technol.* **2018**, *23*, 493–506. [CrossRef] [PubMed]
22. Wang, X.; Zhang, J.; Liu, X.; Wei, B.; Zhan, L. Long noncoding RNAs in endometriosis: Biological functions, expressions, and mechanisms. *J. Cell Physiol.* **2021**, *236*, 6–14. [CrossRef] [PubMed]
23. Qu, S.; Yang, X.; Li, X.; Wang, J.; Gao, Y.; Shang, R.; Sun, W.; Dou, K.; Li, H. Circular RNA: A new star of noncoding RNAs. *Cancer Lett.* **2015**, *365*, 141–148. [CrossRef] [PubMed]
24. Vo, J.N.; Cieslik, M.; Zhang, Y.; Shukla, S.; Xiao, L.; Zhang, Y.; Wu, Y.M.; Dhanasekaran, S.M.; Engelke, C.G.; Cao, X.; et al. The Landscape of Circular RNA in Cancer. *Cell* **2019**, *176*, 869–881.e3. [CrossRef]
25. Pertea, M. The human transcriptome: An unfinished story. *Genes* **2012**, *3*, 344–360. [CrossRef]
26. Hube, F.; Francastel, C. Coding and Non-coding RNAs, the Frontier Has Never Been So Blurred. *Front. Genet.* **2018**, *9*, 140. [CrossRef]

27. Frankish, A.; Diekhans, M.; Jungreis, I.; Lagarde, J.; Loveland, J.E.; Mudge, J.M.; Sisu, C.; Wright, J.C.; Armstrong, J.; Barnes, I.; et al. Gencode 2021. *Nucleic Acids Res.* **2021**, *49*, D916–D923. [CrossRef]
28. van Rossum, D.; Verheijen, B.M.; Pasterkamp, R.J. Circular RNAs: Novel Regulators of Neuronal Development. *Front. Mol. Neurosci* **2016**, *9*, 74. [CrossRef] [PubMed]
29. Greene, J.; Baird, A.M.; Brady, L.; Lim, M.; Gray, S.G.; McDermott, R.; Finn, S.P. Circular RNAs: Biogenesis, Function and Role in Human Diseases. *Front. Mol. Biosci.* **2017**, *4*, 38. [CrossRef]
30. Sun, M.; Kraus, W.L. From discovery to function: The expanding roles of long noncoding RNAs in physiology and disease. *Endocr. Rev.* **2015**, *36*, 25–64. [CrossRef]
31. Statello, L.; Guo, C.J.; Chen, L.L.; Huarte, M. Gene regulation by long non-coding RNAs and its biological functions. *Nat. Rev. Mol. Cell Biol.* **2021**, *22*, 96–118. [CrossRef]
32. Chen, L.; Zhang, Y.H.; Pan, X.; Liu, M.; Wang, S.; Huang, T.; Cai, Y.D. Tissue Expression Difference between mRNAs and lncRNAs. *Int. J. Mol. Sci.* **2018**, *19*, 3416. [CrossRef] [PubMed]
33. Ma, L.; Bajic, V.B.; Zhang, Z. On the classification of long non-coding RNAs. *RNA Biol.* **2013**, *10*, 925–933. [CrossRef]
34. Lou, W.; Ding, B.; Fu, P. Pseudogene-Derived lncRNAs and Their miRNA Sponging Mechanism in Human Cancer. *Front. Cell Dev. Biol.* **2020**, *8*, 85. [CrossRef]
35. Fang, Y.; Fullwood, M.J. Roles, Functions, and Mechanisms of Long Non-coding RNAs in Cancer. *Genom. Proteom. Bioinform.* **2016**, *14*, 42–54. [CrossRef] [PubMed]
36. Shang, Q.; Yang, Z.; Jia, R.; Ge, S. The novel roles of circRNAs in human cancer. *Mol. Cancer* **2019**, *18*, 6. [CrossRef]
37. Ragan, C.; Goodall, G.J.; Shirokikh, N.E.; Preiss, T. Insights into the biogenesis and potential functions of exonic circular RNA. *Sci. Rep.* **2019**, *9*, 2048. [CrossRef] [PubMed]
38. Sun, Y.M.; Chen, Y.Q. Principles and innovative technologies for decrypting noncoding RNAs: From discovery and functional prediction to clinical application. *J. Hematol. Oncol.* **2020**, *13*, 109. [CrossRef]
39. Shoemaker, D.D.; Schadt, E.E.; Armour, C.D.; He, Y.D.; Garrett-Engele, P.; McDonagh, P.D.; Loerch, P.M.; Leonardson, A.; Lum, P.Y.; Cavet, G.; et al. Experimental annotation of the human genome using microarray technology. *Nature* **2001**, *409*, 922–927. [CrossRef]
40. Wang, Z.; Gerstein, M.; Snyder, M. RNA-Seq: A revolutionary tool for transcriptomics. *Nat. Rev. Genet.* **2009**, *10*, 57–63. [CrossRef]
41. Ilott, N.E.; Ponting, C.P. Predicting long non-coding RNAs using RNA sequencing. *Methods* **2013**, *63*, 50–59. [CrossRef]
42. Bertone, P.; Stolc, V.; Royce, T.E.; Rozowsky, J.S.; Urban, A.E.; Zhu, X.; Rinn, J.L.; Tongprasit, W.; Samanta, M.; Weissman, S.; et al. Global identification of human transcribed sequences with genome tiling arrays. *Science* **2004**, *306*, 2242–2246. [CrossRef]
43. Shiraki, T.; Kondo, S.; Katayama, S.; Waki, K.; Kasukawa, T.; Kawaji, H.; Kodzius, R.; Watahiki, A.; Nakamura, M.; Arakawa, T.; et al. Cap analysis gene expression for high-throughput analysis of transcriptional starting point and identification of promoter usage. *Proc. Natl. Acad. Sci. USA* **2003**, *100*, 15776–15781. [CrossRef] [PubMed]
44. Chu, C.; Qu, K.; Zhong, F.L.; Artandi, S.E.; Chang, H.Y. Genomic maps of long noncoding RNA occupancy reveal principles of RNA-chromatin interactions. *Mol. Cell* **2011**, *44*, 667–678. [CrossRef]
45. Mumbach, M.R.; Granja, J.M.; Flynn, R.A.; Roake, C.M.; Satpathy, A.T.; Rubin, A.J.; Qi, Y.; Jiang, Z.; Shams, S.; Louie, B.H.; et al. HiChIRP reveals RNA-associated chromosome conformation. *Nat. Methods* **2019**, *16*, 489–492. [CrossRef] [PubMed]
46. Simon, M.D.; Wang, C.I.; Kharchenko, P.V.; West, J.A.; Chapman, B.A.; Alekseyenko, A.A.; Borowsky, M.L.; Kuroda, M.I.; Kingston, R.E. The genomic binding sites of a noncoding RNA. *Proc. Natl. Acad. Sci. USA* **2011**, *108*, 20497–20502. [CrossRef] [PubMed]
47. Stadhouders, R.; Kolovos, P.; Brouwer, R.; Zuin, J.; van den Heuvel, A.; Kockx, C.; Palstra, R.J.; Wendt, K.S.; Grosveld, F.; van Ijcken, W.; et al. Multiplexed chromosome conformation capture sequencing for rapid genome-scale high-resolution detection of long-range chromatin interactions. *Nat. Protoc.* **2013**, *8*, 509–524. [CrossRef]
48. Engreitz, J.M.; Pandya-Jones, A.; McDonel, P.; Shishkin, A.; Sirokman, K.; Surka, C.; Kadri, S.; Xing, J.; Goren, A.; Lander, E.S.; et al. The Xist lncRNA exploits three-dimensional genome architecture to spread across the X chromosome. *Science* **2013**, *341*, 1237973. [CrossRef]
49. Zhao, J.; Ohsumi, T.K.; Kung, J.T.; Ogawa, Y.; Grau, D.J.; Sarma, K.; Song, J.J.; Kingston, R.E.; Borowsky, M.; Lee, J.T. Genome-wide identification of polycomb-associated RNAs by RIP-seq. *Mol. Cell* **2010**, *40*, 939–953. [CrossRef]
50. Ule, J.; Hwang, H.W.; Darnell, R.B. The Future of Cross-Linking and Immunoprecipitation (CLIP). *Cold Spring Harb. Perspect. Biol.* **2018**, *10*, a032243. [CrossRef] [PubMed]
51. Friedersdorf, M.B.; Keene, J.D. Advancing the functional utility of PAR-CLIP by quantifying background binding to mRNAs and lncRNAs. *Genome Biol.* **2014**, *15*, R2. [CrossRef]
52. McHugh, C.A.; Russell, P.; Guttman, M. Methods for comprehensive experimental identification of RNA-protein interactions. *Genome Biol.* **2014**, *15*, 203. [CrossRef]
53. Rio, D.C. 5′-end labeling of RNA with [gamma-32P]ATP and T4 polynucleotide kinase. *Cold Spring Harb. Protoc.* **2014**, *2014*, 441–443. [CrossRef] [PubMed]
54. Wang, H.V.; Chekanova, J.A. An Overview of Methodologies in Studying lncRNAs in the High-Throughput Era: When Acronyms ATTACK! *Methods Mol. Biol.* **2019**, *1933*, 1–30.
55. Femino, A.M.; Fay, F.S.; Fogarty, K.; Singer, R.H. Visualization of single RNA transcripts in situ. *Science* **1998**, *280*, 585–590. [CrossRef] [PubMed]

56. Chang, K.; Marran, K.; Valentine, A.; Hannon, G.J. RNAi in cultured mammalian cells using synthetic siRNAs. *Cold Spring Harb. Protoc.* **2012**, *2012*, 957–961. [CrossRef]
57. Huarte, M. The emerging role of lncRNAs in cancer. *Nat. Med.* **2015**, *21*, 1253–1261. [CrossRef] [PubMed]
58. Barrangou, R.; Birmingham, A.; Wiemann, S.; Beijersbergen, R.L.; Hornung, V.; Smith, A. Advances in CRISPR-Cas9 genome engineering: Lessons learned from RNA interference. *Nucleic Acids Res.* **2015**, *43*, 3407–3419. [CrossRef]
59. Bassett, A.R.; Akhtar, A.; Barlow, D.P.; Bird, A.P.; Brockdorff, N.; Duboule, D.; Ephrussi, A.; Ferguson-Smith, A.C.; Gingeras, T.R.; Haerty, W.; et al. Considerations when investigating lncRNA function in vivo. *Elife* **2014**, *3*, e03058. [CrossRef]
60. Aparicio-Prat, E.; Arnan, C.; Sala, I.; Bosch, N.; Guigo, R.; Johnson, R. DECKO: Single-oligo, dual-CRISPR deletion of genomic elements including long non-coding RNAs. *BMC Genom.* **2015**, *16*, 846. [CrossRef]
61. Goyal, A.; Myacheva, K.; Gross, M.; Klingenberg, M.; Duran Arque, B.; Diederichs, S. Challenges of CRISPR/Cas9 applications for long non-coding RNA genes. *Nucleic Acids Res.* **2017**, *45*, e12. [CrossRef]
62. Kole, R.; Krainer, A.R.; Altman, S. RNA therapeutics: Beyond RNA interference and antisense oligonucleotides. *Nat. Rev. Drug Discov.* **2012**, *11*, 125–140. [CrossRef]
63. Maracaja-Coutinho, V.; Paschoal, A.R.; Caris-Maldonado, J.C.; Borges, P.V.; Ferreira, A.J.; Durham, A.M. Noncoding RNAs Databases: Current Status and Trends. *Methods Mol. Biol.* **2019**, *1912*, 251–285. [PubMed]
64. Ma, H.; Hao, Y.; Dong, X.; Gong, Q.; Chen, J.; Zhang, J.; Tian, W. Molecular mechanisms and function prediction of long noncoding RNA. *ScientificWorldJournal* **2012**, *2012*, 541786. [CrossRef] [PubMed]
65. Uchida, S. High-Throughput Methods to Detect Long Non-Coding RNAs. *High. Throughput* **2017**, *6*, 12.
66. Carrara, M.; Fuschi, P.; Ivan, C.; Martelli, F. Circular RNAs: Methodological challenges and perspectives in cardiovascular diseases. *J. Cell Mol. Med.* **2018**, *22*, 5176–5187. [CrossRef] [PubMed]
67. Shen, L.; Zhang, Y.; Zhou, W.; Peng, Z.; Hong, X.; Zhang, Y. Circular RNA expression in ovarian endometriosis. *Epigenomics* **2018**, *10*, 559–572. [CrossRef]
68. Bi, J.; Wang, D.; Cui, L.; Yang, Q. RNA sequencing-based long non-coding RNA analysis and immunoassay in ovarian endometriosis. *Am. J. Reprod. Immunol.* **2021**, *85*, e13359. [CrossRef]
69. Li, S.; Teng, S.; Xu, J.; Su, G.; Zhang, Y.; Zhao, J.; Zhang, S.; Wang, H.; Qin, W.; Lu, Z.J.; et al. Microarray is an efficient tool for circRNA profiling. *Brief. Bioinform.* **2019**, *20*, 1420–1433. [CrossRef]
70. Szabo, L.; Salzman, J. Detecting circular RNAs: Bioinformatic and experimental challenges. *Nat. Rev. Genet.* **2016**, *17*, 679–692. [CrossRef]
71. Wu, J.; Huang, H.; Huang, W.; Wang, L.; Xia, X.; Fang, X. Analysis of exosomal lncRNA, miRNA and mRNA expression profiles and ceRNA network construction in endometriosis. *Epigenomics* **2020**, *12*, 1193–1213. [CrossRef]
72. Wang, D.; Luo, Y.; Wang, G.; Yang, Q. Circular RNA expression profiles and bioinformatics analysis in ovarian endometriosis. *Mol. Genet. Genom. Med.* **2019**, *7*, e00756. [CrossRef]
73. Xu, D.; Cai, Y.; Tang, L.; Han, X.; Gao, F.; Cao, H.; Qi, F.; Kapranov, P. A CRISPR/Cas13-based approach demonstrates biological relevance of vlinc class of long non-coding RNAs in anticancer drug response. *Sci. Rep.* **2020**, *10*, 1794. [CrossRef]
74. Holdsworth-Carson, S.J.; Churchill, M.; Donoghue, J.F.; Mortlock, S.; Fung, J.N.; Sloggett, C.; Chung, J.; Cann, L.; Teh, W.T.; Campbell, K.R.; et al. Elucidating the role of long intergenic non-coding RNA 339 in human endometrium and endometriosis. *Mol. Hum. Reprod.* **2021**, *27*, gaab010. [CrossRef] [PubMed]
75. Cabili, M.N.; Dunagin, M.C.; McClanahan, P.D.; Biaesch, A.; Padovan-Merhar, O.; Regev, A.; Rinn, J.L.; Raj, A. Localization and abundance analysis of human lncRNAs at single-cell and single-molecule resolution. *Genome Biol.* **2015**, *16*, 20. [CrossRef]
76. Wang, H.; Sha, L.; Huang, L.; Yang, S.; Zhou, Q.; Luo, X.; Shi, B. LINC00261 functions as a competing endogenous RNA to regulate BCL2L11 expression by sponging miR-132-3p in endometriosis. *Am. J. Transl. Res.* **2019**, *11*, 2269–2279. [PubMed]
77. Brosens, I.A.; Brosens, J.J. Is laparoscopy the gold standard for the diagnosis of endometriosis? *Eur J. Obs. Gynecol. Reprod. Biol.* **2000**, *88*, 117–119. [CrossRef]
78. Tammaa, A.; Fritzer, N.; Strunk, G.; Krell, A.; Salzer, H.; Hudelist, G. Learning curve for the detection of pouch of Douglas obliteration and deep infiltrating endometriosis of the rectum. *Hum. Reprod.* **2014**, *29*, 1199–1204. [CrossRef]
79. Canis, M.; Mage, G.; Wattiez, A.; Pouly, J.L.; Bruhat, M.A. The ovarian endometrioma: Why is it so poorly managed? Laparoscopic treatment of large ovarian endometrioma: Why such a long learning curve? *Hum. Reprod.* **2003**, *18*, 5–7. [CrossRef]
80. Balasch, J.; Creus, M.; Fabregues, F.; Carmona, F.; Ordi, J.; Martinez-Roman, S.; Vanrell, J.A. Visible and non-visible endometriosis at laparoscopy in fertile and infertile women and in patients with chronic pelvic pain: A prospective study. *Hum. Reprod.* **1996**, *11*, 387–391. [CrossRef]
81. Parasar, P.; Ozcan, P.; Terry, K.L. Endometriosis: Epidemiology, Diagnosis and Clinical Management. *Curr. Obs. Gynecol. Rep.* **2017**, *6*, 34–41. [CrossRef] [PubMed]
82. Savelli, L. Transvaginal sonography for the assessment of ovarian and pelvic endometriosis: How deep is our understanding? *Ultrasound Obs. Gynecol.* **2009**, *33*, 497–501. [CrossRef] [PubMed]
83. Wang, W.T.; Sun, Y.M.; Huang, W.; He, B.; Zhao, Y.N.; Chen, Y.Q. Genome-wide Long Non-coding RNA Analysis Identified Circulating LncRNAs as Novel Non-invasive Diagnostic Biomarkers for Gynecological Disease. *Sci. Rep.* **2016**, *6*, 23343. [CrossRef]
84. Cui, D.; Ma, J.; Liu, Y.; Lin, K.; Jiang, X.; Qu, Y.; Lin, J.; Xu, K. Analysis of long non-coding RNA expression profiles using RNA sequencing in ovarian endometriosis. *Gene* **2018**, *673*, 140–148. [CrossRef] [PubMed]

85. Huang, H.; Zhu, Z.; Song, Y. Downregulation of lncrna uca1 as a diagnostic and prognostic biomarker for ovarian endometriosis. *Rev. Assoc. Med. Bras.* **2019**, *65*, 336–341. [CrossRef] [PubMed]
86. Xu, X.X.; Jia, S.Z.; Dai, Y.; Zhang, J.J.; Li, X.Y.; Shi, J.H.; Leng, J.H.; Lang, J.H. Identification of Circular RNAs as a Novel Biomarker for Ovarian Endometriosis. *Chin. Med. J.* **2018**, *131*, 559–566. [CrossRef]
87. Xu, X.; Jia, S.Z.; Dai, Y.; Zhang, J.J.; Li, X.; Shi, J.; Leng, J.; Lang, J. The Relationship of Circular RNAs With Ovarian Endometriosis. *Reprod. Sci.* **2018**, *25*, 1292–1300. [CrossRef]
88. Khalaj, K.; Miller, J.E.; Lingegowda, H.; Fazleabas, A.T.; Young, S.L.; Lessey, B.A.; Koti, M.; Tayade, C. Extracellular vesicles from endometriosis patients are characterized by a unique miRNA-lncRNA signature. *JCI Insight* **2019**, *4*, e128846. [CrossRef]
89. Qiu, J.J.; Lin, Y.Y.; Tang, X.Y.; Ding, Y.; Yi, X.F.; Hua, K.Q. Extracellular vesicle-mediated transfer of the lncRNA-TC0101441 promotes endometriosis migration/invasion. *Exp. Cell Res.* **2020**, *388*, 111815. [CrossRef] [PubMed]
90. Liu, S.; Xin, W.; Tang, X.; Qiu, J.; Zhang, Y.; Hua, K. LncRNA H19 Overexpression in Endometriosis and its Utility as a Novel Biomarker for Predicting Recurrence. *Reprod. Sci.* **2020**, *27*, 1687–1697. [CrossRef] [PubMed]
91. Vlassov, A.V.; Magdaleno, S.; Setterquist, R.; Conrad, R. Exosomes: Current knowledge of their composition, biological functions, and diagnostic and therapeutic potentials. *Biochim. Biophys. Acta* **2012**, *1820*, 940–948. [CrossRef]
92. Anfossi, S.; Babayan, A.; Pantel, K.; Calin, G.A. Clinical utility of circulating non-coding RNAs—An update. *Nat. Rev. Clin. Oncol.* **2018**, *15*, 541–563. [CrossRef]
93. Pardini, B.; Sabo, A.A.; Birolo, G.; Calin, G.A. Noncoding RNAs in Extracellular Fluids as Cancer Biomarkers: The New Frontier of Liquid Biopsies. *Cancers* **2019**, *11*, 1170. [CrossRef]
94. Sukowati, C.H.C.; Cabral, L.K.D.; Tiribelli, C.; Pascut, D. Circulating Long and Circular Noncoding RNA as Non-Invasive Diagnostic Tools of Hepatocellular Carcinoma. *Biomedicines* **2021**, *9*, 90. [CrossRef] [PubMed]
95. Yuan, L.; Xu, Z.Y.; Ruan, S.M.; Mo, S.; Qin, J.J.; Cheng, X.D. Long non-coding RNAs towards precision medicine in gastric cancer: Early diagnosis, treatment, and drug resistance. *Mol. Cancer* **2020**, *19*, 96. [CrossRef]
96. Lessey, B.A.; Kim, J.J. Endometrial receptivity in the eutopic endometrium of women with endometriosis: It is affected, and let me show you why. *Fertil. Steril.* **2017**, *108*, 19–27. [CrossRef]
97. Xu, X.; Li, Z.; Liu, J.; Yu, S.; Wei, Z. MicroRNA expression profiling in endometriosis-associated infertility and its relationship with endometrial receptivity evaluated by ultrasound. *J. Xray Sci. Technol.* **2017**, *25*, 523–532. [CrossRef]
98. Mari-Alexandre, J.; Barcelo-Molina, M.; Belmonte-Lopez, E.; Garcia-Oms, J.; Estelles, A.; Braza-Boils, A.; Gilabert-Estelles, J. Micro-RNA profile and proteins in peritoneal fluid from women with endometriosis: Their relationship with sterility. *Fertil. Steril.* **2018**, *109*, 675–684.e2. [CrossRef] [PubMed]
99. Li, X.; Zhang, W.; Fu, J.; Xu, Y.; Gu, R.; Qu, R.; Li, L.; Sun, Y.; Sun, X. MicroRNA-451 is downregulated in the follicular fluid of women with endometriosis and influences mouse and human embryonic potential. *Reprod. Biol. Endocrinol.* **2019**, *17*, 96. [CrossRef]
100. Pearce, C.L.; Templeman, C.; Rossing, M.A.; Lee, A.; Near, A.M.; Webb, P.M.; Nagle, C.M.; Doherty, J.A.; Cushing-Haugen, K.L.; Wicklund, K.G.; et al. Association between endometriosis and risk of histological subtypes of ovarian cancer: A pooled analysis of case-control studies. *Lancet Oncol.* **2012**, *13*, 385–394. [CrossRef]
101. Nakamura, N.; Terai, Y.; Nunode, M.; Kokunai, K.; Konishi, H.; Taga, S.; Nakamura, M.; Yoo, M.; Hayashi, M.; Yamashita, Y.; et al. The differential expression of miRNAs between ovarian endometrioma and endometriosis-associated ovarian cancer. *J. Ovarian Res.* **2020**, *13*, 51. [CrossRef]
102. Suryawanshi, S.; Vlad, A.M.; Lin, H.M.; Mantia-Smaldone, G.; Laskey, R.; Lee, M.; Lin, Y.; Donnellan, N.; Klein-Patel, M.; Lee, T.; et al. Plasma microRNAs as novel biomarkers for endometriosis and endometriosis-associated ovarian cancer. *Clin. Cancer Res.* **2013**, *19*, 1213–1224. [CrossRef]
103. Arun, G.; Diermeier, S.D.; Spector, D.L. Therapeutic Targeting of Long Non-Coding RNAs in Cancer. *Trends Mol. Med.* **2018**, *24*, 257–277. [CrossRef]
104. Winkle, M.; El-Daly, S.M.; Fabbri, M.; Calin, G.A. Noncoding RNA therapeutics—Challenges and potential solutions. *Nat. Rev. Drug Discov.* **2021**, *20*, 629–651. [CrossRef]
105. Ghazal, S.; McKinnon, B.; Zhou, J.; Mueller, M.; Men, Y.; Yang, L.; Mueller, M.; Flannery, C.; Huang, Y.; Taylor, H.S. H19 lncRNA alters stromal cell growth via IGF signaling in the endometrium of women with endometriosis. *EMBO Mol. Med.* **2015**, *7*, 996–1003. [CrossRef]
106. Gu, Z.Y.; Jia, S.Z.; Leng, J.H. Establishment of endometriotic models: The past and future. *Chin. Med. J.* **2020**, *133*, 1703–1710. [CrossRef] [PubMed]
107. Romano, A.; Xanthoulea, S.; Giacomini, E.; Delvoux, B.; Alleva, E.; Vigano, P. Endometriotic cell culture contamination and authenticity: A source of bias in in vitro research? *Hum. Reprod.* **2020**, *35*, 364–376. [CrossRef] [PubMed]
108. Huan, Q.; Cheng, S.C.; Du, Z.H.; Ma, H.F.; Li, C. LncRNA AFAP1-AS1 regulates proliferation and apoptosis of endometriosis through activating STAT3/TGF-beta/Smad signaling via miR-424-5p. *J. Obs. Gynaecol. Res.* **2021**, *47*, 2394–2405. [CrossRef] [PubMed]
109. Lin, D.; Huang, Q.; Wu, R.; Dai, S.; Huang, Z.; Ren, L.; Huang, S.; Chen, Q. Long non-coding RNA AFAP1-AS1 promoting epithelial-mesenchymal transition of endometriosis is correlated with transcription factor ZEB1. *Am. J. Reprod Immunol.* **2019**, *81*, e13074. [CrossRef] [PubMed]

110. Liu, Y.; Huang, X.; Lu, D.; Feng, Y.; Xu, R.; Li, X.; Yin, C.; Xue, B.; Zhao, H.; Wang, S.; et al. LncRNA SNHG4 promotes the increased growth of endometrial tissue outside the uterine cavity via regulating c-Met mediated by miR-148a-3p. *Mol. Cell Endocrinol.* **2020**, *514*, 110887. [CrossRef] [PubMed]
111. Liu, Y.; Ma, J.; Cui, D.; Fei, X.; Lv, Y.; Lin, J. LncRNA MEG3-210 regulates endometrial stromal cells migration, invasion and apoptosis through p38 MAPK and PKA/SERCA2 signalling via interaction with Galectin-1 in endometriosis. *Mol. Cell Endocrinol.* **2020**, *513*, 110870. [CrossRef]
112. Cakmak, H.; Seval-Celik, Y.; Arlier, S.; Guzeloglu-Kayisli, O.; Schatz, F.; Arici, A.; Kayisli, U.A. p38 Mitogen-Activated Protein Kinase is Involved in the Pathogenesis of Endometriosis by Modulating Inflammation, but not Cell Survival. *Reprod. Sci.* **2018**, *25*, 587–597. [CrossRef] [PubMed]
113. Chetry, M.; Thapa, S.; Hu, X.; Song, Y.; Zhang, J.; Zhu, H.; Zhu, X. The Role of Galectins in Tumor Progression, Treatment and Prognosis of Gynecological Cancers. *J. Cancer* **2018**, *9*, 4742–4755.
114. Mondal, T.; Subhash, S.; Vaid, R.; Enroth, S.; Uday, S.; Reinius, B.; Mitra, S.; Mohammed, A.; James, A.R.; Hoberg, E.; et al. Author Correction: MEG3 long noncoding RNA regulates the TGF-beta pathway genes through formation of RNA-DNA triplex structures. *Nat. Commun.* **2019**, *10*, 5290. [CrossRef] [PubMed]
115. Hawkins, S.M.; Creighton, C.J.; Han, D.Y.; Zariff, A.; Anderson, M.L.; Gunaratne, P.H.; Matzuk, M.M. Functional microRNA involved in endometriosis. *Mol. Endocrinol.* **2011**, *25*, 821–832. [CrossRef]
116. Dong, L.; Zhang, L.; Liu, H.; Xie, M.; Gao, J.; Zhou, X.; Zhao, Q.; Zhang, S.; Yang, J. Circ_0007331 knock-down suppresses the progression of endometriosis via miR-200c-3p/HiF-1alpha axis. *J. Cell Mol. Med.* **2020**, *24*, 12656–12666. [CrossRef]
117. He, X.; Liu, N.; Mu, T.; Lu, D.; Jia, C.; Wang, S.; Yin, C.; Liu, L.; Zhou, L.; Huang, X.; et al. Oestrogen induces epithelial-mesenchymal transition in endometriosis via circ_0004712/miR-148a-3p sponge function. *J. Cell. Mol. Med.* **2020**, *24*, 9658–9666. [CrossRef] [PubMed]
118. Schmitt, A.M.; Chang, H.Y. Long Noncoding RNAs in Cancer Pathways. *Cancer Cell* **2016**, *29*, 452–463. [CrossRef]
119. Chang, C.Y.; Tseng, C.C.; Lai, M.T.; Chiang, A.J.; Lo, L.C.; Chen, C.M.; Yen, M.J.; Sun, L.; Yang, L.; Hwang, T.; et al. Genetic impacts on thermostability of onco-lncRNA HOTAIR during the development and progression of endometriosis. *PLoS ONE* **2021**, *16*, e0248168. [CrossRef]
120. Du, H.; Taylor, H.S. The Role of Hox Genes in Female Reproductive Tract Development, Adult Function, and Fertility. *Cold Spring Harb. Perspect. Med.* **2015**, *6*, a023002. [CrossRef]
121. Gupta, R.A.; Shah, N.; Wang, K.C.; Kim, J.; Horlings, H.M.; Wong, D.J.; Tsai, M.C.; Hung, T.; Argani, P.; Rinn, J.L.; et al. Long non-coding RNA HOTAIR reprograms chromatin state to promote cancer metastasis. *Nature* **2010**, *464*, 1071–1076. [CrossRef]
122. Ozes, A.R.; Miller, D.F.; Ozes, O.N.; Fang, F.; Liu, Y.; Matei, D.; Huang, T.; Nephew, K.P. NF-kappaB-HOTAIR axis links DNA damage response, chemoresistance and cellular senescence in ovarian cancer. *Oncogene* **2016**, *35*, 5350–5361. [CrossRef] [PubMed]
123. Zhang, C.; Wu, W.; Zhu, H.; Yu, X.; Zhang, Y.; Ye, X.; Cheng, H.; Ma, R.; Cui, H.; Luo, J.; et al. Knockdown of long noncoding RNA CCDC144NL-AS1 attenuates migration and invasion phenotypes in endometrial stromal cells from endometriosisdagger. *Biol. Reprod.* **2019**, *100*, 939–949. [CrossRef]
124. Kennedy, S.; Bergqvist, A.; Chapron, C.; D'Hooghe, T.; Dunselman, G.; Greb, R.; Hummelshoj, L.; Prentice, A.; Saridogan, E.; Soriano, D.; et al. ESHRE guideline for the diagnosis and treatment of endometriosis. *Hum. Reprod.* **2005**, *20*, 2698–2704. [CrossRef] [PubMed]
125. Krakowsky, R.H.; Tollefsbol, T.O. Impact of Nutrition on Non-Coding RNA Epigenetics in Breast and Gynecological Cancer. *Front. Nutr.* **2015**, *2*, 16. [CrossRef]
126. Agrawal, S.; Tapmeier, T.; Rahmioglu, N.; Kirtley, S.; Zondervan, K.; Becker, C. The miRNA Mirage: How Close Are We to Finding a Non-Invasive Diagnostic Biomarker in Endometriosis? A Systematic Review. *Int. J. Mol. Sci* **2018**, *19*, 599. [CrossRef] [PubMed]
127. Becker, C.M.; Laufer, M.R.; Stratton, P.; Hummelshoj, L.; Missmer, S.A.; Zondervan, K.T.; Adamson, G.D.; Group, W.E.W. World Endometriosis Research Foundation Endometriosis Phenome and Biobanking Harmonisation Project: I. Surgical phenotype data collection in endometriosis research. *Fertil. Steril.* **2014**, *102*, 1213–1222. [CrossRef]
128. Ciebiera, M.; Esfandyari, S.; Siblini, H.; Prince, L.; Elkafas, H.; Wojtyla, C.; Al-Hendy, A.; Ali, M. Nutrition in Gynecological Diseases: Current Perspectives. *Nutrients* **2021**, *13*, 1178. [CrossRef]
129. Kalra, E.K. Nutraceutical—Definition and introduction. *AAPS PharmSci.* **2003**, *5*, E25. [CrossRef]
130. Machairiotis, N.; Vasilakaki, S.; Kouroutou, P. Natural products: Potential lead compounds for the treatment of endometriosis. *Eur. J. Obs. Gynecol. Reprod. Biol.* **2020**, *245*, 7–12. [CrossRef]

Article

Endometriosis Susceptibility to Dapsone-Hydroxylamine-Induced Alterations Can Be Prevented by Licorice Intake: In Vivo and In Vitro Study

Chiara Sabbadin [1], Alessandra Andrisani [2], Gabriella Donà [3], Elena Tibaldi [3], Anna Maria Brunati [3], Stefano Dall'Acqua [4], Eugenio Ragazzi [4], Guido Ambrosini [2], Decio Armanini [1,*] and Luciana Bordin [3,*]

1. Department of Medicine—Endocrinology, University of Padova, 35121 Padova, Italy; ChiaraSabbadin@libero.it
2. Department of Women's and Children's Health, University of Padova, 35121 Padova, Italy; alessandra.andrisani@unipd.it (A.A.); guido.ambrosini@unipd.it (G.A.)
3. Department of Molecular Medicine-Biological Chemistry, University of Padova, 35131 Padova, Italy; gabriella.dona@hotmail.com (G.D.); elena.tibaldi@unipd.it (E.T.); annamaria.brunati@unipd.it (A.M.B.)
4. Department of Pharmaceutical and Pharmacological Sciences, University of Padova, 35131 Padova, Italy; stefano.dallacqua@unipd.it (S.D.); eugenio.ragazzi@unipd.it (E.R.)
* Correspondence: decio.armanini@unipd.it (D.A.); luciana.bordin@unipd.it (L.B.)

Abstract: Endometriosis, an estrogen-dependent chronic gynecological disease, is characterized by a systemic inflammation that affects circulating red blood cells (RBC), by reducing anti-oxidant defenses. The aim of this study was to investigate the potential beneficial effects of licorice intake to protect RBCs from dapsone hydroxylamine (DDS-NHOH), a harmful metabolite of dapsone, commonly used in the treatment of many diseases. A control group (CG, $n = 12$) and a patient group (PG, $n = 18$) were treated with licorice extract (25 mg/day), for a week. Blood samples before (T_0) and after (T_1) treatment were analyzed for: i) band 3 tyrosine phosphorylation and high molecular weight aggregates; and ii) glutathionylation and carbonic anhydrase activity, in the presence or absence of adjunctive oxidative stress induced by DDS-NHOH. Results were correlated with plasma glycyrrhetinic acid (GA) concentrations, measured by HPLC–MS. Results showed that licorice intake decreased the level of DDS-NHOH-related oxidative alterations in RBCs, and the reduction was directly correlated with plasma GA concentration. In conclusion, in PG, the inability to counteract oxidative stress is a serious concern in the evaluation of therapeutic approaches. GA, by protecting RBC from oxidative assault, as in dapsone therapy, might be considered as a new potential tool for preventing further switching into severe endometriosis.

Keywords: endometriosis; dapsone; DDS-NHOH; red blood cell; glycyrrhetinic acid

1. Introduction

One of the most common gynecological pathologies in reproductive age women is endometriosis, characterized by the presence of endometrial-like tissue in the uterine cavity [1,2].

Both heme and cellular debris contribute consistently to the formation of local [3] and systemic [4] inflammation status, thus promoting the increased production of reactive oxygen species (ROS) and reactive nitrogen species, cytokines, growth factors, and prostaglandins [5].

The presence of oxidative stress status markers in circulating red blood cells (RBCs) has been recently pointed out as a systemic feature of endometriosis [4]. Due to their fundamental role in oxygen transport, RBCs are particularly exposed to the oxidant threat, which represents a limiting factor of the lifespan of RBCs because no new proteins can be synthesized [6]. Therefore, oxidative-related damage is critical in the regulation of RBC's proper functioning and aging.

Besides ensuring deformability, which is determined by membrane protein-protein and lipid-protein interactions, membranes also provide cellular ion exchange and the expression of aging-related epitopes for RBC senescence recognition and removal.

In the RBC membrane, one of the most important integral proteins is protein band 3 (or anion exchanger, AE1), a 100 kDa protein with 12–14 transmembrane segments, mainly involved in the maintaining of the biconcave-shape and the CO_2/HCO_3^- homeostasis through chloride and bicarbonate (Cl^-/HCO_3^-) anion exchange [7]. The presence of phosphorylatable residues in the cytoplasmic domain (including both the N- and C-terminal ends of the molecule) provides band 3 the peculiarity of being considered as a redox stress sensor [8] in many prooxidant disorders [8–10], such as in glucose-6-phosphate dehydrogenase deficiency (G6PDd) [10,11]. The band 3 Tyr-P level regulates many of the physiological processes in RBCs, from glycolysis [12] to morphology [13], but it is also involved in erythrocyte aging [11,14] and antibody recognition [15].

Dapsone (DDS) is an aniline compound commonly used for many indications [16,17], including the treatment of leprosy, varied skin conditions, *Pneumocystis carinii* infection, and a variety of immuno-related conditions [18,19]. Unfortunately, DDS shares a well-documented toxicity, related to its routes of biotransformation [20,21] leading to the formation of dapsone hydroxylamine (DDS-NHOH), the powerful oxidizing dapsone metabolite [20,22]. In in vitro studies, DDS-NHOH has been demonstrated to shorten RBC lifespan through the progressive oxidative alteration pathway starting from methemoglobin formation, glutathione oxidation, [22–25], and band 3 high molecular weight aggregates (HMWA) [26], which leads to autologous antibody recognition [24].

Among the antioxidants assumed with the diet, such as vitamins, carotenoids, and minerals, which have been shown to contribute to maintaining the redox homeostasis, glycyrrhizin, the glycoside extracted from roots of the liquorice, known for its characteristic sweetness (about 30–50 times sweeter than sucrose), is widely used in the treatment of many diseases, such as chronic hepatitis [27], erythrodermic psoriasis [28], a variety of human viruses such as avian infectious bronchitis virus [29], HIV [30,31], and SARS-CoV-2 [32,33], as a few examples. Orally administered glycyrrhizin is metabolized by intestinal bacteria into 18β-glycyrrhetinic acid (GA) [34], a pentacyclic triterpenoid, whose structure is similar to those of the mineralocorticoid and glucocorticoid hormones secreted by the adrenal cortex. In in vitro experiments in human RBCs, GA prevented oxidative-induced alterations, greatly reducing both band 3 Tyr-P and band 3 high molecular weight aggregate (HMWA) formation [35].

The aim of this study was to evaluate the effect of the licorice intake on the oxidative stress generated by DDS-NHOH in RBCs from PG by monitoring band 3 Tyr-P levels and HMWA as parameters for the detection of RBC membrane denaturation. In addition, we analyzed the state and the activity of cytosolic carbonic anhydrase (CA), to investigate if GA could mitigate DDS-NHOH side-effects involving this enzyme, a useful parameter of the potential worsening of RBC oxidative status [36].

2. Results

2.1. Evaluation of the RBC Oxidative Status (Diamide) and Response to DDS-NHOH before Licorice Intake

Cytosolic compartments of PG RBC showed much higher monomeric CAII isoform (30 kDa) than CG RBC ($35 \pm 3.7\%$ compared to $12 \pm 3\%$, respectively, $p < 0.001$). Being the activity of CA strictly depending on its monomerization [36], a CA activity assay was performed, with PG RBC exhibiting almost six times higher values compared to CG RBC (Figure 1). When RBCs were treated with diamide, the amount of the 30 kDa band of CA increased to 24% and 49%, in CG and PG RBC, respectively, ($p < 0.001$), with a parallel activity increase (5.2 ± 2 in CG and 32.7 ± 8.0 in PG, $p < 0.001$). In addition, in the presence of DDS-NHOH, if the process of formation of the 30 kDa isoform was more evident (26% in CG, 68% in PG), the correspondent values of CA activity were not so drastically increased as expected (3.3 ± 0.6 and 12.2 ± 3.1 in CG and PG, respectively).

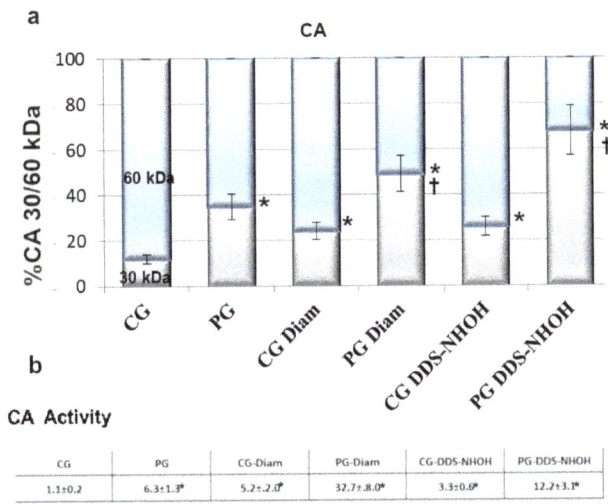

CA Activity

CG	PG	CG-Diam	PG-Diam	CG-DDS-NHOH	PG-DDS-NHOH
1.1±0.2	6.3±1.3*	5.2±2.0*	32.7±.8.0*	3.3±0.6*	12.2±3.1*

Figure 1. Fresh blood was collected from CG and PG RBCs (isolated as described in the Methods section) and was incubated with and without 1.5 mM diamide or 0.3 mM DDS-NHOH. (**a**) Diluted cytosol from 1 µL of packed cells, underwent Western blotting in non-reducing conditions. Bands immunostained with anti-CA antibodies were densitometrically analyzed, and the sum of the 30 and 60 kDa bands was arbitrarily calculated as 100%, taking into account that amount of proteolytic 30 kDa bands accounts for half the larger bands. Values were expressed as the means ± SD of $n = 12$ CG and $n = 18$ PG patients. * $p < 0.001$, comparison of CA 30 kDa isoform before and after treatments within groups, Student's t-test for paired data; † $p < 0.001$, comparison of the 30 kDa band between CG and PG groups, in both experimental conditions (diamide and DDS-NHOH treatments), Student's t-test. (**b**) CA activity: 300 µL of diluted cytosol from CG or PG RBCs, previously incubated with and without 1.5 mM diamide or 0.3 mM DDS-NHOH, were assayed for activity as described in the Methods section. The activity was calculated as the ratio to activity observed in untreated CG (chosen as arbitrary comparison unit, experimentally determined as 1 ± 0.23, mean value ± SD). Data show the means ± SD of $n = 12$ CG and $n = 18$ PG patients. * $p < 0.001$, comparison of CA activity to CG, before and after diamide treatment, Student's t-test for paired data.

2.2. Effect of Licorice Intake on the Membrane and Cytosol Oxidative Status

In both CG and PG, RBC membranes at T0 (before licorice intake) showed a similar pattern of B3 Tyr-P levels (which remained practically undetectable) and HMWA content (Figure 2, panel b).

In the presence of diamide, RBCs from PG showed a much higher Tyr-P level in RBC membranes compared to that from CG (221 ± 26 and 100 ± 9 for PG and CG membranes, respectively, $p < 0.005$). Similarly, membrane band 3 HMWA content also increased to double the basal amount in CG but reached almost four times the basal value in PG (196 ± 19 and 349 ± 45, for membranes from CG and PG, respectively, $p < 0.001$) (Figure 2, panel a, lanes T_0 and Figure 3, panels a and b, compare CG and PG at T_0, diamide) [4]. When diamide was replaced by DDS-NHOH, the average increment in the Tyr-P level was almost 6 times in RBCs from PG compared to CG ($p < 0.001$) (Figure 3, panel a). Similarly, in PG, DDS-NHOH treatment induced a higher increase in band 3 HMWA content (average PG increase of about 471 ± 37 % compared to CG, $p < 0.001$), much higher than that evidence in the RBC membranes of CG (196 ± 35 and 135 ± 29 for diamide and DDS-NHOH treatment, respectively, $p < 0.01$) (Figure 3, panels a and b, compare CG and PG at T_0, DDS-NHOH).

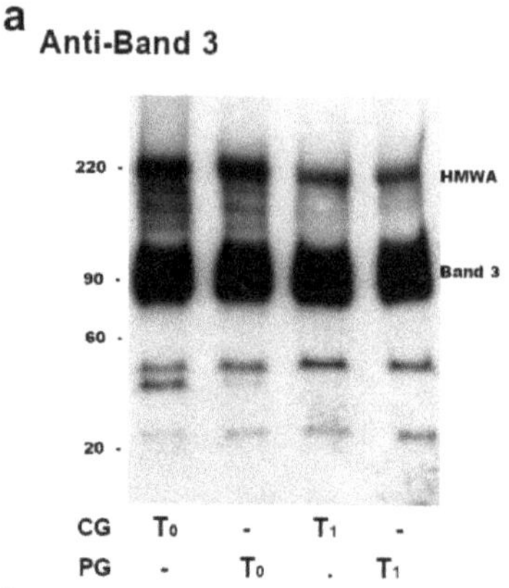

a
Anti-Band 3

	220 -				
					HMWA
	90 -				Band 3
	60 -				
	20 -				
CG	T₀	-	T₁	-	
PG	-	T₀	.	T₁	

b

Samples		Tyr-P level	HMWA content (% compared to CG T0)	GS-SP (% compared to CGT0)
CG	T0	nd	100±5	102±7
	T1	nd	67±6*‡	89±12*‡
PG	T0	nd	105±8	109±5
	T1	nd	75±9*‡	69±6*‡

Figure 2. The membranes (10 µg) obtained, as described in the Methods section, were analyzed by Western blotting in non-reducing conditions (panel **a**) and immunostained with anti-band 3 P-Tyr antibodies or in non-reducing conditions and immunostained with anti-band 3 (panel **a** and **b**), anti-P-Tyr or anti-GSH antibodies (panel **b**). For each immunostaining, bands corresponding to the relative proteins were densitometrically estimated and statistically analyzed (panel **b**). The Tyr-P value of both CG and PG RBCs were undetectable. The band 3 HMWA or GSH values were calculated as the ratio to band 3 HMWA or GSH obtained in basal (T_0) samples of CG (chosen as arbitrary comparison unit, experimentally determined as $100 \pm 5\%$ and $102 \pm 7\%$, respectively). Data shows the means ± SD of $n = 12$ CG and $n = 18$ PG patients. Comparison from respective baseline values: * $p < 0.001$, Student's t-test for paired data. Comparison CG vs PG: ‡ $p < 0.001$, Student t-test for unpaired data.

The increased oxidative status of the membrane was also evaluated by glutathionylated protein content (average increase of about 145% and 140% for diamide and DDS-NHOH, respectively, $p < 0.001$) (panel c).

After 1 week of licorice intake (T_1), RBCs from both groups were reanalyzed and the HMWA anti-Tyr-P and anti-GSH content from PG were compared to those from CG (Figure 2).

Results showed that both the HMWA and protein-bound GSH (GS-SG) contents were reduced after licorice intake (T_1), both in CG (with an average decrease of about 30% in HMWA and 10% in GS-SP) and PG (average decrease of 25% in HMWA, but almost 40 % in the GS-SP). Either in CG or PG, no alterations were detectable in the Tyr-P level.

Interestingly, at T_1, the PG RBCs also showed a net reduction in both diamide- and DDS-NHOH-induced alterations compared with their own values at T_0, with an average decrease ranging from $35 \pm 15\%$ (diamide-induced Tyr-P level) to $61 \pm 5\%$ (decrease of DDS-NHOH-induced glutathionylation) (panel f). All the other parameters ranged between these two values, with a reduction higher than 50%. CG RBCs showed a slight decrease only in diamide-induced Tyr-P values ($7 \pm 7\%$), but in all the other parameters the average decrease ranged from a minimum of $17 \pm 9\%$ (DDS-NHOH-induced HMWA formation) to a maximum of $48 \pm 6\%$ (the decrease in membrane glutathionylation was induced by DDS-NHOH). The variations of all parameters observed between T_0 and T_1 were statistically different, both in the CG and PG groups ($p < 0.005$). Also, the average values were statistically different between the CG and PG groups ($p < 0.001$) in all conditions (panels a–c), except for DDS-NHOH-induced glutathionylation, because, following licorice intake (T_1), the higher level of glutathionylated protein in PG RBCs was almost completely lowered, thus resembling the level in the CG RBCs (panel c, T_1).

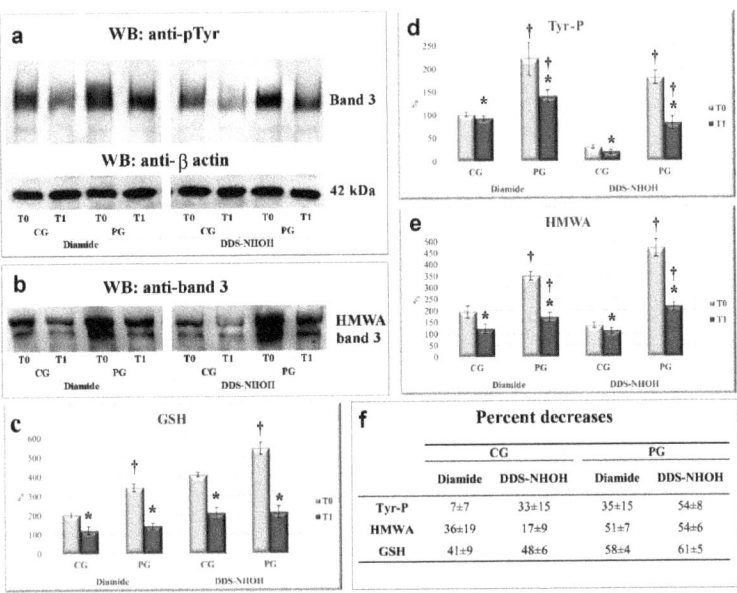

Figure 3. The effect of 1-week licorice intake on the Tyr-P level (**a**), HMWA, (**b**) and membrane GSH contents (**c**), following diamide or DDS-NHOH stimulation, in the CG and PG groups. RBCs from CG and PG were incubated with 1.5 mM diamide or 0.30 mM DDS-NHOH. The membranes (10 µg) obtained, as described in Methods, were analyzed by Western blotting and immunostained with the anti-P-Tyr antibody and then with anti-β actin as a loading control (Panel **a**). The membranes were also analyzed in non-reducing conditions and immunostained with anti-band 3 (Panel **b**) or anti-GSH (not shown) antibodies, in order to evidence the band 3 high molecular weight aggregate (HMWA) and bound glutathione, respectively. The figure is representative of the study population. For each immunostaining, bands corresponding to the relative proteins were densitometrically estimated and statistically analyzed GSH values of diamide or DDS-NHOH treated RBCs were calculated as the ratio percentage to GSH levels obtained in the basal samples of CG at T_0 (chosen as an arbitrary comparison unit, experimentally determined as $101 \pm 3\%$) (Panel **c**). The Tyr-P value of diamide—or DDS-NHOH—treated RBCs before (T_0) and after a week of licorice intake (T_1) was calculated as: Tyr-P% = (Tyr-P(x)/Tyr-P(CG) diamide T_0%, with the Tyr-P value obtained in diamide samples of CG at T_0 chosen as an arbitrary comparison unit (experimentally determined as $100 \pm 5\%$) (Panel **d**). The band 3 HMWA of diamide or DDS-NHOH treated RBCs were calculated as the ratio percentage to band 3 HMWA obtained in the basal samples of CG at T_0 (chosen as an arbitrary comparison unit, experimentally determined as 100 ± 4 and) (Panel **e**). (Panel **f**) average percent decrease for each parameter, referring to the corresponding values at T_0, were calculated and reported. Data show the means $\pm$ SD of $n = 12$ healthy subjects (CG) and $n = 18$ patients (PG). Comparison from the respective T_0 values: * $p < 0.005$, Student's t-test for paired data. Comparison CG vs PG: † $p < 0.001$, Student t-test for unpaired data.

2.3. Licorice Intake and CA Monomerization and Activity in RBC Cytosol

The cytosolic oxidative status was also evaluated, and the monomerization and activity of CA and the variation of GSH contents were compared between the two groups in the presence of diamide or DDS-NHOH at T_0 and T_1. As expected, in PG, at T_0 the monomeric form of this enzyme, representative of increased oxidation [26,36], was much higher compared to that of CG (35 ± 5 % of the 30 kDa isoform in PG compared to 12 ± 4 % present in CG, $p < 0.001$), and, consequently, also the CA activity was by far higher (Figure 2, $p < 0.001$).

What is interesting is that, following licorice intake, net decreases of both monomerization and activity were observed. By evaluating the average decrease in both values between T_1 and T_0, at T_1 the percentage of CA activity reduction was 8.5 ± 7 and 50.7 ± 4.3, in CG at basal or DDS-NHOH conditions, respectively ($p < 0.005$). In PG, CA activity reduction was 61.7 ± 16 and 79.1 ± 8.7, at basal or DDS-NHOH conditions, respectively ($p < 0.005$) (Table 1).

Table 1. The effect of 1-week licorice intake on CA activity and monomerization and ΔGSH in the cytosol of RBCs, in the presence of diamide or DDS-NHOH in in vitro treatment. Panel **a**: CA activity and monomerization values, obtained at T_0 and T_1, were expressed as the decrease after licorice intake, in the absence (basal), or presence of DDS-NHOH. The activity of CA was assayed in the RBC cytosol as described in the Methods. The decrease following the licorice intake (ΔCA activity %) was calculated as: (1-activity T_1/ activity T_0)%. The monomerization of CA was assayed in diluted cytosol from 1 μL of packed RBCs, obtained as described in the Methods. The cytosol underwent Western blotting in non-reducing conditions and was immunostained with an anti-CA antibody. Densitometrical analysis of the CA bands was carried out and the sum of the 30 and 60 kDa bands was arbitrarily calculated as 100%, taking into account that amount of proteolytic 30 kDa bands accounts for half the larger [36]. Panel **b**: Total glutathione was determined according to the Tietze method [4], as described in the Methods. The total decrease of glutathione content after diamide or DDS-NHOH treatment (ΔGSH) was expressed as 1-GSH(Diam or DDS-NHOH)/GSH(Basal) [4,36].

a		ΔCA activity %	CA 30 kDa (T_1-T_0 %)
CG	Diamide	8.5 ± 7.0	−0.42 ± 0.79
	DDS-NHOH	50.7 ± 4.3 *	−12.08 ± 2.84 *
PG	Diamide	61.7 ± 16.0 †	−16.28 ± 4.27 †
	DDS-NHOH	79.1 ± 8.7 † *	−45.00 ± 6.94 † *
b		ΔGSH (diamide)	ΔGSH (DDS-NHOH)
CG	T_0	0.08 ± 0.03	0.20 ± 0.01 *
	T_1	0.08 ± 0.03	0.08 ± 0.03 ‡
PG	T_0	0.54 ± 0.10 †	0.85 ± 0.08 † *
	T_1	0.36 ± 0.08 † ‡	0.38 ± 0.08 † * ‡

Values are expressed as the mean ± SD of $n = 12$ healthy subjects (CG) and $n = 18$ patients (PG). Comparison from respective basal values: * $p < 0.005$, Student's t-test for paired data. Comparison CG vs. PG: † $p < 0.001$, Student's t-test for unpaired data. Comparison between T_0 and T_1 within each group: ‡ $p < 0.001$, Student's t-test for paired data.

When the cytosol was analyzed for the GSH content, DDS-NHOH treatment induced a drop in the total glutathione content of about a mean value of 0.85 ± 0.08 in PG RBCs (Table 1, panel b, T_0). In CG only, a slight decrease in the glutathione content was observed after both diamide and DDS-NHOH treatments, 0.08 ± 0.03 and 0.20 ± 0.01, respectively, thus confirming that the band 3 Tyr-P level and HMWA formation involved cell GSH-related anti-oxidant defenses, with the depletion of cytosolic pools to implement the membrane protein glutathionylation. Also, in this case, licorice intake induced a net reduction of the GSH lost, as indicated by the lowering of ΔGSH values in both CG and PG (Table 1).

2.4. Correlation between Plasma GA Content and Reduction of RBC Oxidative Parameters

To assess if these licorice intake-related improvements and GA metabolites were correlated, we quantified the plasma GA content following the licorice intake (Figure 4). Plasma GA concentrations ranged from a minimum of 484 to1546 ng/mL in both groups, representative of great subjectivity in metabolizing licorice to yield GA. No significant difference was found between the mean GA plasma concentrations in the two groups (886.7 ± 329.3 ng/mL in CG vs. 1087.8 ± 261.6 ng/mL in PG; $p = 0.0734$). What is noteworthy is that we found a direct proportionality between the plasma GA content and a reduction in both diamide and DDS-NHOH-induced alterations (Figure 4), which resulted in highly significant for all parameters in CG, and less in PG (see correlation coefficients reported in Figure 4).

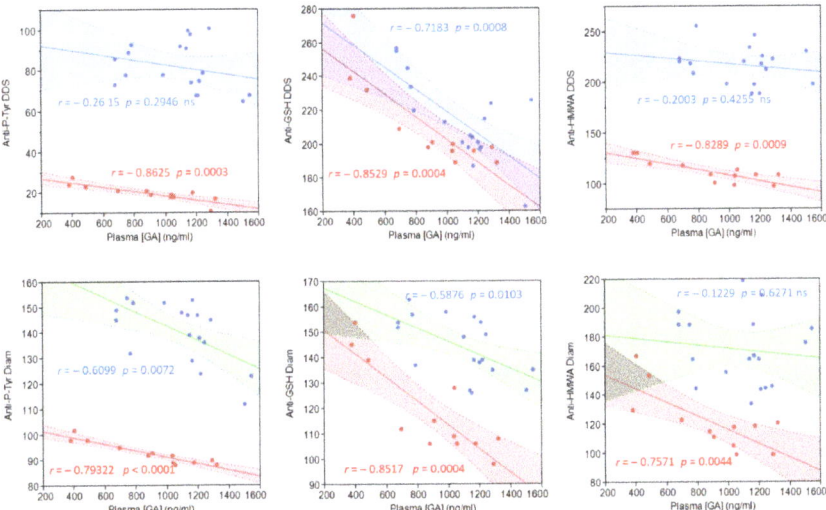

Figure 4. Correlation between the plasma GA concentration and measured parameters, after 1-week of licorice treatment, in both CG (red points) and PG (blue points) groups. Upper graphs: stimulation with DDS-NHOH. Lower graphs: basal values (not stimulated). For each regression line, Pearson's correlation coefficient r is indicated, together with the corresponding p-value. To obtain the plasma GA concentration, an HPLC–MS full scan method was used as described in the Methods.

The highly significant proportionality between the plasmatic GA content and the reduction of diamide-induced alterations was consistent with previous in vitro observations [35], but only for the Tyr-P parameter. Compared to DDS-NHOH, GA was not so efficacious in reducing diamide-induced membrane glutathionylation and HMWA formation. On the contrary, the GA plasma concentration better fitted with the improvements of both membrane and cytosol parameters following DDS-NHOH treatment, thus evidencing those alterations induced by the two compounds were different and, so, differently affected by GA.

3. Discussion

In this study, we investigated the effect of licorice intake on RBC improvements towards oxidative stress in endometriosis.

Dapsone-induced hemolytic anemia is closely related to erythrocyte membrane alterations, leading to premature cell removal, which can occur both extra-vascularly (witness hyperbilirubinemia), or intravascularly by dapsone-induced cell fragility. All hematological side effects reported for dapsone therapy are due to the N-hydroxy metabolite of the drug, dapsone hydroxylamine (DDS-NHOH) [20,25,37].

These alterations should be taken into account in choosing therapy for endometriosis patients. Endometriosis is a chronic inflammatory disease with a genetic, epigenetic, and environmental background [38]. It has been recently shown that the presence of endometriosis susceptibility genes whose wide variations of penetrance would be seriously influenced by phenotypic alterations [39]. Environmental changes, such as iron overload during menstruation, can induce a Fenton-mediated oxidative assault, which would affect

DNA hypermethylation and chromatin remodeling, thus stressing gene instability by introducing point mutations and/or DNA single- and double-strand breaks, all leading to a significant increase in cancer risk [39]. For these reasons, redox and inflammatory modifications, which can accumulate in endometriosis patients, may be not only at the origin of endometriosis but also responsible for the further development/worsening of the disease [39].

In this study, we addressed the potential effect of licorice in ameliorating PG RBC tolerance to dapsone treatments. We have previously demonstrated that GA, one of the licorice intestinal metabolism products, was able to prevent diamide-induced band 3 Tyr-P levels and HMWA formation, as well as band 3 proteolytic degradation in in vitro experiments performed with normal RBCs [35]. To investigate if this important GA shielding effect could be efficacious also in endometriosis to lower potential oxidant injuries, we analyzed the same parameters in RBCs after volunteers were given one week of licorice intake. Interestingly, all parameters resulted in positively affected PG RBCs, with net reductions in DDS-NHOH-induced alterations ranging from 35 to 61%, compared to T_0. That this effect was due to the GA licorice component was confirmed by the correlation between the plasma GA content and diamide, used as a reference, with its effects amply studied and described in previous studies [35,40], or DDS-NHOH effects. Only with diamide, for bound GSH and HMWA formation parameters, it seemed that weak a correlation was present in PG, but not in CG. This could be explained by the fact that diamide-induced alterations are different from those by DDS-NHOH. Diamide is known to induce disulfide bond formation, thus clustering membrane band 3 and leading to HMWA formation. Band 3 is normally distributed between detergent soluble (66%) and detergent-insoluble (33%) fractions of RBC membranes, and following diamide treatment, band 3 aggregated in HMWA increased only in the detergent soluble fraction [41]. On the contrary, DDS-NHOH induces a complete rearrangement of HMWA, which starts at the soluble fraction but slowly migrates to increase the insoluble counterpart [26].

Among the cytosolic enzymes, an important role is played by CA, a metallo-enzyme, converting CO_2 to HCO_3- and $H+$, which regulates many physiological processes such as acid–base balance homeostasis, respiration, carbon dioxide, ion transport, and bone resorption [42]. To date, their biological functioning has not been clarified, but recent evidence has pointed out how abnormal levels or activities [34] of many CA isoforms were associated with different diseases such as cancer (overexpression of CA IX/XII due to the hypoxia cascade activation), epilepsy (abnormal levels/activities of brain CA isoforms), and obesity (dysregulation of the mitochondrial isoforms CA VA/B) [42].

In human RBCs, the upregulation or high activity level of CA 2, the main isoform [36], has been related to glaucoma [42], and for this its functioning could represent an important parameter to be evaluated, mainly due to the recent finding showing an oxidative-related net increase of CA 2 activity in endometriosis patients. In fact, by increasing oxidative conditions, CA 2, normally present as an inactive dimer, can be activated following a monomerization process [36]. In the present study, the mean CA activity from PG was about 30 times higher than that from CG with a mean monomerization three times superior compared with CG, and 5 times lower GSH (ΔGSH). These data identify CA as an important parameter in the evaluation of the oxidative status in endometriosis, as well as a novel paradigm in the prevention of potential clinical complications.

In PG, one week of GA intake succeeded in considerably reducing both untreated and, much more interestingly, DDS-NHOH treated RBC effects on CA, with 5 times activity reduction and 3 times less monomerization, whereas in CG, both CA activity and monomerization, and GSH drop, returned to the level of the DDS-NHOH untreated RBC.

GA, a licorice metabolite, mitigates DDS-NHOH-induced side effects by lowering membrane sensitivity to oxidative stress and preserving cell GSH content.

For a long time, licorice has been considered in many natural medical resources, and these findings emphasize how GA can protect RBCs from strong oxidant-induced denaturation, thus preventing risks from extensive and prolonged exposure to oxidative stress in impaired anti-oxidant conditions.

4. Materials and Methods

4.1. Materials

Reagents were purchased from Sigma (Milan, Italy), and an anti-phospho-tyrosine (P-Tyr) (clone PY20) mouse monoclonal antibody was obtained from Biosource-Invitrogen (Camarillo, CA, USA). Anti-mouse secondary antibody conjugated with horseradish peroxidase (HRP) was obtained from BioRad Laboratories (Irvine, CA, USA), and DDS-NHOH from Toronto Research Chemicals Inc. (North York, ON, Canada).

4.2. Participants

Between December 2011 and December 2016, patients, presenting with pelvic pain and an ultrasonographically that identified an adnexal ovarian mass, were referred to our endometriosis care unit for laparoscopy. Only women classified as having endometriosis by histological examination of surgical specimens were put in the endometriosis group ($n = 18$, aged 34.1 ± 8.5 years). Following surgery, the stage of the disease was defined according to the classification system of the revised American Society for Reproductive Medicine (rASRM) as stage I (minimal, $n = 4$), stage II (mild, $n = 7$), stage III (moderate, $n = 4$), and stage IV (severe, $n = 3$).

Patients met the following criteria: no hormone therapy for at least 3 months; regular menstruation; non-smoker; no signs of other inflammatory disease (as assessed by leucocytes, body temperature, or other specific symptoms). Fresh blood was collected from patients undergoing laparoscopy and also from a group of 12 volunteers, mean age 34.9 (SD 9.2) years, whose clinical and ultrasound tests identified as being healthy (Table S1).

Clinical data and peripheral blood samples were collected from both PG and CG subjects only after explaining the objectives of the study and obtaining signed informed consent, according to the Italian Law for Privacy 675/96 prior to enrolment.

All participants were asked to take licorice sweets containing licorice extract up to 25 mg/day, a dose by far lower than what is recommended by the Scientific Committee which considered it prudent that regular ingestion should not exceed 100 mg/day [43].

This study was conducted in accordance with the ethical standards of the Ethics Committee for Research and Clinical Trials of our University (Em. n. 7, 13 February 2012) and in accordance with the Helsinki Declaration.

4.2.1. Treatment of Erythrocytes

RBCs were pelleted at $3750\times g$ for 3 min. After removal of the supernatant, packed RBCs were washed three times at $3750\times g$ for 3 min in 5 volumes of Dulbecco's Phosphate Buffered Saline (D-PBS) to avoid contamination by leucocytes and platelets. Packed cells (50 µL) were suspended (at 20% hematocrit) in D-PBS and treated at 35 °C for 30 min in the absence (Basal) or presence of 1.5 mM diamide (dissolved in D-PBS) (Diamide), or 0.3 mM DDS-NHOH dissolved in acetone (DDS-NHOH).

After washing, RBCs underwent hemolysis in 1.5 mL of hypotonic buffer (5 mM sodium phosphate, pH 8, 0.02 % sodium azide (NaN_3), 30 µM phenylmethylsulphonyl fluoride (PMSF), 1 mM sodium orthovanadate, and a protease inhibitor cocktail) [24].

Membranes were separated from the cytosol by centrifugation ($16,100\times g$ for 20 min in an Eppendorf centrifuge) and washed once in a hypotonic buffer. Aliquots of membranes and the cytosol were analyzed by Western blotting in reducing or non-reducing conditions and immunostained with appropriate antibodies.

4.2.2. Determination of GSH

Total glutathione was determined according to [10]. Briefly, 10 µL of cytosol obtained from differently treated erythrocytes were added to 2 mL of a reaction mixture containing 1.9 mL of phosphate 0.1 M/ EDTA 0.6 mM buffer, pH 7.4, 30 µL of 5,5'-dithio-bis(2-

nitrobenzoic acid) (DTNB) 10 mM, 100 µL of NADPH 5 mM, and 10 µg glutathione reductase (GR), and analyzed spectrophotometrically at 412 nm. The total decrease of glutathione content after diamide or DDS-NHOH treatment (ΔGSH) was expressed as 1-GSH (Diam or DDS-NHOH)/GSH(Basal) [24].

4.2.3. Esterase Activity Assay

The activity of CA was assayed in RBC cytosols by following the change in absorbance at 348 nm from the 4-nitrophenylacetate (NPA) to the 4-nitrophenylate (PNP) ion over a period of 10 min at 25 °C with a spectrophotometer (CHEBIOS UV–VIS), according to [36]. The enzymatic reaction was carried out in a total volume of 3.0 mL, containing 1.4 mL 0.05 M Tris–SO_4 buffer (pH 7.4), 1 mL 3 mM NPA, 0.5 mL H_2O, and 0.1 mL diluted cytosol. A reference measurement was obtained by preparing the same cuvette with a sample solution in the absence of incubation. One unit of CA activity was defined as the amount of enzyme which catalyzes the formation of 1 pmol PNP/min in standard conditions of incubation. The following formula incorporating the extinction coefficient was used to calculate: CA units $\times$ 10^{-3}/µL packed RBC = OD $\times$ sample dilution factor/(min $\times$ 667), with an extinction coefficient of 667 [28,35]. The decrease following the licorice intake (ΔCA activity %) was calculated as: (1- activity T_1/ activity T_0)%.

4.2.4. HPLC–MS Plasma Analysis

To obtain a metabolic profiling of plasma, an HPLC–MS full scan method was used, according to [44]. A Varian MS 500 equipped with a Prostar 430 autosampler and binary chromatograph 212 series (Varian, Palo Alto, CA, USA), was used as the HPLC–MS system. An Agilent (Milan, Italy) Eclipse XDB C−8 column (2.1 $\times$ 150 mm 3.5 µm) was used as a stationary phase. The mobile phase was composed of solvent A (acetonitrile with 0.5% acetic acid) and solvent B (water with 2% formic acid). Linear gradients of A and B were used as follows: 0 min, 10% A; 20 min, 85% A; 21 min, 100% A, 21.30 min, 10% A; 27 min, 10% A. The flow rate was 200 µL/min and the injection volume was 10 µL. The mass range explored was 50–1000 m/z. The mass spectra were recorded both in positive standard mode and in turbo data depending scanning (tdds) mode that allows the elucidation of the fragmentation patterns of the detected ions. Collected plasma samples were centrifuged (13,000$\times$ g for 10 min) and directly injected in the HPLC. Each HPLC–MS data set was processed with the MZmine 2.9 software; from the raw data files, a data set composed of 102 variables was obtained. The Median Fold Change normalization was applied to take into account the effects of sample dilution. Data were log-transformed and mean-centered.

4.3. Statistical Analysis

Data are expressed as the mean $\pm$ SD. Differences between the groups were compared with the Student's t-test (two-tailed). Comparisons before and after treatment with licorice within each group of subjects were obtained with the Student's t-test for paired data. The paired t-test was also used to compare values before and after DDS-NHOH treatment.

Relationships between pairs of variables were tested by least-squares linear regression. Pearson's correlation coefficient r was used to quantify the strength of relationships. The statistical significance of r was determined using a t-test (two-tailed).

A p-value < 0.05 was considered as statistically significant.

5. Conclusions

Endometriosis RBC membranes are characterized by high oxidative levels, which impairs the RBC response to a potential high oxidant therapy, such as in the case of DDS, commonly used for the treatments of leprosy, malaria, and autoimmune diseases. DDS-NHOH, a DDS metabolite, exasperates the oxidative status of the patients' RBCs. The resulting condition leads to a premature RBC removal from circulation as an index of reduced RBC life-span due to the overwhelming oxidative assault [24]. It is also involved in a potential further worsening of patients' conditions by increasing the oxidative stress which, in turn, may also trigger genetic/epigenetic cell transformation [38,39]. The DDS-NHOH-related further drop in the total glutathione content was also responsible for the serious increase of CA activity, thus bringing new concerns for the development of further complications, such as glaucoma [45].

After licorice intake, the GSH loss was clearly reduced, showing a net improvement of the cell anti-oxidant defenses, as confirmed by the related reduction of CA monomerization and activation. A similar protective effect of GA also mitigated DDS-NHOH induced side effects by lowering membrane sensitivity to oxidative stress and preserving the cell GSH content.

In conclusion, the results demonstrate that licorice intake prevented/ameliorated the oxidative stress generated by a strong oxidizing agent, a byproduct of a commonly used therapy, in RBCs already seriously struggling with an endometriosis-related inflammatory status—but it is far from being an endometriosis therapy. Our study represents a promising pilot study that would request further investigations to better evaluate licorice potential in inflammatory diseases.

Supplementary Materials: The following are available online at https://www.mdpi.com/article/10.3390/ijms22168476/s1.

Author Contributions: Conceptualization D.A. and L.B.; data curation, C.S., A.A., G.D., E.T., A.M.B., S.D., E.R. and L.B.; formal analysis, C.S., A.A., G.D., E.T., A.M.B., E.R., D.A. and L.B.; funding acquisition, D.A.; investigation, C.S., A.A., G.D., S.D. and L.B.; methodology, C.S., A.A., G.D., E.T., A.M.B., S.D., E.R., D.A. and L.B.; project administration, D.A. and L.B.; supervision, G.A. and D.A.; validation, E.R.; writing—original draft, C.S., A.A., G.D., E.T., A.M.B., S.D., E.R., G.A., D.A. and L.B.; writing—review and editing, C.S., A.A., G.D., E.R., G.A., D.A. and L.B. All authors have read and agreed to the published version of the manuscript.

Funding: This work was supported by the Italian Ministero dell'Università e della Ricerca Scientifica e Tecnologica (MURST, grant N. 60A06-0558/12). Doctors C. Sabbadin and G. Donà were partially supported by grants from Katjes Fassin GmbH + Co. KG, Emmerich (Germany).

Institutional Review Board Statement: This study was conducted in accordance with the ethical standards of the Ethics Committee for Research and Clinical Trials of our University (Em. n. 7, 13 February 2012) and with the Helsinki Declaration.

Informed Consent Statement: Informed consent was obtained from all subjects involved in the study.

Data Availability Statement: The data presented in this study are available in the article.

Conflicts of Interest: The authors declare no conflict of interest.

References

1. Vercellini, P.; Degiorgi, O.; Aimi, G.; Panazza, S.; Uglietti, A.; Crosignani, P. Menstrual Characteristics in Women with and without Endometriosis. *Obstet. Gynecol.* **1997**, *90*, 264–268. [CrossRef]
2. Zondervan, K.T.; Becker, C.M.; Missmer, S.A. Endometriosis. *N. Engl. J. Med.* **2020**, *382*, 1244–1256. [CrossRef]
3. Santanam, N.; Murphy, A.A.; Parthasarathy, S. Macrophages, Oxidation, and Endometriosis. *Ann. N. Y. Acad. Sci.* **2002**, *955*, 183–198. [CrossRef]
4. Bordin, L.; Fiore, C.; Donà, G.; Andrisani, A.; Ambrosini, G.; Faggian, D.; Plebani, M.; Clari, G.; Armanini, D. Evaluation of Erythrocyte Band 3 Phosphotyrosine Level, Glutathione Content, CA-125, and Human Epididymal Secretory Protein E4 as Combined Parameters in Endometriosis. *Fertil. Steril.* **2010**, *94*, 1616–1621. [CrossRef] [PubMed]
5. Augoulea, A.; Alexandrou, A.; Creatsa, M.; Vrachnis, N.; Lambrinoudaki, I. Pathogenesis of Endometriosis: The Role of Genetics, Inflammation and Oxidative Stress. *Arch. Gynecol. Obstet.* **2012**, *286*, 99–103. [CrossRef]
6. D'Alessandro, A.; Hansen, K.C.; Eisenmesser, E.Z.; Zimring, J.C. Protect, Repair, Destroy or Sacrifice: A Role of Oxidative Stress Biology in Inter-Donor Variability of Blood Storage? *Blood Transfus.* **2019**, *17*, 281. [CrossRef]
7. Reithmeier, R.A.F.; Casey, J.R.; Kalli, A.C.; Sansom, M.S.P.; Alguel, Y.; Iwata, S. Band 3, the Human Red Cell Chloride/Bicarbonate Anion Exchanger (AE1, SLC4A1), in a Structural Context. *Biochim. Biophys. Acta* **2016**, *1858*, 1507–1532. [CrossRef]
8. Pantaleo, A.; Ferru, E.; Pau, M.C.; Khadjavi, A.; Mandili, G.; Mattè, A.; Spano, A.; De Franceschi, L.; Pippia, P.; Turrini, F. Band 3 Erythrocyte Membrane Protein Acts as Redox Stress Sensor Leading to Its Phosphorylation by p^{72} Syk. *Oxid. Med. Cell. Longev.* **2016**, *2016*, 6051093. [CrossRef]

9. Pantaleo, A.; De Franceschi, L.; Ferru, E.; Vono, R.; Turrini, F. Current Knowledge about the Functional Roles of Phosphorylative Changes of Membrane Proteins in Normal and Diseased Red Cells. *J. Proteom.* **2010**, *73*, 445–455. [CrossRef]
10. Bordin, L.; Zen, F.; Ion-Popa, F.; Barbetta, M.; Baggio, B.; Clari, G. Band 3 Tyr-Phosphorylation in Normal and Glucose-6-Phospate Dehydrogenase-Deficient Human Erythrocytes. *Mol. Membr. Biol.* **2005**, *22*, 411–420. [CrossRef]
11. Pantaleo, A.; Ferru, E.; Giribaldi, G.; Mannu, F.; Carta, F.; Matte, A.; de Franceschi, L.; Turrini, F. Oxidized and Poorly Glycosylated Band 3 Is Selectively Phosphorylated by Syk Kinase to Form Large Membrane Clusters in Normal and G6PD-Deficient Red Blood Cells. *Biochem. J.* **2009**, *418*, 359–367. [CrossRef]
12. Puchulu-Campanella, E.; Chu, H.; Anstee, D.J.; Galan, J.A.; Tao, W.A.; Low, P.S. Identification of the Components of a Glycolytic Enzyme Metabolon on the Human Red Blood Cell Membrane. *J. Biol. Chem.* **2013**, *288*, 848–858. [CrossRef]
13. Bordin, L.; Clari, G.; Moro, I.; Dalla Vecchia, F.; Moret, V. Functional Link between Phosphorylation State of Membrane Proteins and Morphological Changes of Human Erythrocytes. *Biochem. Biophys. Res. Commun.* **1995**, *213*, 249–257. [CrossRef]
14. Bordin, L.; Fiore, C.; Bragadin, M.; Brunati, A.M.; Clari, G. Regulation of Membrane Band 3 Tyr-Phosphorylation by Proteolysis of P72(Syk) and Possible Involvement in Senescence Process. *Acta Biochim. Biophys. Sin.* **2009**, *41*, 846–851. [CrossRef]
15. Pantaleo, A.; Giribaldi, G.; Mannu, F.; Arese, P.; Turrini, F. Naturally Occurring Anti-Band 3 Antibodies and Red Blood Cell Removal under Physiological and Pathological Conditions. *Autoimmun. Rev.* **2008**, *7*, 457–462. [CrossRef]
16. Wozel, G.; Blasum, C. Dapsone in Dermatology and Beyond. *Arch. Dermatol. Res.* **2014**, *306*, 103–124. [CrossRef]
17. Kurien, G.; Jamil, R.T.; Preuss, C.V. *Dapsone*; StatPearls Publishing: Treasure Island, FL, USA, 2021.
18. Bahadir, S.; Cobanoglu, U.; Cimsit, G.; Yayli, S.; Alpay, K. Erythema Dyschromicum Perstans: Response to Dapsone Therapy. *Int. J. Dermatol.* **2004**, *43*, 220–222. [CrossRef] [PubMed]
19. Ujiie, H.; Shimizu, T.; Ito, M.; Arita, K.; Shimizu, H. Lupus Erythematosus Profundus Successfully Treated With Dapsone: Review of the Literature. *Arch. Dermatol.* **2006**, *142*, 393–403. [CrossRef]
20. Coleman, M.D.; Simpson, J.; Jacobus, D.P. Reduction of Dapsone Hydroxylamine to Dapsone during Methaemoglobin Formation in Human Erythrocytes in Vitro III: Effect of Diabetes. *Biochem. Pharmacol.* **1994**, *48*, 1341–1347. [CrossRef]
21. Swartzentruber, G.S.; Yanta, J.H.; Pizon, A.F. Methemoglobinemia as a Complication of Topical Dapsone. *N. Engl. J. Med.* **2015**, *372*, 491–492. [CrossRef]
22. Don, G.; Ragazzi, E.; Clari, G.; Bordin, L. *Hemolysis and Anemia Induced by Dapsone Hydroxylamine*; Silverberg, D., Ed.; InTech: London, UK, 2012; ISBN 978-953-51-0138-3.
23. Albuquerque, R.V.; Malcher, N.S.; Amado, L.L.; Coleman, M.D.; dos Santos, D.C.; Borges, R.S.; Valente, S.A.S.; Valente, V.C.; Monteiro, M.C. In Vitro Protective Effect and Antioxidant Mechanism of Resveratrol Induced by Dapsone Hydroxylamine in Human Cells. *PLoS ONE* **2015**, *10*, e0134768. [CrossRef]
24. Bordin, L.; Fiore, C.; Zen, F.; Coleman, M.D.; Ragazzi, E.; Clari, G. Dapsone Hydroxylamine Induces Premature Removal of Human Erythrocytes by Membrane Reorganization and Antibody Binding: DDS-NHOH and Human Erythrocytes. *Br. J. Pharmacol.* **2010**, *161*, 1186–1199. [CrossRef]
25. Schiff, D.E.; Roberts, W.D.; Sue, Y.-J. Methemoglobinemia Associated with Dapsone Therapy in a Child with Pneumonia and Chronic Immune Thrombocytopenic Purpura. *J. Pediatr. Hematol. Oncol.* **2006**, *28*, 395–398. [CrossRef]
26. Andrisani, A.; Donà, G.; Sabbadin, C.; Dall'Acqua, S.; Tibaldi, E.; Roveri, A.; Bosello Travain, V.; Brunati, A.M.; Ambrosini, G.; Ragazzi, E.; et al. Dapsone Hydroxylamine-Mediated Alterations in Human Red Blood Cells from Endometriotic Patients. *Gynecol. Endocrinol.* **2017**, *33*, 928–932. [CrossRef]
27. Li, J.; Cao, H.; Liu, P.; Cheng, G.; Sun, M. Glycyrrhizic Acid in the Treatment of Liver Diseases: Literature Review. *BioMed Res. Int.* **2014**, *2014*, 872139. [CrossRef]
28. Yu, J.J.; Zhang, C.S.; Coyle, M.E.; Du, Y.; Zhang, A.L.; Guo, X.; Xue, C.C.; Lu, C. Compound Glycyrrhizin plus Conventional Therapy for Psoriasis Vulgaris: A Systematic Review and Meta-Analysis of Randomized Controlled Trials. *Curr. Med. Res. Opin.* **2017**, *33*, 279–287. [CrossRef]
29. Li, J.; Yin, J.; Sui, X.; Li, G.; Ren, X. Comparative Analysis of the Effect of Glycyrrhizin Diammonium and Lithium Chloride on Infectious Bronchitis Virus Infection in Vitro. *Avian Pathol. J. WVPA* **2009**, *38*, 215–221. [CrossRef]
30. Ito, M.; Sato, A.; Hirabayashi, K.; Tanabe, F.; Shigeta, S.; Baba, M.; De Clercq, E.; Nakashima, H.; Yamamoto, N. Mechanism of Inhibitory Effect of Glycyrrhizin on Replication of Human Immunodeficiency Virus (HIV). *Antivir. Res.* **1988**, *10*, 289–298. [CrossRef]
31. Bailly, C.; Vergoten, G. Glycyrrhizin: An Alternative Drug for the Treatment of COVID-19 Infection and the Associated Respiratory Syndrome? *Pharmacol. Ther.* **2020**, *214*, 107618. [CrossRef]
32. Armanini, D.; Fiore, C.; Bielenberg, J.; Sabbadin, C.; Bordin, L. Coronavirus-19: Possible Therapeutic Implications of Spironolactone and Dry Extract of *Glycyrrhiza glabra* L. (Licorice). *Front. Pharmacol.* **2020**, *11*, 558418. [CrossRef]
33. Ng, S.L.; Khaw, K.-Y.; Ong, Y.S.; Goh, H.P.; Kifli, N.; Teh, S.P.; Ming, L.C.; Kotra, V.; Goh, B.H. Licorice: A Potential Herb in Overcoming SARS-CoV-2 Infections. *J. Evid. Based Integr. Med.* **2021**, *26*. [CrossRef]
34. Ishiuchi, K.; Morinaga, O.; Ohkita, T.; Tian, C.; Hirasawa, A.; Mitamura, M.; Maki, Y.; Kondo, T.; Yasujima, T.; Yuasa, H.; et al. 18β-Glycyrrhetyl-3-O-Sulfate Would Be a Causative Agent of Licorice-Induced Pseudoaldosteronism. *Sci. Rep.* **2019**, *9*, 1587. [CrossRef]
35. Fiore, C.; Bordin, L.; Pellati, D.; Armanini, D.; Clari, G. Effect of Glycyrrhetinic Acid on Membrane Band 3 in Human Erythrocytes. *Arch. Biochem. Biophys.* **2008**, *479*, 46–51. [CrossRef] [PubMed]

36. Andrisani, A.; Donà, G.; Brunati, A.M.; Clari, G.; Armanini, D.; Ragazzi, E.; Ambrosini, G.; Bordin, L. Increased Oxidation-Related Glutathionylation and Carbonic Anhydrase Activity in Endometriosis. *Reprod. Biomed. Online* **2014**, *28*, 773–779. [CrossRef] [PubMed]
37. Orion, E.; Matz, H.; Wolf, R. The Life-Threatening Complications of Dermatologic Therapies. *Clin. Dermatol.* **2005**, *23*, 182–192. [CrossRef] [PubMed]
38. Kobayashi, H.; Higashiura, Y.; Shigetomi, H.; Kajihara, H. Pathogenesis of Endometriosis: The Role of Initial Infection and Subsequent Sterile Inflammation (Review). *Mol. Med. Rep.* **2014**, *9*, 9–15. [CrossRef]
39. Kobayashi, H.; Imanaka, S.; Nakamura, H.; Tsuji, A. Understanding the Role of Epigenomic, Genomic and Genetic Alterations in the Development of Endometriosis (Review). *Mol. Med. Rep.* **2014**, *9*, 1483–1505. [CrossRef]
40. Bordin, L.; Ion-Popa, F.; Brunati, A.M.; Clari, G.; Low, P.S. Effector-Induced Syk-Mediated Phosphorylation in Human Erythrocytes. *Biochim. Biophys. Acta* **2005**, *1745*, 20–28. [CrossRef]
41. Bordin, L.; Quartesan, S.; Zen, F.; Vianello, F.; Clari, G. Band 3 Tyr-Phosphorylation in Human Erythrocytes from Non-Pregnant and Pregnant Women. *Biochim. Biophys. Acta* **2006**, *1758*, 611–619. [CrossRef]
42. Abdel Gawad, N.M.; Amin, N.H.; Elsaadi, M.T.; Mohamed, F.M.M.; Angeli, A.; De Luca, V.; Capasso, C.; Supuran, C.T. Synthesis of 4-(Thiazol-2-Ylamino)-Benzenesulfonamides with Carbonic Anhydrase I, II and IX Inhibitory Activity and Cytotoxic Effects against Breast Cancer Cell Lines. *Bioorg. Med. Chem.* **2016**, *24*, 3043–3051. [CrossRef]
43. Scientific Committee on Food. *Opinion of the Scientific Committee on Food on Glycyrrhizinic Acid and Its Ammonium Salt*; Report SCF/CS/ADD/EDUL/225; Health Consumer Protection Directorate-General, European Commission: Brussels, Belgium, 2003.
44. Dall'Acqua, S.; Stocchero, M.; Boschiero, I.; Schiavon, M.; Golob, S.; Uddin, J.; Voinovich, D.; Mammi, S.; Schievano, E. New Findings on the in Vivo Antioxidant Activity of Curcuma Longa Extract by an Integrated 1H NMR and HPLC–MS Metabolomic Approach. *Fitoterapia* **2016**, *109*, 125–131. [CrossRef] [PubMed]
45. Bozdag, M.; Ferraroni, M.; Nuti, E.; Vullo, D.; Rossello, A.; Carta, F.; Scozzafava, A.; Supuran, C.T. Combining the Tail and the Ring Approaches for Obtaining Potent and Isoform-Selective Carbonic Anhydrase Inhibitors: Solution and X-ray Crystallographic Studies. *Bioorg. Med. Chem.* **2014**, *22*, 334–340. [CrossRef] [PubMed]

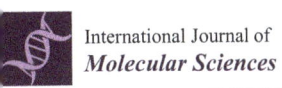

Article

LINC01133 Inhibits Invasion and Promotes Proliferation in an Endometriosis Epithelial Cell Line

Iveta Yotova [1,*], Quanah J. Hudson [1], Florian M. Pauler [2], Katharina Proestling [1], Isabella Haslinger [1], Lorenz Kuessel [1], Alexandra Perricos [1], Heinrich Husslein [1] and René Wenzl [1,*]

1 Department of Obstetrics and Gynecology, Medical University of Vienna, Waehringer Guertel 18-20, A-1090 Vienna, Austria; quanah.hudson@univie.ac.at (Q.J.H.); katharina.proestling@meduniwien.ac.at (K.P.); isabella.haslinger@meduniwien.ac.at (I.H.); lorenz.kuessel@meduniwien.ac.at (L.K.); alexandra.perricos@meduniwien.ac.at (A.P.); heinrich.husslein@meduniwien.ac.at (H.H.)
2 Institute of Science and Technology Austria, Am Campus 1, 3400 Klosterneuburg, Austria; florian.pauler@ist.ac.at
* Correspondence: iveta.yotova@meduniwien.ac.at (I.Y.); rene.wenzl@meduniwien.ac.at (R.W.)

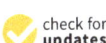

Citation: Yotova, I.; Hudson, Q.J.; Pauler, F.M.; Proestling, K.; Haslinger, I.; Kuessel, L.; Perricos, A.; Husslein, H.; Wenzl, R. *LINC01133* Inhibits Invasion and Promotes Proliferation in an Endometriosis Epithelial Cell Line. *Int. J. Mol. Sci.* **2021**, *22*, 8385. https://doi.org/10.3390/ijms22168385

Academic Editor: Antonio Simone Laganà

Received: 23 June 2021
Accepted: 1 August 2021
Published: 4 August 2021

Publisher's Note: MDPI stays neutral with regard to jurisdictional claims in published maps and institutional affiliations.

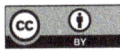

Copyright: © 2021 by the authors. Licensee MDPI, Basel, Switzerland. This article is an open access article distributed under the terms and conditions of the Creative Commons Attribution (CC BY) license (https://creativecommons.org/licenses/by/4.0/).

Abstract: Endometriosis is a common gynecological disorder characterized by ectopic growth of endometrium outside the uterus and is associated with chronic pain and infertility. We investigated the role of the long intergenic noncoding RNA 01133 (*LINC01133*) in endometriosis, an lncRNA that has been implicated in several types of cancer. We found that *LINC01133* is upregulated in ectopic endometriotic lesions. As expression appeared higher in the epithelial endometrial layer, we performed a siRNA knockdown of *LINC01133* in an endometriosis epithelial cell line. Phenotypic assays indicated that *LINC01133* may promote proliferation and suppress cellular migration, and affect the cytoskeleton and morphology of the cells. Gene ontology analysis of differentially expressed genes indicated that cell proliferation and migration pathways were affected in line with the observed phenotype. We validated upregulation of p21 and downregulation of Cyclin A at the protein level, which together with the quantification of the DNA content using fluorescence-activated cell sorting (FACS) analysis indicated that the observed effects on cellular proliferation may be due to changes in cell cycle. Further, we found testis-specific protein kinase 1 (TESK1) kinase upregulation corresponding with phosphorylation and inactivation of actin severing protein Cofilin, which could explain changes in the cytoskeleton and cellular migration. These results indicate that endometriosis is associated with *LINC01133* upregulation, which may affect pathogenesis via the cellular proliferation and migration pathways.

Keywords: endometriosis; long noncoding RNAs; lncRNAs; epithelial to mesenchymal transition; EMT; proliferation; migration; cytoskeleton

1. Introduction

Endometriosis is a disorder characterized by the presence of endometrial tissue outside of the uterine cavity, most often attached to organs of the peritoneal cavity [1]. As a common gynecological disorder affecting 6–10% of reproductive age women, endometriosis presents a significant burden on affected patients and society. However, the pathogenesis of the disease is still not well defined. The most accepted explanation for the origin of the cells from which endometriosis lesions develop is retrograde menstruation, whereby endometrial cells flow out into the peritoneal cavity via the fallopian tubes [1]. In order to establish a lesion, endometrial cells in the peritoneal cavity must adhere, implant, and differentiate while avoiding the immune system. Thus, complex interactions between molecular, humoral, immune, genetic and epigenetic signals must occur to support the development, growth and persistence of a lesion [2].

The advent of next-generation sequencing has accelerated identification of changes in the transcriptome, genome and epigenome in the pathogenesis of human diseases including endometriosis. In recent years, it has become clear that interactions between protein-coding (mRNA) and non-coding transcripts such as long-non-coding RNAs (LncRNAs) can influence the development of disease.

LncRNAs are a class of RNAs greater than 200 nucleotides in length that show similar RNA biology features to mRNAs but do not code for a protein [3]. LncRNA can be transcribed from different genomic regions, including introns, exons, and intergenic regions. Around 30,000 lncRNAs have been identified in humans and mice [4], but only a fraction of these have so far been demonstrated to be functional. LncRNAs are less evolutionarily conserved than mRNA [5], and are thought to form a complex tertiary structure when binding DNA, RNA and proteins that may be required for their function [6]. They may act as epigenetic gene regulators by affecting biological functions in the cell such as the assembly and function of nuclear bodies, the stability and translation of cytoplasmic mRNAs, and signaling pathways [7,8]. LncRNAs have been reported to regulate gene expression in a number of different ways, including targeting chromatin modifiers such as Polycomb repressive complex 2 (PRC2), or by acting as so-called miRNA sponges to bind miRNAs that would otherwise bind other targets thereby affecting their expression [9]. Several studies using patient samples and animal models have reported aberrant expression of long non-coding RNAs in endometriosis [10,11]. A growing body of evidence has identified lncRNAs that can alter cell proliferation, migration, invasion and apoptosis of endometriosis cells [12–14]. The molecular mechanism by which these lncRNAs cause these phenotypes has not been shown in all cases. LncRNAs have also been associated with endometriosis-associated angiogenesis [15], infertility [12] and epithelial to mesenchymal transition (EMT) [16]. EMT is a cellular process where epithelial cells acquire a more invasive mesenchymal phenotype and is associated with the loss of E-cadherin (CDH1) and a gain of N-cadherin (CDH2), and the presence of EMT promoting factors such as TWIST1, SNAIL, SLUG and TGFβ [17,18]. In a pathogenic context, it has been established that EMT is a key process in carcinogenesis, but also plays a less well-characterized role in endometriosis lesion development [19]. Hence, clarifying the role of EMT in endometriosis, and its regulation by pathways that may include lncRNAs remains an important issue in the field.

LINC01133 is an lncRNA that has recently been identified as a putative prognostic marker for endometrial cancer [20]. It has also been associated with the regulation of EMT in several cancers including cervical [21], breast [22], colorectal [23] and gastric [24]. Given that EMT is also a feature of endometriosis [25] we reasoned that LINC01133 may also be involved in the pathogenesis of endometriosis, and sought to investigate this in our study.

2. Results

2.1. LINC01133 Is Upregulated in Ectopic Endometriosis Lesions

In order to identify changes that may occur in LINC01133 expression levels during endometriosis pathogenesis, we compared control eutopic endometrium from women without endometriosis with eutopic endometrium from endometriosis patients, and ectopic endometriosis lesions using quantitative reverse transcription PCR (qRT-PCR). This showed that LINC01133 expression is significantly upregulated in endometriosis lesions compared to eutopic tissue of both patients and controls (Figure 1A). These changes were independent of disease stage and menstrual cycle phase (Figure 1B,C). We next used RNA Scope in situ hybridization to determine LINC01133 spatial localization within endometrium tissue. We found that LINC01133 is expressed in both stromal and epithelial cells of the eutopic endometrium of women with endometriosis, but appeared to show higher levels in glandular epithelial cells (Figure S1A). Quantification confirmed this observation, with positive glandular epithelial cells around five times more frequent than positive stroma cells ($p = 0.0012$) (Figure S1B).

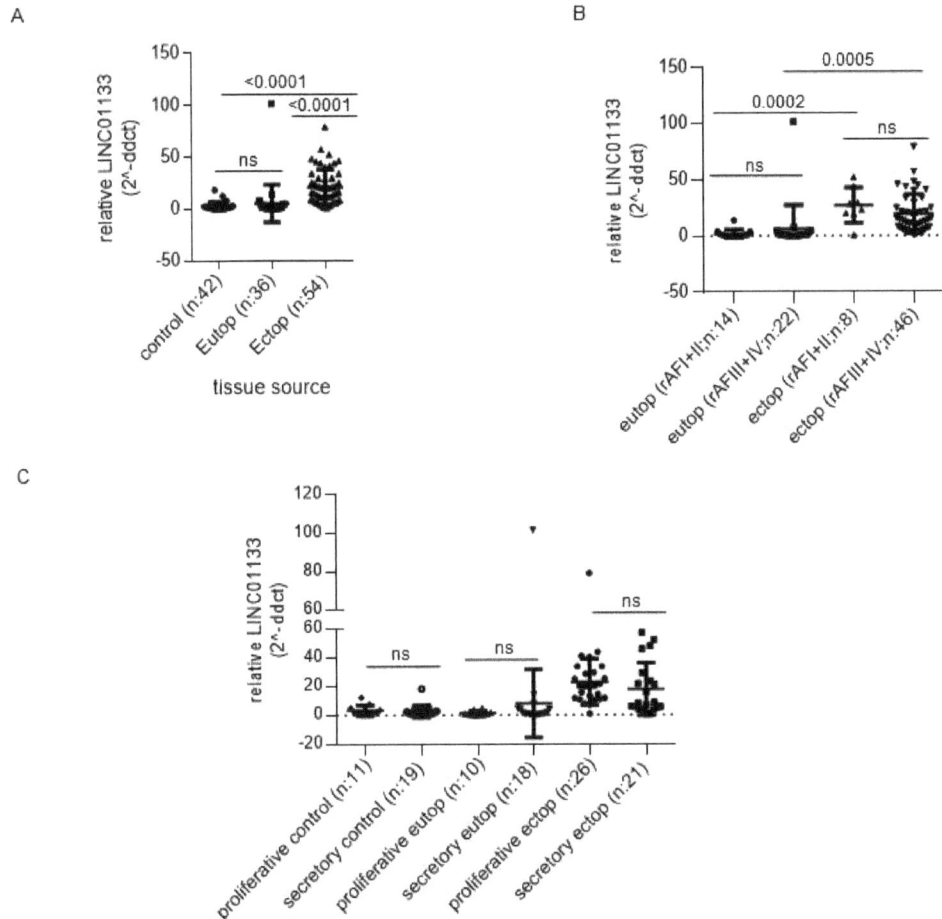

Figure 1. *LINC01133* expression is upregulated in endometriosis lesions. (**A**) Relative expression of *LINC01133* is significantly increased in ectopic endometriotic lesions compared to the eutopic endometrium of women with and without endometriosis. Expression in the eutopic endometrium does not differ between women with and without the disease. (**B**) In endometriosis patients, *LINC01133* expression does not significantly differ between mild (rAF I + II) and more severe (rAF III + IV) disease stages, in either the eutopic endometrium or ectopic lesions. (**C**) *LINC01133* expression does not significantly differ between the proliferative and secretory stages of the menstrual cycle in control eutopic endometrium, eutopic endometrium from patients, or ectopic lesions. Data in (**A–C**) are presented as dot plots including the mean relative expression levels and standard deviation in each group As the sample sizes were not equal, data were analyzed by fitting a mixed model, rather than repeated measures ANOVA (which requires equal sample size). Adjusted *p*-values values (adjp) < 0.05 were considered significant with non-significant differences indicated by ns. Control: endometrial tissue of women without endometriosis, Eutop: endometrial tissue of women with endometriosis, Ectop: endometriosis lesions.

2.2. LINC01133 siRNA Knockdown in 12Z Endometriosis Epithelial Cells Leads to Transcriptional Deregulation of 1210 Genes

To evaluate the role of *LINC01133* within the epithelial cell compartment of endometriosis lesions, we performed transient siRNAs-based knockdown of *LINC01133* in the 12Z endometriosis epithelial cell line, followed by RNA-sequencing. First, using qRT-PCR we confirmed the efficiency of *LINC01133* knockdown using three independent siRNA oligos. Significant knockdown was achieved for all 3 oligos ($p \leq 0.0001$), with the most efficient siRNA *LINC01133a* reducing *LINC01133* expression by more than 90% 72 h after transfection (Figure 2A). In order to identify any genes and pathways affected by *LINC01133* knockdown, we then conducted RNA-sequencing comparing *LINC01133a* knockdown cells with non-targeting siRNA control cells 72 h after transfection (3 biological replicates each). We identified four *LINC01133* transcript isoforms that are expressed in 12Z cells and confirmed that all were efficiently targeted by the *LINC01133a* siRNA oligo (Figure 2B). Further, analysis revealed 1210 differentially expressed (DE) transcripts in 12Z knockdown cells, compared to controls using a fold change cutoff of >1.5 and adjp < 0.05. From those DE genes, 703 were down-regulated and 507 up-regulated in knockdown cells (Table S4). These transcriptional changes enabled a clear separation of *LINC01133* knockdown and control samples by unsupervised hierarchical clustering (Figure 2C).

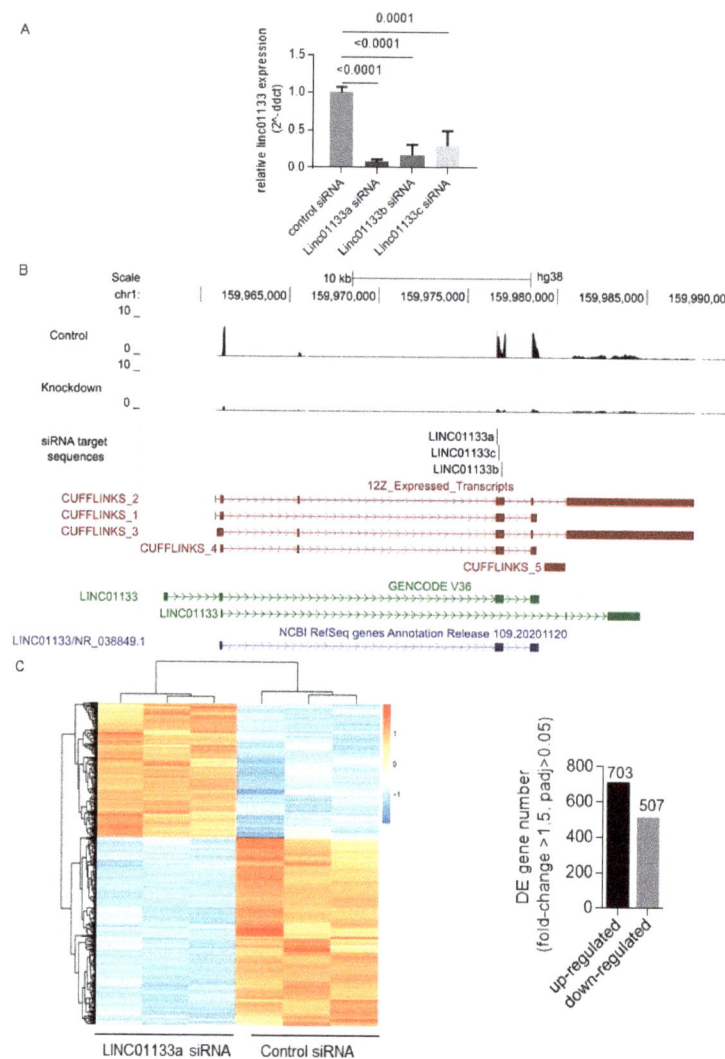

Figure 2. *LINC01133* knockdown leads to the deregulation of hundreds of genes in an endometriosis epithelial cell line.

(**A**) qRT-PCR shows relative expression of *LINC01133* is significantly reduced in 12Z cells for all 3 siRNA oligos that were used. (**B**) Tissue-specific *LINC01133* isoforms are efficiently knocked down in 12Z cells. Top: A UCSC genome browser screenshot shows RNA sequencing reads mapping to *LINC01133* are dramatically reduced in a knockdown with siRNA oligo *LINC01133a*. Bottom: Genome assembly using Cufflinks reveals multiple *LINC01133* isoforms in 12Z cells that differ from the annotated GENCODE and Refseq transcripts. (**C**) Left: Hierarchical clustering of differentially expressed genes from RNA sequencing biological replicates shows that the control and *LINC01133a* siRNA samples cluster separately. Right: Hundreds of genes are up- or down-regulated in the *LINC01133a* knockdown in 12Z cells.

2.3. The Knockdown of LINC01133 in 12Z Cells Effects Genes and Pathways with a Known Function in Endometriosis Lesion Formation

To gain insight into the function of the genes being regulated by *LINC01133*, we carried out gene ontology enrichment analysis (GOEA) (http://bioinformatics.sdstate.edu/go/) (accessed on 2 December 2020) [26] and gene set enrichment analysis (GSEA) (http://www.gsea-msigdb.org/gsea) (accessed on 2 December 2020) [27,28]. The GOEA showed enrichment in genes that control cell proliferation, migration and angiogenesis (Figure S2A and Table S5), all processes to be involved in the pathogenesis of the disease. GSEA enrichment in targets of the mammalian histone methyltransferase EZH2, adult tissue stem cells and mesenchymal cells (Figure S2B and Table S6), Together these results suggest that *LINC01133* may be involved in the regulation of epithelial cell proliferation, invasion and cell fate conversion (EMT), processes that are known to support ectopic lesion growth.

2.4. LINC01133 Regulates Proliferation and Invasion of Endometriosis Epithelial Cells In Vitro

To determine if the phenotypic changes predicted by GOEA and GSEA analysis following *LINC01133* knockdown in 12Z cells occur, we evaluated changes in cell proliferation and invasion in 12Z cells 72 h post knockdown. The results showed that *LINC01133* knockdown leads to a slight, but significant downregulation of 12Z proliferation (Figure 3A) and significantly enhances the invasion phenotype of knockdown cells (Figure 3B). The relative proliferation rate of *LINC01133* knockdown cells was 30% lower (adjp < 0.0001), and the invasion rate was 1.5 times higher (adjp < 0.05) when compared to cells transfected with the siRNA control oligo.

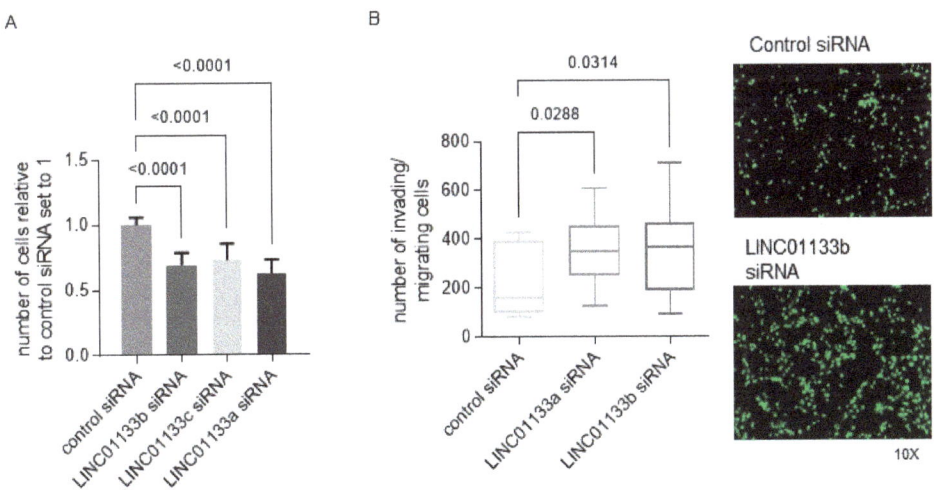

Figure 3. *LINC01133* knockdown reduces proliferation and increases invasion of 12Z endometriosis epithelial cells.

(**A**) Relative number of proliferating cells is significantly reduced in *LINC01133* knockdowns using 3 different siRNA oligos. Data are presented as bar plots of mean values from three biological replicates +SD. (**B**) Invading cells are significantly increased following *LINC01133* knockdown using 2 different siRNA oligos. Left: Quantification of the number of invading cells after *LINC01133* knockdown analyzed by the trans-well method. Right: Representative images of control and knockdown cells at 10× magnification stained with CyQuant fluorescence dye (green), which shows fluorescence enrichment when bound to cellular nucleic acids. Data are presented as a box plot ranging from minimum to maximum, including the median and box boundaries at the 25th and 75th percentiles from three biological replicates. Six independent fields were counted and the mean values taken for analysis. Statistical analysis of the data between the groups in A and B was done using Kruskal–Wallis ANOVA test with Dunn's test for multiple comparison. Adjp < 0.05 were considered significant.

2.5. LINC01133 Regulates Cell Cycle and the Levels of Expression of Cell Cycle Regulatory Proteins p21 and Cyclin A

We further examined the viability of 12Z cells following *LINC01133* knockdown using an AnnexinV/Propidium Iodide FACS assay. We found that *LINC01133* knockdown did not influence the survival of the cells (Figure 4A). The mean percent of early apoptotic AnnexinV positive cells was about 25% for both cells transfected with a control or *LINC01133a* oligo. Analysis of the DNA profiles of the *LINC01133* siRNA transfected cells showed a slight but significant enrichment of the number of cells in the G1 phase (7%, adjp < 0.005), and a concomitant down-regulation of the number of cells entering S-phase of the cell cycle (5%, adjp < 0.05), compared to control siRNA transfected cells (Figure 4B). This effect on cell cycle in knockdown cells was associated with significant up-regulation of the levels of expression of the cell cycle checkpoint regulatory protein p21 (~2.5-fold, adjp < 0.005) and down-regulation of Cyclin A (~2-fold, adjp < 0.05) (Figure 4C), compared to control oligo transfected cells. These findings were consistent with the results of our RNA-seq (see Table S4), further indicating that changes in expression of these genes may be responsible for the cell cycle phenotype.

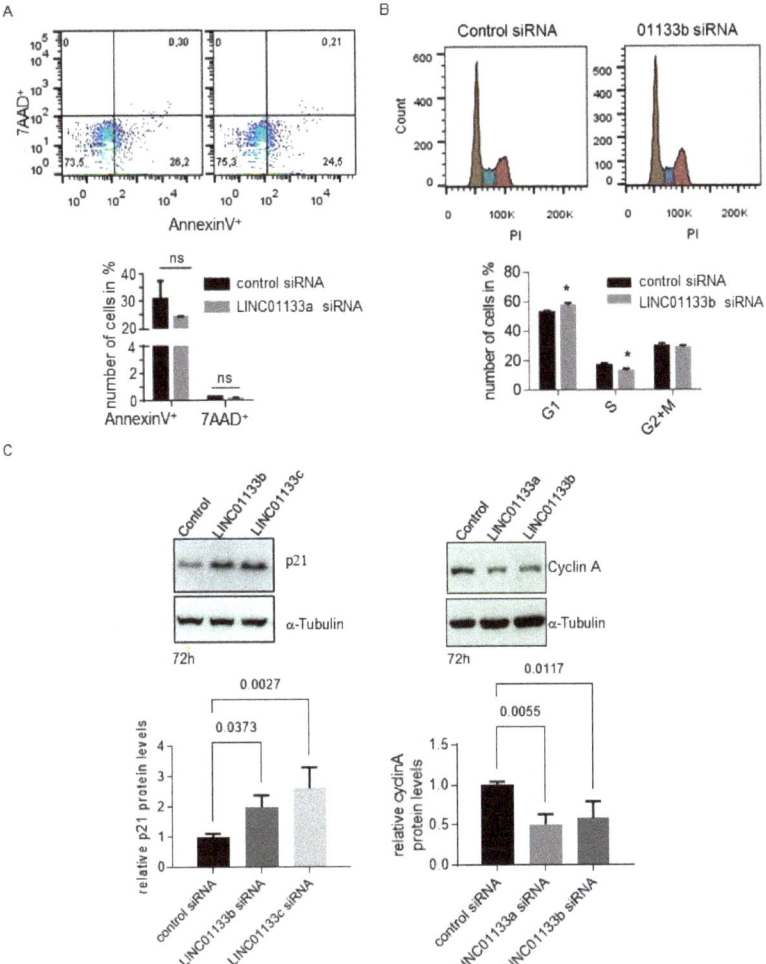

Figure 4. *LINC01133* knockdown leads to an increase in cells in the G1 phase and a decrease in cells in the S phase associated with an increase in p21 and a decrease in Cyclin A levels. (**A**) No significant changes in the number of apoptotic cells are seen 72 h after *LINC01133* knockdown. Top: Representative flow cytometry scatter plots for AnnexinV+ versus 7-AAD+ cells. Bottom: No significant change in the number of AnnexinV+ or 7AAD+ cells was observed between *LINC01133a* knockdown and control siRNA transfected cells. Mean values + SD of three biological replicates are shown. (**B**) *LINC01133* knockdown leads to an increase in cells in the G1 phase and a decrease in cells in the S phase. Top: Representative DNA profiles obtained from flow cytometry analysis of PI stained 12Z cells 72 h after transfection with *LINC01133b* siRNA or control siRNA (brown G1 peak, blue S phase, purple G2 + M). Bottom: The percentage of cells in each cell cycle phase are plotted as mean + SD of three independent experiments. Statistically significant differences between the groups in A and B are indicated with a star on the top of each panel. *—adjp < 0.05 (two-way ANOVA test with Sidak's for multiple comparison), ns-not significant. (**C**) p21 protein is significantly upregulated and Cyclin A protein significantly down-regulated following *LINC01133* knockdown. Top: Representative examples of Western blot analysis following *LINC01133* knockdown of p21 (left) and Cyclin A (right) together with the α-tubulin loading control. Bottom: Densitometric analysis of p21 (left) and cyclin A (right) levels from Western blots normalized to the α-tubulin loading control. Data are displayed as bar graphs with the level from the control siRNA set to 1, and mean and + SD of biological triplicates shown. Statistically significant differences between the groups are indicated with adj *p*-values on the top of each graph (ANOVA, with Dunnett's multiple comparison test).

2.6. LINC01133 Is Not a Regulator of EMT in 12Z Endometriosis Epithelial Cells

The enrichment of differentially expressed genes associated with a mesenchymal phenotype (Figure S2, Table S6A,B) and an increased invasion of 12Z cells following *LINC01133* knockdown (Figure 3B) indicated that these cells may be converted to a more mesenchymal phenotype. To evaluate the role of *LINC01133* in epithelial to mesenchymal transition (EMT) in endometriosis, we further investigated expression of selected EMT regulatory proteins indicated to be differentially expressed in our RNA-seq data (Table S7). qRT-PCR and Western blot analysis confirmed the loss of CDH1 (E-cadherin) following *LINC01133* knockdown (Figure S3A). The levels of *CDH1* transcription correlated with the efficiency of the *LINC01133* knockdown in 12Z cells (Figure 2A, Figure S3A left panel), further supporting the involvement of *LINC01133* in its regulation. Specifically, a knockdown of *LINC01133* to about 10% of the levels of controls (*LINC01133a* siRNA, adjp < 0.0001), led to reduction of the relative levels of *CDH1* expression to 20% of the controls (adjp < 0.0001), whereas *LINC01133* knockdown to 35% (*LINC01133b* siRNA, adjp < 0.0001) led to a 30% reduction of *CDH1* transcript ($p = 0.007$) compared to controls. However, we did not see a classical EMT-associated Cadherin switch in *LINC01133* knockdown cells. The levels of *CDH2* (*N-cadherin*) transcript were downregulated to 53% of normal level in cells with high efficiency of *LINC01133* knockdown (*LINC01133a* oligo, adjp = 0.002), but were not changed in cells with a less efficient knockdown of *LINC01133* (*LINC01133b* siRNA oligo, adjp > 0.05) (Figure S3A, left panel). Further, we validated the significant downregulation of VCAM-1 ($p = 0.029$, Figure S3B), and significant upregulation of *SOX4* ($p = 0.02$, Figure S3C) and *TGFβ2* ($p = 0.0014$, Figure S3D) in *LINC01133* knockdown cells compared to controls for both the *LINC01133a* and *LINC01133b* oligos. However, we could not validate the reduction of *KRT7* and *KRT19* (Figure S3E,F) in cells with *LINC01133* knockdown, when compared to siRNA controls. Given that we did not see a classic E-cadherin to N-cadherin switch, and that expression changes for some EMT markers could not be validated, these data suggest that *LINC01133* does not play a significant role in regulating EMT in endometriosis epithelial cells.

2.7. Active Cytoskeleton Remodeling in 12Z Cells Following LINC01133 Knockdown

LINC01133 knockdown led to the deregulation of genes involved in cell adhesion and EMT, and was associated with changes in the cellular phenotype of 12Z knockdown cells, which appeared to have a more flattened, larger phenotype with an increased number of actin stress fibers (Figure 5A). This was supported by analysis of cell area and fluorescence intensity in *LINC01133* knockdown cells compared to controls. We confirmed that the cross-sectional cellular area of *LINC01133* knockdown cells was greater, with knockdown cells 1.7 fold the size of control siRNA treated cells (adjp = 0.006, Figure S4A). Further, analysis of Phalloidin fluorescence intensity showed that *LINC01133* knockdown cells had 4.5-fold higher corrected total cell fluorescence (CTCF) than cells transfected with control siRNA oligo ($p < 0.0001$) (Figure S4B). This data indicated that active actin remodeling may occur following *LINC01133* knockdown. Therefore, we further evaluated the expression and/or activity of some proteins involved in the regulation of actin filaments, stress fibers formation and focal adhesions such as TESK1 and Cofilin. TESK1 phosphorylates and thereby inactivates the Actin severing protein Cofilin at Ser3, thus regulating the organization of the Actin cytoskeleton [29]. We identified *TESK1* as being differentially expressed in 12Z knockdown cells by RNA-seq (Table S4) and confirmed that the protein was significantly increased following *LINC01133* knockdown (1.5-times higher, adjp < 0.05) (Figure 5B). These changes in TESK1 expression were associated with a significant increase in Cofilin phosphorylation to 2.2-fold higher (adjp < 0.05) following *LINC01133* knockdown (Figure 5C). Together this data indicates that *LINC01133* may regulate actin remodeling in endometriosis epithelial cells via this pathway.

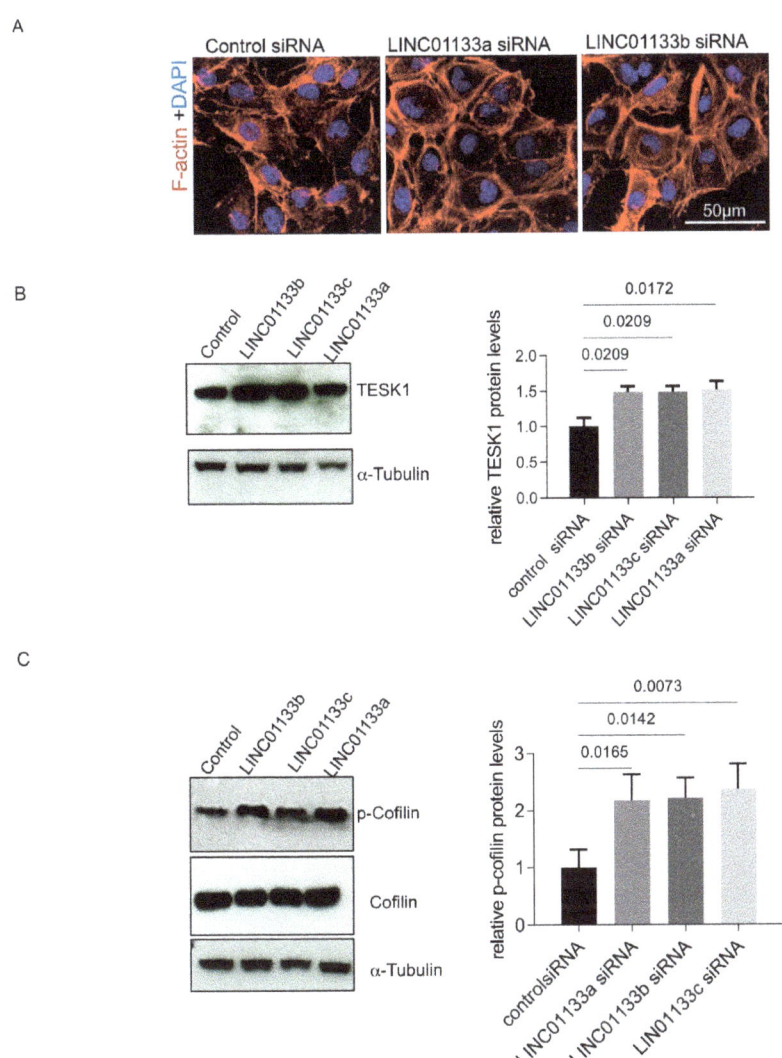

Figure 5. *LINC01133* knockdown affects cellular morphology of 12Z cells (**A**) Immunofluorescence of F-actin 72 h after transfection with siRNA control and 2 different *LINC01133* oligos shows a more flattened phenotype and an increase in the number of actin stress fibers. Representative confocal images are shown (three independent experiments were analyzed). Cell nuclei were visualized with DAPI. The magnification scale of 50 µm is indicated with white line on the figure. (**B**) *LINC01133* knockdown leads to upregulation of the levels of TESK1 protein. Left: Representative Western blot showing TESK1 levels together with the α-tubulin loading control. Right: TESK1 relative protein levels normalized to α-tubulin determined by densitometric analysis of Western blots. The relative levels of TESK1 from three independent experiments are shown as bar graphs with the control set to 1 and the mean and + SD of protein shown (**C**) *LINC01133* knockdown increases the levels of Cofilin phosphorylation. Left: Representative example of *p*-Cofilin and Cofilin levels detected by Western blot with α-tubulin loading control. Right: Phosphorylated Cofilin relative levels normalized to α-tubulin determined by densitometric analysis of Western blots. The relative levels of phosphorylated Cofilin from three independent experiments are shown as bar graphs with the control set to 1, and the mean and +SD of protein shown. Statistically significant differences between the groups are indicated by adj *p*-values on the top of each graph (ANOVA, with Dunnett's multiple comparison test).

3. Discussion

LncRNAs are epigenetic regulators that have been implicated in development and disease, but whose role in the pathogenesis of endometriosis remains relatively unknown. Endometriosis shares some features with cancer, including EMT, therefore we chose to investigate the role of *LINC01133* in endometriosis, a well-characterized lncRNA that has been associated with EMT in cervical [21], breast [22], colorectal [23] and gastric [24] cancer. We found that *LINC01133* is significantly upregulated in ectopic endometriosis lesions, and that knockdown in an epithelial endometriosis cell line indicates that it promotes cell proliferation and suppresses cell migration and invasion in endometriosis, but that it does not regulate EMT in this disease. Our results indicate that *LINC01133* affects cell proliferation by affecting the cell cycle via the p21/cyclin pathway, and cellular invasion and cytoskeleton remodeling due to Cofilin phosphorylation and inactivation by the TESK1 kinase. A caveat of our study is that we used the immortalized endometriosis epithelial cell line 12Z for our functional experiments, although this cell line is widely accepted in the field as a cell model of endometriosis [30].

The effects on cell proliferation were associated with cell cycle arrest in G1 and impaired S-phase entry due to significant up-regulation of cell cycle checkpoint protein p21 and concomitant downregulation of Cyclin A. The mechanism by which *LINC01133* may regulate these genes in endometriosis remains unclear. In non-small cell lung carcinoma *LINC01133* suppresses the transcription of *CDKN1A (p21)* via a direct EZH2-mediated chromatin remodeling mechanism [31]. In another context, *LINC01133* promotes the progression of cervical cancer by sponging miR-4784 to cause the up-regulation of AT-hook DNA-binding motif-containing protein 1 (AHDC1) promoting EMT [21]. The high basal level of p21 expression and moderate transcriptional activation upon *LINC01133* knockdown (~2.5-fold) indicates that sponging rather than an EZH2 mediated p21 activation may be a more likely mechanism of regulation, although this remains to be tested.

Impaired expression of *LINC01133* has been associated with the regulation of EMT in cancer [23,31,32]. EMT is a multi-stage process leading to the gradual remodeling of the epithelial into a mesenchymal phenotype. This includes the loss of epithelial markers and concomitant acquisition of mesenchymal markers, an increase in cell migration and invasion, disruption of cell-cell contacts, impaired adhesion and the remodeling of the cytoskeleton [19]. This molecular remodeling also takes place during the establishment of endometriosis lesions [17]. However, although we saw an enrichment of some mesenchymal gene sets among differentially expressed genes in 12Z endometriosis epithelial cells following *LINC01133* knockdown, we found little phenotypic evidence for EMT. Our data showed a significant upregulation of *TGFβ2* following *LINC01133* knockdown is associated with an increase in the levels of expression of the master regulator of EMT, *SOX4* [33,34] and subsequent down-regulation of *CDH1* and *CDH2*. However, expression of the epithelial markers *KDR7* and *KDR19* [35], along with the EMT regulators *TWIST*, *SNAIL*, *ZEB1* and *ZEB2* [36] were not significantly affected by *LINC01133* knockdown. CDH1 is a tumor suppressor and cell polarity regulator [37] and the loss of CDH1 promotes motility and invasion. There is also some evidence that in endometriosis lesions the loss of CDH2 expression may be associated with increased invasive capacity of endometrial epithelial cells. Matsuzaki et al. [38] have shown that deep infiltrating endometriosis lesions express less CDH2, compared to early peritoneal lesions. In normal endometrial tissue high levels of CDH2 were associated with the proliferative phase of the cycle [39]. However, whether activation of CDH2 by *LINC01133* is responsible for the loss of proliferation capacity and increased invasiveness of endometriosis epithelial cells needs to be tested.

Recently, we have shown that the levels of expression of *VCAM-1* are increased in tissue samples of women with endometriosis, compared to women without the disease [40]. The loss of *VCAM-1* was shown to attenuate the TGF-β1 induced proliferation, migration and invasion of endometriosis stroma cells derived from ovarian endometriomas [41]. Our data showed that the function of the protein as a regulator of cell invasion of epithelial endometriosis cells might differ from those in stroma, while downregulation of *VCAM-1* following *LINC01133* knockdown was associated with an increase of cellular invasion. As up-regulation of *VCAM-1* in malignant cells is associated with recruitment of tumor-associated monocytes and macrophages and immune escape of the tumors [42,43], we postulate that *LINC01133* dependent *VCAM-1* regulation in endometriosis epithelial cells may be related to immune surveillance of the lesions.

A central event in cellular invasion is the dynamic cytoskeleton remodeling leading to changes in cellular morphology. We [44] and others [45,46] have shown that the dysregulation of cytoskeleton dynamics and related signaling pathways are linked to pathogenesis of endometriosis and disease-associated infertility. Actin filaments, microtubules, and intermediate filaments involved in the formation of cytoskeletal structures, such as stress fibers and pseudopodia promote the invasion of normal cells and invasion and metastasis of tumor cells. Here we showed that the increase in the invasion capacity of 12Z cell under *LINC01133* knockdown is associated with changes in cellular morphology to more flattened and larger phenotype with an increased number of stress fibers, provoked by the activation of TESK1 expression and inactivation of Cofilin. TESK1 is a serine/threonine kinase with kinase domain similar to those of LIM-kinases and a unique C-terminal proline-rich domain [47] known to phosphorylate Cofilin at Ser-3 [29]. Cofilin plays an essential role in actin filament dynamics by enhancing depolymerization and severance of actin filaments [48]. These activities of Cofilin are abolished by phosphorylation at Ser-3. Therefore, the changes in Cofilin phosphorylation at Ser-3 are regarded as one of the most important mechanisms for regulating Cofilin activity and actin filament dynamics. It has been shown that induction of stress fibers require an active Rho-ROCK signaling pathway independent of TESK1 [29]. Several studies also indicate that the balance between Rho and Rac activity in cells determines the patterns of actin organization, cell morphology and motility [49]. Thus, the effects of *LINC01133* on the cellular filament and cytoskeleton dynamics may not be restricted only to the TESK1/Cofilin pathway.

Overall, in this study, we found that *LINC01133* is overexpressed in ectopic endometriosis lesions compared to the eutopic endometrium of women both with and without the disease. By knocking down *LINC01133* in endometriosis epithelial cells we were able to show that the lncRNA promotes cellular proliferation and inhibits cell invasion in these cells, and to identify components of these pathways that were affected, including p21, Cyclin A and TESK. These results indicate that *LINC01133* may be a clinically relevant player in endometriosis, although this remains to be tested in vivo.

4. Materials and Methods

4.1. Study Population

For this study, tissue samples were collected in accordance with the protocols of the Endometriosis Marker Austria (EMMA) study, a prospective cohort study conducted at the Tertiary Endometriosis Referral Center of the Medical University of Vienna. Premenopausal women 18–50 years of age undergoing a laparoscopic procedure due to suspected endometriosis, infertility, chronic pelvic pain, benign adnexal masses or uterine leiomyoma were invited to participate in the EMMA study. Women who had acute inflammation, known or suspected infectious disease, chronic autoimmune disease or malignancy were excluded from the study. Ethics approval for this study was provided by the institutional ethics committee of the Medical University of Vienna (EK 545/2010). Verbal and written informed consent was obtained from each participant prior to inclusion into the study. The detailed baseline characteristics of the participants are summarized in Table S1. Briefly, from a total number of $n = 95$ participating women, $n = 42$ were defined as controls and $n = 53$ were patients suffering from endometriosis. The control group consisted of women undergoing laparoscopy for uterine fibroids, benign ovarian cysts, fallopian tube disorders or diagnostic laparoscopy due to unexplained infertility or chronic pelvic pain. Each participating woman contributed only one sample of eutopic endometrium and some of the women with endometriosis contributed samples of diverse types of endometriotic lesions. All tissue samples were collected during laparoscopic surgical intervention for diagnosis and/or therapy of endometriosis. All samples were collected in accordance to Endometriosis Phenome and Biobanking Harmonization Project guidelines [50].

4.2. Cell Line for In Vitro Evaluation of LINC01133 Function

Endometriotic epithelial cell line 12Z established and characterized by the laboratory of Professor Starzinski-Powitz [51,52] was kindly provided for our in vitro studies. The cells were cultured in Dulbecco's modified Eagle's medium (DMEM-F12) containing penicillin/streptomycin in final concentrations of 50 U/mL and 50 µg/mL, respectively and 10% v/v fetal calf serum (FCS). The cells were maintained in a 37 °C CO_2-humified incubator. Cells were tested and found to be negative for mycoplasm infection. All cell culture reagents were purchased from Thermo Fisher Scientific (Waltham, MA, USA) or Sarstedt (Nümbrecht, Germany).

4.3. RNA-Scope

To visualize the subcellular localization of *LINC01133* RNA in tissue samples of women with endometriosis we used the RNAscope® 2.5 HD Red assay on formalin-fixed paraffin-embedded eutopic endometrial tissues of women with endometriosis ($n = 5$), according to the manufacturer's protocol (Advanced Cell Diagnostics (ACD), Hayward, CA, USA). This method uses a signal amplification method and double Z probe design provides high sensitivity and specificity suitable for detecting relatively lowly expressed RNAs, such as lncRNAs. The system visualizes target RNA as a single dot, where each dot is an amplified signal of an individual RNA molecule. We used the probe Hs-LINC01133 designed by ACD to specifically detect *LINC01133*, and probe dapB (bacterial dihydrodipicolinate reductase, PN310043) as a negative control.

4.4. LINC01133 Knockdown

The 12Z cells were seeded in complete culture cell medium 12 h prior to transfection on 6-well culture plates (Nunc, Thermo Fisher Scientific, Waltham, MA, USA) at a concentration of 1×10^5 cells/well and allowed to grow to approximately 40% confluency. The cells were then transfected with one of three different LINC0133 targeting siRNA oligos at a final concentration of 10 nM (Table S2A) or a non-targeting control siRNA oligo (Cat.4390846, Ambion, Austin, Texas, USA) using Lipofectamine RNAiMAX transfection reagent according to the manufacturer's protocol (Invitrogen by Life Technology, Waltham, MA, USA). Phenotypic analysis of *LINC01133* knockdown cells for changes in cellular proliferation and invasion/migration was conducted 48 h post-transfection. RNA-sequencing, qRT-PCR and Western blot analysis were conducted 72 h post-transfection. The 3 siRNAs had similar *LINC01133* knockdown efficiencies (Figure 2A). Therefore, for each experiment, we first checked *LINC01133* knockdown efficiency by qRT-PCR, and then proceeded with the 2 siRNAs that showed the greatest knockdown efficiency.

4.5. RNA Isolation

Frozen tissue samples were homogenized with a Precellys 24 homogenizer (PEQLAB, Erlangen, Germany). Subsequently, total RNA was isolated from eutopic and ectopic endometrium using the Agilent Absolutely RNA kit in accordance with the manufacturer's instructions (DNase I treatment included), and total RNA from the 12Z cell line was isolated using the RNeasy mini kit (Qiagen). To remove DNA contamination the RNA samples were subsequently treated with DNAseI using RapidOut DNA removal Kit (Thermo Fisher Scientific, Waltham, MA, USA). RNA concentration and purity were determined by measuring optical density using a NanoDrop ND-1000 spectrophotometer (NanoDrop Technologies, Wilmington, DE, USA). We defined the quality of the RNA samples to be sufficient when the ratios of OD260/280 and OD260/230 were around 2.00. Additionally, for RNA-sequencing we confirmed that RNA integrity was RIN > 7 on a Bio Analyzer (Agilent Technologies, Santa Clara, CA, USA).

4.6. RNA-Sequencing and Data Analysis

RNA sequencing was performed by the Next Generation Sequencing Facility at Vienna BioCenter Core Facilities (VBCF), a member of the Vienna BioCenter (VBC), Austria. From the total RNA, we provided they conducted poly-A enrichment for mRNAs and prepared libraries using the Illumina TruSeq RNA kit. The six libraries (3 control oligo, 3 *LINC01133* knock-down) were multiplexed on a single lane and subjected to 125 bp paired-end sequencing on an Illumina HiSeq2500 machine. The facility provided de-multiplexed BAM files containing the raw reads, which we converted to fastq using Samtools (v1.10) for alignment with STAR using the parameters: –outFilterMultimapNmax 1 –outSAMstrandField intronMotif –outFilterIntronMotifs RemoveNoncanonical –outSAMtype BAM SortedByCoordinate –quantMode GeneCounts. On average 38M reads (94% of all reads) mapped uniquely to the human genome (Table S2B). Annotation files and genome sequences were downloaded from https://www.gencodegenes.org (accessed on 2 December 2020). Index for alignments was prepared using STAR (2.7.6a_patch_2020-11-17) [53] with FASTA files from the GRCh38.p13 assembly and Gencode (v36) gene annotation in GTF format.

Differential gene expression analysis was performed in the R statistical computing environment (v4.0.3) [54] using the DESeq2 package (v1.30.0) [55] with count tables produced by STAR during alignment (*ReadsPerGene.out.tab files).

4.7. Assembly of LINC01133 Isoforms Expressed in the 12Z Cell Line

Aligned reads from the genomic positions chr1:159955239-15998963, were extracted using Samtools for all downstream analyses [56]. For that region, read coverage was calculated using bam2wig (v4.0.0) (https://github.com/MikeAxtell/bam2wig) accessed on 3 December 2020. Read coverage at each informative genomic position was normalized for sequencing depth and averaged over all control siRNA transfected and knock-down *LINC01133a* siRNA samples. Transcript assembly was performed using Cufflinks (v2.2.1) [57] with the parameter: -F 0.05. Note that for transcript assembly only the control siRNA samples were used and the resulting GTF files were merged using Cuffmerge to obtain the final *LINC01133* annotation.

4.8. Gene Set Enrichment Analysis (GSEA) and Gene Ontology Enrichment Analysis (GOEA)

To test whether the differentially expressed genes identified by our cutoff criteria (fold change > 1.5, adjusted *p*-value (adjp) < 0.05) are associated with specific biological functions we performed gene ontology enrichment analysis (GOEA http://bioinformatics.sdstate.edu/go/) (accessed on 25 November 2020) [26] and gene set enrichment analysis (GSEA, Broad Institute http://www.gsea-msigdb.org/gsea) [27] accessed on 26 December 2020) [28]. For GOEA annotation Fisher's exact test is used to determine if different annotation terms are enriched among the differentially expressed genes. Gene ontology (GO) terms showing a Fisher's exact *p*-value < 0.05 were considered significantly enriched. To calculate GSEA we used the Molecular Signature Database (MSigDB) to investigate the overlap between our gene lists and known annotated gene sets. Gene sets showing a false discovery rate (FDR) <0.05 were considered as significantly enriched among differentially expressed genes. We considered the biological processes associated with significantly enriched GO terms or MSigDB gene sets as being potentially relevant for endometriosis.

4.9. Quantitative Reverse Transcription PCR (qRT-PCR) for Measuring mRNA Expression

Total RNA was reverse transcribed with SuperScript® III First-Strand Synthesis Reverse Transcriptase using a mixture of oligo-d (T) and random hexamer primers (Life Sciences Advance Technology, St. Petersburg, FL, USA). These cDNA preparations were then diluted 2 fold with water before being assayed. qRT-PCR was performed in triplicate in 96-well optical plates with 6 biological replicates. Each reaction contained 1X TaqMan PCR master mix (Applied Biosystems, Waltham, MA, USA with ROX reference dye) and 0.2 µM of each specific primer pair-probe set listed in Table S3. qRT-PCR was performed using a 7500 Fast Real-Time PCR System (Applied Biosystems, Waltham, MA, USA), with an initial denaturation for 10 minutes at 95 °C, primer annealing at 50 °C for 2 min, followed by 40 cycles of 15 seconds at 95 °C and 1 minute at 60 °C. The relative expression of target genes was calculated using the delta-CT method as described [58], and normalized to *GAPDH* expression. The average Ct values were ≤ 30 except for *SOX4* transcripts that showed an average Ct-value of 35 cycles.

4.10. Protein Isolation and Western Blot

Cells for Western Blot analysis were harvested and lysed in a whole-cell lysis buffer composed of 1% Triton-X 100, 10 mM Tris-HCl, pH7.4, 150 mM NaCl and 5 mM EDTA. Prior to use, the lysis buffer was supplemented with phosphatase and protease inhibitor cocktail (phosStop, cOmplete mini, EDTA free, Thermo Fisher Scientific, Waltham, MA, USA). The protein concentration was determined by the standard Bradford assay. The normalized samples were immunoblotted as previously described [59] and incubated with primary antibodies for the proteins of interest (Table S3). The secondary antibodies were diluted in a Tris pH 8.0, 0.1% Tween 20 buffer and incubated for 1 h at room temperature. Bound antibodies were detected by the horseradish peroxidase chemiluminescent substrate Luminata^{TM} (Millipore Corporation, Burlington, MA, USA). X-ray films (GE Healthcare, Frankfurt am Main, Germany) were used for chemiluminescence detection. The levels of protein expression on the blot were quantified using ImageJ Software (http://rsbweb.nih.gov/ij) (accessed on 15 March 2021).

4.11. Analysis of Cell Cycle and Cell Death Using Fluorescence-Activated Cell Scanning (FACS) Flow Cytometry

For FACS based analysis of the cell cycle changes upon *LINC01133* knockdown, we used standard propidium iodide (PI) DNA staining protocol. In brief, transfected cells were harvested 72 h after siRNA knockdown and 1×10^6 cells were fixed in 70% precooled ethanol for 2 h on ice. After washing with PBS (Thermo Fisher Scientific, Waltham, MA, USA) the cells were re-suspended in 0.5 mL PI/RNAse containing staining buffer (550825), BD Pharminogen™, Heidelberg, Germany) supplemented with 10 µL PI staining solution (51-6621-1E, BD Pharmingen™, Heidelberg, Germany). After incubation for 15 minutes at room temperature, the number of PI positive cells was measured by flow cytometry. The effect of *LINC01133* on cellular apoptotic rate was evaluated using staining with AnnexinV (FITC-conjugated antibody (640906), BioLegend, San Diego, CA, USA; Annexin V Binding Buffer, (422201), BioLegend, San Diego, CA, USA) in conjunction with the vital dye 7-amino-actomycin D (00-6993-50) eBioscience, San Diego, CA, USA) followed by flow cytometry measurement. A total of 1×10^6 cells 72 h after transfection was used in the analysis, with a total of 10,000 events recorded for each sample, and unstained cells being used as assay control.

4.12. Proliferation Assay

The proliferation rate of 12Z cells 72 h after LINC01133 knockdown was analyzed using the CyQuant direct cell proliferation Assay (Invitrogen, Waltham, MA, USA) according to the manufacture's protocol. Prior to the assay, transfected cells were trypsinized 48 h after transfection with targeting and control siRNA oligos, seeded on 96 flat-bottom cell culture plates (Thermo Fisher Scientific, Roskilde, Denmark) at a concentration of 15,000 cells/well and allowed to grow for an additional 12 h. The level of fluorescence was accessed with the Clariostar^{plus} microplate reader (BMG Labtech, Ortenberg, Germany) with filters appropriate for 480 nm excitation and 520 nm emission maxima. The observed fluorescence values were first corrected for the background fluorescence determined with a cell- free sample, and a standard curve was used to estimate cell number. All measurements were performed in technical triplicates, and the average number of proliferating cells relative to control siRNA-treated cells was set to 1.

4.13. Matrigel-Invasion Assay

The ability of cells to migrate or invade through a Matrigel barrier was measured in a Boyden chamber assay with polycarbonate membranes. After 48 h of siRNA knockdown, an equal number of 12Z cells (2×10^4) were re-suspended in 100 µL of growing media supplemented with 1% v/v FCS and antibiotics and plated on top of matrigel coated filter (Corning Matrigel growth factor reduced (354230); Corning Incorporated, Corning, NY, USA, 1% matrigel solution in PBS, filter: 6.5 mm diameter, 8 µm-pores, Corning Incorporated, Corning, NY, USA). The cells were allowed to migrate/invade for 12 h toward the bottom of the well, which contained media supplemented with 10% FCS. Cells on the lower surface of the filter were fixed with 4% PFA and stained with CyQUANT™ Direct Red nucleic acid stain (Invitrogen, Thermo Fisher Scientific, Waltham, MA, USA) and photographed with an ×10 objective under the microscope. The values for invasion were taken as the average number of invaded cells per photographic field over five independent fields per experiment and expressed as averages of triplicate experiments.

4.14. Immunofluorescence, Cell Size and Stress Fiber Analysis

12Z cells were seeded in 6-well plates and subject to siRNA knockdown for a non-targeting control, *LINC01133a* and *LINC01133b* oligos, as described above. The cells were trypsinized 48 h after transfection, 20,000 cells from each treatment re-plated on 8-well chamber slides, and then 24 h later the cells were fixed and processed for immunofluorescence as previously described [60]. Cells were stained for F-actin (Rhodamine conjugated Phalloidin, Invitrogen Cat. R415) and counterstained for DAPI. Cells were then imaged with a Leica SP8 confocal microscope using an ×63 glycerol objective and images processed using ImageJ.

We measured cell area in ImageJ using a previously described protocol (https://www.youtube.com/watch?v=IeicxaeMUwA) (accessed on 15 March 2021). First, we used the line tool to draw a line over a scale bar on one image and selected "measure" under the analyze menu. Next, we selected "set scale" under the analyze menu, and entered the number of pixels for 20 µM, a known distance of 20, and µM as the unit of length, and ticked the "Global" box so that this scale would be applied to all images. To measure the cross-sectional area of cells we chose the free-hand selection tool, mapped the outline of the first cells with the computer mouse, and pressed "measure" under the analyze menu. We then repeated this for all cells in each image.

We used ImageJ to measure fluorescence intensity in control and *LINC01133a* knockdown cells followed an established technique https://theolb.readthedocs.io/en/latest/imaging/measuring-cell-fluorescence-using-imagej.html (accessed on 15 March 2021) [61]. Briefly, we used drawing tools to select cells, chose "area integrated intensity" and "mean grey value" in the "set measurements" menu, and then "measure" from the analyze menu. We then measured an area near the cell with no fluorescence as a background control. We then repeated this process until all cells in the field had been measured. We then calculated the corrected total cell fluorescence (CTCF) for each cell in each image using the following formula (Equation (1)):

$$\text{CTCF} = \text{Integrated Density} - (\text{area of selected cell} \times \text{mean fluorescence background}) \quad (1)$$

4.15. Statistics

All statistical tests were performed using SPSS version 27.0 (IBM, SPSS statistics 27.0, Armonk, NY, USA: IBM Corp.) for patient cohort characterization and Prism (GraphPad Prism 9.0 software, La Jolla, CA, USA) for the remaining experimental settings. The exact statistical procedures for each analysis are described in the corresponding figure legends.

4.16. Websites and Software

The following websites were used for analysis and to download software for this study: http://bioinformatics.sdstate.edu/go/, http://www.gsea-msigdb.org/gsea, https://www.gencodegenes.org, https://github.com/MikeAxtell/bam2wig, https://www.R-project.org/ (accessed on 25 November 2020).

Supplementary Materials: The following are available online at https://www.mdpi.com/article/10.3390/ijms22168385/s1.

Author Contributions: Conceptualization, I.Y. and Q.J.H.; Methodology, I.Y., Q.J.H., F.M.P. and I.H.; Resources, L.K., A.P., H.H. and R.W.; Formal Analysis, I.Y., Q.J.H. and F.M.P.; Data Curation, Q.J.H., F.M.P., K.P., L.K., A.P., H.H. and R.W.; Writing—Original Draft Preparation, I.Y. and Q.J.H.; Writing—Review & Editing, F.M.P., K.P., L.K., A.P., H.H. and R.W.; Visualization, I.Y., Q.J.H., F.M.P. and K.P.; Supervision and Project Administration, I.Y.; Funding Acquisition, H.H. and R.W. All authors have read and agreed to the published version of the manuscript.

Funding: This research received no external funding.

Institutional Review Board Statement: The study was conducted according to the guidelines of the Declaration of Helsinki, and approved by the Institutional Review Board (or Ethics Committee) of Medical University of Vienna (EK 545/2010, approved 9 February 2017).

Informed Consent Statement: Informed consent was obtained from all subjects involved in the study.

Data Availability Statement: RNA-sequencing data and processed files from this study are available from GEO database under the accession number GSE174741 (https://www.ncbi.nlm.nih.gov/geo/query/acc.cgi?acc=GSE174741) (accessed on 15 March 2021).

Acknowledgments: Open access funding provided by Medical University of Vienna. The authors would like to thank all the participants and health professionals involved in the present study. We want to thank our technical assistants Barbara Widmar and Matthias Witzmann-Stern for their diligent work and constant assistance. We would like to thank Simon Hippenmeyer for access to bioinformatic infrastructure and resources.

Conflicts of Interest: The authors declare no conflict of interest.

References

1. Zondervan, K.T.; Becker, C.M.; Missmer, S.A. Endometriosis. *N. Engl. J. Med.* **2020**, *382*, 1244–1256. [CrossRef] [PubMed]
2. Hogg, C.; Horne, A.W.; Greaves, E. Endometriosis-Associated Macrophages: Origin, Phenotype, and Function. *Front. Endocrinol.* **2020**, *11*, 7. [CrossRef]
3. Kapranov, P.; Cheng, J.; Dike, S.; Nix, D.A.; Duttagupta, R.; Willingham, A.T.; Stadler, P.F.; Hertel, J.; Hackermuller, J.; Hofacker, I.L.; et al. RNA maps reveal new RNA classes and a possible function for pervasive transcription. *Science* **2007**, *316*, 1484–1488. [CrossRef]
4. Frankish, A.; Diekhans, M.; Ferreira, A.M.; Johnson, R.; Jungreis, I.; Loveland, J.; Mudge, J.M.; Sisu, C.; Wright, J.; Armstrong, J.; et al. GENCODE reference annotation for the human and mouse genomes. *Nucleic Acids Res.* **2019**, *47*, D766–D773. [CrossRef]
5. Ponting, C.P.; Oliver, P.L.; Reik, W. Evolution and functions of long noncoding RNAs. *Cell* **2009**, *136*, 629–641. [CrossRef] [PubMed]
6. Wang, K.C.; Chang, H.Y. Molecular mechanisms of long noncoding RNAs. *Mol. Cell* **2011**, *43*, 904–914. [CrossRef] [PubMed]
7. Uszczynska-Ratajczak, B.; Lagarde, J.; Frankish, A.; Guigo, R.; Johnson, R. Towards a complete map of the human long non-coding RNA transcriptome. *Nat. Rev. Genet.* **2018**, *19*, 535–548. [CrossRef]
8. Statello, L.; Guo, C.J.; Chen, L.L.; Huarte, M. Gene regulation by long non-coding RNAs and its biological functions. *Nat. Rev. Mol. Cell Biol.* **2021**, *22*, 96–118. [CrossRef] [PubMed]
9. Geisler, S.; Coller, J. RNA in unexpected places: Long non-coding RNA functions in diverse cellular contexts. *Nat. Rev. Mol. Cell Biol.* **2013**, *14*, 699–712. [CrossRef] [PubMed]
10. Sun, P.R.; Jia, S.Z.; Lin, H.; Leng, J.H.; Lang, J.H. Genome-wide profiling of long noncoding ribonucleic acid expression patterns in ovarian endometriosis by microarray. *Fertil. Steril.* **2014**, *101*, 1038–1046 e7. [CrossRef]
11. Cai, H.; Zhu, X.; Li, Z.; Zhu, Y.; Lang, J. lncRNA/mRNA profiling of endometriosis rat uterine tissues during the implantation window. *Int. J. Mol. Med.* **2019**, *44*, 2145–2160. [CrossRef] [PubMed]

12. Li, Y.; Liu, Y.D.; Chen, S.L.; Chen, X.; Ye, D.S.; Zhou, X.Y.; Zhe, J.; Zhang, J. Down-regulation of long non-coding RNA MALAT1 inhibits granulosa cell proliferation in endometriosis by up-regulating P21 via activation of the ERK/MAPK pathway. *Mol. Hum. Reprod.* **2019**, *25*, 17–29. [CrossRef] [PubMed]
13. Liu, Y.; Ma, J.; Cui, D.; Fei, X.; Lv, Y.; Lin, J. LncRNA MEG3-210 regulates endometrial stromal cells migration, invasion and apoptosis through p38 MAPK and PKA/SERCA2 signalling via interaction with Galectin-1 in endometriosis. *Mol. Cell. Endocrinol.* **2020**, *513*, 110870. [CrossRef]
14. Zhang, C.; Wu, W.; Zhu, H.; Yu, X.; Zhang, Y.; Ye, X.; Cheng, H.; Ma, R.; Cui, H.; Luo, J.; et al. Knockdown of long noncoding RNA CCDC144NL-AS1 attenuates migration and invasion phenotypes in endometrial stromal cells from endometriosisdagger. *Biol. Reprod.* **2019**, *100*, 939–949. [CrossRef]
15. Qiu, J.J.; Lin, X.J.; Zheng, T.T.; Tang, X.Y.; Zhang, Y.; Hua, K.Q. The Exosomal Long Noncoding RNA aHIF is Upregulated in Serum From Patients With Endometriosis and Promotes Angiogenesis in Endometriosis. *Reprod. Sci.* **2019**, *26*, 1590–1602. [CrossRef]
16. Wang, X.; Zhang, J.; Liu, X.; Wei, B.; Zhan, L. Long noncoding RNAs in endometriosis: Biological functions, expressions, and mechanisms. *J. Cell. Physiol.* **2021**, *236*, 6–14. [CrossRef]
17. Proestling, K.; Birner, P.; Gamperl, S.; Nirtl, N.; Marton, E.; Yerlikaya, G.; Wenzl, R.; Streubel, B.; Husslein, H. Enhanced epithelial to mesenchymal transition (EMT) and upregulated MYC in ectopic lesions contribute independently to endometriosis. *Reprod. Biol. Endocrinol.* **2015**, *13*, 75. [CrossRef]
18. Zondervan, K.T.; Becker, C.M.; Koga, K.; Missmer, S.A.; Taylor, R.N.; Vigano, P. Endometriosis. *Nat. Rev. Dis. Primers* **2018**, *4*, 9. [CrossRef] [PubMed]
19. Konrad, L.; Dietze, R.; Riaz, M.A.; Scheiner-Bobis, G.; Behnke, J.; Horne, F.; Hoerscher, A.; Reising, C.; Meinhold-Heerlein, I. Epithelial-Mesenchymal Transition in Endometriosis-When Does It Happen? *J. Clin. Med.* **2020**, *9*, 1915. [CrossRef]
20. Yang, W.; Yue, Y.; Yin, F.; Qi, Z.; Guo, R.; Xu, Y. LINC01133 and LINC01243 are positively correlated with endometrial carcinoma pathogenesis. *Arch. Gynecol. Obstet.* **2021**, *303*, 207–215. [CrossRef] [PubMed]
21. Feng, Y.; Qu, L.; Wang, X.; Liu, C. LINC01133 promotes the progression of cervical cancer by sponging miR-4784 to up-regulate AHDC1. *Cancer Biol. Ther.* **2019**, *20*, 1453–1461. [CrossRef]
22. Song, Z.; Zhang, X.; Lin, Y.; Wei, Y.; Liang, S.; Dong, C. LINC01133 inhibits breast cancer invasion and metastasis by negatively regulating SOX4 expression through EZH2. *J. Cell Mol. Med.* **2019**, *23*, 7554–7565. [CrossRef] [PubMed]
23. Kong, J.; Sun, W.; Li, C.; Wan, L.; Wang, S.; Wu, Y.; Xu, E.; Zhang, H.; Lai, M. Long non-coding RNA LINC01133 inhibits epithelial-mesenchymal transition and metastasis in colorectal cancer by interacting with SRSF6. *Cancer Lett.* **2016**, *380*, 476–484. [CrossRef]
24. Yang, X.Z.; Cheng, T.T.; He, Q.J.; Lei, Z.Y.; Chi, J.; Tang, Z.; Liao, Q.X.; Zhang, H.; Zeng, L.S.; Cui, S.Z. LINC01133 as ceRNA inhibits gastric cancer progression by sponging miR-106a-3p to regulate APC expression and the Wnt/beta-catenin pathway. *Mol. Cancer* **2018**, *17*, 126. [CrossRef] [PubMed]
25. Yang, Y.-M.; Yang, W.-X. Epithelial-to-mesenchymal transition in the development of endometriosis. *Oncotarget* **2017**, *8*, 41679–41689. [CrossRef]
26. Ge, S.X.; Jung, D.; Yao, R. ShinyGO: A graphical gene-set enrichment tool for animals and plants. *Bioinformatics* **2020**, *36*, 2628–2629. [CrossRef] [PubMed]
27. Subramanian, A.; Tamayo, P.; Mootha, V.K.; Mukherjee, S.; Ebert, B.L.; Gillette, M.A.; Paulovich, A.; Pomeroy, S.L.; Golub, T.R.; Lander, E.S.; et al. Gene set enrichment analysis: A knowledge-based approach for interpreting genome-wide expression profiles. *Proc. Natl. Acad. Sci. USA* **2005**, *102*, 15545–15550. [CrossRef]
28. Mootha, V.K.; Lindgren, C.M.; Eriksson, K.F.; Subramanian, A.; Sihag, S.; Lehar, J.; Puigserver, P.; Carlsson, E.; Ridderstrale, M.; Laurila, E.; et al. PGC-1alpha-responsive genes involved in oxidative phosphorylation are coordinately downregulated in human diabetes. *Nat. Genet.* **2003**, *34*, 267–273. [CrossRef]
29. Toshima, J.; Toshima, J.Y.; Amano, T.; Yang, N.; Narumiya, S.; Mizuno, K. Cofilin phosphorylation by protein kinase testicular protein kinase 1 and its role in integrin-mediated actin reorganization and focal adhesion formation. *Mol. Biol. Cell* **2001**, *12*, 1131–1145. [CrossRef]
30. Klemmt, P.A.B.; Starzinski-Powitz, A. Molecular and Cellular Pathogenesis of Endometriosis. *Curr. Womens Health Rev.* **2018**, *14*, 106–116. [CrossRef]
31. Zang, C.; Nie, F.Q.; Wang, Q.; Sun, M.; Li, W.; He, J.; Zhang, M.; Lu, K.H. Long non-coding RNA LINC01133 represses KLF2, P21 and E-cadherin transcription through binding with EZH2, LSD1 in non small cell lung cancer. *Oncotarget* **2016**, *7*, 11696–11707. [CrossRef]
32. Liu, Y.; Tang, T.; Yang, X.; Qin, P.; Wang, P.; Zhang, H.; Bai, M.; Wu, R.; Li, F. Tumor-derived exosomal long noncoding RNA LINC01133, regulated by Periostin, contributes to pancreatic ductal adenocarcinoma epithelial-mesenchymal transition through the Wnt/beta-catenin pathway by silencing AXIN2. *Oncogene* **2021**, *40*, 3164–3179. [CrossRef] [PubMed]
33. Hanieh, H.; Ahmed, E.A.; Vishnubalaji, R.; Alajez, N.M. SOX4: Epigenetic regulation and role in tumorigenesis. *Semin. Cancer Biol.* **2020**, *67 Pt 1*, 91–104. [CrossRef]
34. Tiwari, N.; Tiwari, V.K.; Waldmeier, L.; Balwierz, P.J.; Arnold, P.; Pachkov, M.; Meyer-Schaller, N.; Schubeler, D.; van Nimwegen, E.; Christofori, G. Sox4 is a master regulator of epithelial-mesenchymal transition by controlling Ezh2 expression and epigenetic reprogramming. *Cancer Cell* **2013**, *23*, 768–783. [CrossRef] [PubMed]

35. Hazan, R.B.; Qiao, R.; Keren, R.; Badano, I.; Suyama, K. Cadherin switch in tumor progression. *Ann. N. Y. Acad. Sci.* **2004**, *1014*, 155–163. [CrossRef] [PubMed]
36. Thiery, J.P.; Acloque, H.; Huang, R.Y.; Nieto, M.A. Epithelial-mesenchymal transitions in development and disease. *Cell* **2009**, *139*, 871–890. [CrossRef]
37. Wheelock, M.J.; Jensen, P.J. Regulation of keratinocyte intercellular junction organization and epidermal morphogenesis by E-cadherin. *J. Cell Biol.* **1992**, *117*, 415–425. [CrossRef]
38. Matsuzaki, S.; Darcha, C. Epithelial to mesenchymal transition-like and mesenchymal to epithelial transition-like processes might be involved in the pathogenesis of pelvic endometriosis. *Hum. Reprod.* **2012**, *27*, 712–721. [CrossRef]
39. Van Patten, K.; Parkash, V.; Jain, D. Cadherin expression in gastrointestinal tract endometriosis: Possible role in deep tissue invasion and development of malignancy. *Mod. Pathol.* **2010**, *23*, 38–44. [CrossRef] [PubMed]
40. Kuessel, L.; Wenzl, R.; Proestling, K.; Balendran, S.; Pateisky, P.; Yotova, S.; Yerlikaya, G.; Streubel, B.; Husslein, H. Soluble VCAM-1/soluble ICAM-1 ratio is a promising biomarker for diagnosing endometriosis. *Hum. Reprod.* **2017**, *32*, 770–779. [CrossRef]
41. Zhang, J.; Li, H.; Yi, D.; Lai, C.; Wang, H.; Zou, W.; Cao, B. Knockdown of vascular cell adhesion molecule 1 impedes transforming growth factor beta 1-mediated proliferation, migration, and invasion of endometriotic cyst stromal cells. *Reprod. Biol. Endocrinol.* **2019**, *17*, 69. [CrossRef]
42. Wu, T.C. The role of vascular cell adhesion molecule-1 in tumor immune evasion. *Cancer Res.* **2007**, *67*, 6003–6006. [CrossRef] [PubMed]
43. Schlesinger, M.; Bendas, G. Vascular cell adhesion molecule-1 (VCAM-1)–an increasing insight into its role in tumorigenicity and metastasis. *Int. J. Cancer* **2015**, *136*, 2504–2514. [CrossRef]
44. Yotova, I.; Quan, P.; Gaba, A.; Leditznig, N.; Pateisky, P.; Kurz, C.; Tschugguel, W. Raf-1 levels determine the migration rate of primary endometrial stromal cells of patients with endometriosis. *J. Cell. Mol. Med.* **2012**, *16*, 2127–2139. [CrossRef]
45. Morris, K.; Ihnatovych, I.; Ionetz, E.; Reed, J.; Braundmeier, A.; Strakova, Z. Cofilin and slingshot localization in the epithelium of uterine endometrium changes during the menstrual cycle and in endometriosis. *Reprod. Sci.* **2011**, *18*, 1014–1024. [CrossRef]
46. Yuge, A.; Nasu, K.; Matsumoto, H.; Nishida, M.; Narahara, H. Collagen gel contractility is enhanced in human endometriotic stromal cells: A possible mechanism underlying the pathogenesis of endometriosis-associated fibrosis. *Hum. Reprod.* **2007**, *22*, 938–944. [CrossRef]
47. Toshima, J.; Ohashi, K.; Okano, I.; Nunoue, K.; Kishioka, M.; Kuma, K.; Miyata, T.; Hirai, M.; Baba, T.; Mizuno, K. Identification and characterization of a novel protein kinase, TESK1, specifically expressed in testicular germ cells. *J. Biol. Chem.* **1995**, *270*, 31331–31337. [CrossRef]
48. Bamburg, J.R.; McGough, A.; Ono, S. Putting a new twist on actin: ADF/cofilins modulate actin dynamics. *Trends Cell Biol.* **1999**, *9*, 364–370. [CrossRef]
49. Sander, E.E.; ten Klooster, J.P.; van Delft, S.; van der Kammen, R.A.; Collard, J.G. Rac downregulates Rho activity: Reciprocal balance between both GTPases determines cellular morphology and migratory behavior. *J. Cell. Biol.* **1999**, *147*, 1009–1022. [CrossRef]
50. Fassbender, A.; Rahmioglu, N.; Vitonis, A.F.; Vigano, P.; Giudice, L.C.; D'Hooghe, T.M.; Hummelshoj, L.; Adamson, G.D.; Becker, C.M.; Missmer, S.A.; et al. World Endometriosis Research Foundation Endometriosis Phenome and Biobanking Harmonisation Project: IV. Tissue collection, processing, and storage in endometriosis research. *Fertil. Steril.* **2014**, *102*, 1244–1253. [CrossRef]
51. Zeitvogel, A.; Baumann, R.; Starzinski-Powitz, A. Identification of an invasive, N-cadherin-expressing epithelial cell type in endometriosis using a new cell culture model. *Am. J. Pathol.* **2001**, *159*, 1839–1852. [CrossRef]
52. Banu, S.K.; Lee, J.; Starzinski-Powitz, A.; Arosh, J.A. Gene expression profiles and functional characterization of human immortalized endometriotic epithelial and stromal cells. *Fertil. Steril.* **2008**, *90*, 972–987. [CrossRef]
53. Dobin, A.; Davis, C.A.; Schlesinger, F.; Drenkow, J.; Zaleski, C.; Jha, S.; Batut, P.; Chaisson, M.; Gingeras, T.R. STAR: Ultrafast universal RNA-seq aligner. *Bioinformatics* **2013**, *29*, 15–21. [CrossRef]
54. R Core Team. *R: A Language and Environment for Statistical Computing*; R Foundation for Statistical Computing: Vienna, Austria, 2020.
55. Love, M.I.; Huber, W.; Anders, S. Moderated estimation of fold change and dispersion for RNA-seq data with DESeq2. *Genome Biol.* **2014**, *15*, 550. [CrossRef] [PubMed]
56. Li, H.; Handsaker, B.; Wysoker, A.; Fennell, T.; Ruan, J.; Homer, N.; Marth, G.; Abecasis, G.; Durbin, R. The Sequence Alignment/Map format and SAMtools. *Bioinformatics* **2009**, *25*, 2078–2079. [CrossRef]
57. Trapnell, C.; Roberts, A.; Goff, L.; Pertea, G.; Kim, D.; Kelley, D.R.; Pimentel, H.; Salzberg, S.L.; Rinn, J.L.; Pachter, L. Differential gene and transcript expression analysis of RNA-seq experiments with TopHat and Cufflinks. *Nat. Protoc.* **2012**, *7*, 562–578. [CrossRef] [PubMed]
58. Livak, K.J.; Schmittgen, T.D. Analysis of relative gene expression data using real-time quantitative PCR and the 2(-Delta Delta C(T)) Method. *Methods* **2001**, *25*, 402–408. [CrossRef]
59. Rubiolo, C.; Piazzolla, D.; Meissl, K.; Beug, H.; Huber, J.C.; Kolbus, A.; Baccarini, M. A balance between Raf-1 and Fas expression sets the pace of erythroid differentiation. *Blood* **2006**, *108*, 152–159. [CrossRef] [PubMed]

60. Yotova, I.; Hsu, E.; Do, C.; Gaba, A.; Sczabolcs, M.; Dekan, S.; Kenner, L.; Wenzl, R.; Tycko, B. Epigenetic alterations affecting transcription factors and signaling pathways in stromal cells of endometriosis. *PLoS ONE* **2017**, *12*, e0170859. [CrossRef]
61. Hammond, L. Measuring cell fluoresecence using ImageJ. In *The Open Lab Book, Release 1.0*; Fitzpatrick, M., Ed.; The University of Queensland: Brisbane, Australia, 2020; pp. 50–53.

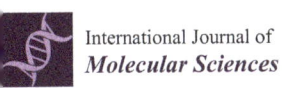

Article

Peritoneal Fluid from Patients with Ovarian Endometriosis Displays Immunosuppressive Potential and Stimulates Th2 Response

Joanna Olkowska-Truchanowicz [1], Agata Białoszewska [2], Aneta Zwierzchowska [3,4], Alicja Sztokfisz-Ignasiak [2], Izabela Janiuk [2], Filip Dąbrowski [3,5], Grażyna Korczak-Kowalska [6], Ewa Barcz [3,4], Katarzyna Bocian [6,*] and Jacek Malejczyk [2,7,*]

1. Department of Transplantology and Central Tissue Bank, Centre of Biostructure Research, Medical University of Warsaw, 02-004 Warsaw, Poland; joanna.olkowska-truchanowicz@wum.edu.pl
2. Department of Histology and Embryology, Centre of Biostructure Research, Medical University of Warsaw, 02-004 Warsaw, Poland; agata.bialoszewska@wum.edu.pl (A.B.); ala.sztokfisz@gmail.com (A.S.-I.); izabela.janiuk@wum.edu.pl (I.J.)
3. 1st Department of Obstetrics and Gynecology, Medical University of Warsaw, 02-015 Warsaw, Poland; teksanskamasakra@o2.pl (A.Z.); fil.dabrowski@gmail.com (F.D.); ewa.barcz@interia.pl (E.B.)
4. Department of Obstetrics and Gynecology, Multidisciplinary Hospital Warsaw-Miedzylesie, 04-749 Warsaw, Poland
5. Department of Gynecology and Obstetrics, Medical University of Silesia, 40-778 Katowice, Poland
6. Department of Immunology, Faculty of Biology, University of Warsaw, 02-096 Warsaw, Poland; gkorczak-k@biol.uw.edu.pl
7. Laboratory of Experimental Immunology, Military Institute of Hygiene and Epidemiology, 01-163 Warsaw, Poland
* Correspondence: kbocian@biol.uw.edu.pl (K.B.); jacek.malejczyk@wum.edu.pl (J.M.)

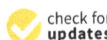

Citation: Olkowska-Truchanowicz, J.; Białoszewska, A.; Zwierzchowska, A.; Sztokfisz-Ignasiak, A.; Janiuk, I.; Dąbrowski, F.; Korczak-Kowalska, G.; Barcz, E.; Bocian, K.; Malejczyk, J. Peritoneal Fluid from Patients with Ovarian Endometriosis Displays Immunosuppressive Potential and Stimulates Th2 Response. *Int. J. Mol. Sci.* **2021**, *22*, 8134. https://doi.org/10.3390/ijms22158134

Academic Editors: Antonio Simone Laganà and Alfonso Baldi

Received: 23 May 2021
Accepted: 27 July 2021
Published: 29 July 2021

Publisher's Note: MDPI stays neutral with regard to jurisdictional claims in published maps and institutional affiliations.

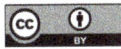

Copyright: © 2021 by the authors. Licensee MDPI, Basel, Switzerland. This article is an open access article distributed under the terms and conditions of the Creative Commons Attribution (CC BY) license (https://creativecommons.org/licenses/by/4.0/).

Abstract: Endometriosis is a common gynaecological disorder characterized by the ectopic growth of endometrial tissue outside the uterine cavity. It is associated with chronic pelvic inflammation and autoimmune reactivity manifesting by autoantibody production and abrogated cellular immune responses. Endometriotic peritoneal fluid contains various infiltrating leucocyte populations and a bulk of proinflammatory and immunoregulatory cytokines. However, the nature and significance of the peritoneal milieu in women with endometriosis still remains obscure. Therefore, the aim of the present study was to investigate the immunoregulatory activity of the peritoneal fluid (PF) from women with endometriosis. The peritoneal fluid samples were collected during laparoscopic surgery from 30 women with and without endometriosis. Immunoregulatory cytokines (IL-2, IL-4, IL-6, IL-10, IL-17A, IFN-γ and TNF) and chemokines (CCL2, CCL5, CXCL8 and CXCL9) were evaluated in PF and culture supernatants generated by unstimulated and CD3/CD28/IL-2-stimulated CD4$^+$ T cells cultured in the presence of PF. The effect of PF on the generation of Treg and Th17 cells in CD4$^+$ T cell cultures, as well as the natural cytotoxic activity of peripheral blood mononuclear cells, was also investigated. Concentrations of IL-6, IL-10, CCL2, CXCL8 and CXCL9 were significantly upregulated in the PF from women with endometriosis when compared to control women, whereas concentrations of other cytokines and chemokines were unaffected. The culturing of unstimulated and CD3/CD28/IL-2-stimulated CD4$^+$ T cells in the presence of endometriotic PF resulted in the downregulation of their IL-2, IFN-γ, IL-17A and TNF production as compared to culture medium alone. On the other side, endometriotic PF significantly stimulated the production of IL-4 and IL-10. Endometriotic PF also stimulated the release of CCL2 and CXCL8, whereas the production of CCL5 and CXCL9 was downregulated. Endometriotic PF stimulated the generation of Treg cells and had an inhibitory effect on the generation of Th17 cells in cultures of CD4$^+$ T cells. It also inhibited the NK cell cytotoxic activity of the peripheral blood lymphocytes. These results strongly imply that the PF from patients with endometriosis has immunoregulatory/immunosuppressive activity and shifts the Th1/Th2 cytokine balance toward the Th2 response, which may account for deviation of local and systemic immune responses. However, a similar trend, albeit not a statistically significant one, was also observed in case of PF from women without endometriosis, thus suggesting that peritoneal milieu may in general display some immunoregulatory/immunosuppressive properties. It should be stressed, however, that our present observations were made on a relatively small number of PF samples and further studies are needed to reveal possible mechanism(s) responsible for this phenomenon.

Keywords: endometriosis; peritoneal fluid; cytokines; chemokines; Th1 cells; Th2 cells; Treg cells; Th17 cells

1. Introduction

Endometriosis is a common gynecological disorder affecting ca. 10% women of reproductive age. The disease is related to the endometrial-like tissue (endometrial glands and stroma) located outside the uterine cavity, mainly on the pelvic viscera and/or ovaries. Endometriosis is associated with chronic pelvic inflammation and manifests with dysmenorrhea, dyspareunia or chronic pelvic pain. It also accounts for ca. 50% of women's infertility. Endometriosis is a debilitating disorder having a significant impact on patients' quality of life. Nevertheless, the etiopathogenesis of this disease is still poorly understood [1–4].

There are several theories on the origin of the endometriosis; however, the most accepted cause of this disease is retrograde menstrual blood flow [5]. In this mechanism shed endometrial cells enter the peritoneal cavity, where they survive and form ectopic foci of the endometriotic tissue. This may be possible owing to the resistance of endometriotic cells to apoptosis and their increased adhesiveness and invasiveness [6–9]. It is also plausible that the formation of ectopic endometriotic lesions may also be facilitated by a permissive local peritoneal milieu as well as abrogated elimination of endometriotic cells by the cells of the local immune system, e.g., NK cells and macrophages [10,11].

Due to chronic pelvic inflammation and the elevated production of a variety of autoantibodies such as anti-nuclear, anti-phospholipid, and anti-endometrial antibodies, endometriosis may be considered as an autoimmune/autoinflammatory disorder [11–14]. The disease manifests with the local and systemic abnormal lymphocyte responses and abrogated NK cell cytotoxicity [10,13,15–17]. Pelvic inflammation includes peritoneal infiltration with a variety of immune cells including various subsets of lymphocytes, activated macrophages and granulocytes [18,19]. The endometriotic peritoneal milieu is also characterized by a local excessive production and accumulation of a bulk of proinflammatory and regulatory cytokines [20,21].

The role of the peritoneal milieu and the peritoneal fluid (PF) in the immunopathogenesis of endometriosis still remains obscure. Although endometriosis is considered to be an inflammatory disorder there is a growing body of evidence that the local peritoneal milieu may display, rather, an immunosuppressive character. Indeed, it has been reported that endometriosis is characterized by increased numbers of the peritoneal Treg cells displaying immunosuppressive and anti-inflammatory activity [22–25]. Furthermore, the PF from women with endometriosis also contains increased levels of suppressive anti-inflammatory cytokines such as TGF-β and IL-10 [20,26]. Thus, it is plausible that the PF from women with endometriosis may display some immunoregulatory properties. These properties, however, are still poorly characterized. Therefore, the present study was aimed at testing the immunomodulatory effects of the PF from women with endometriosis in comparison to control women without the disease. We investigated the effects of the PF on the immunoregulatory cytokine and chemokine production by the isolated CD4$^+$ T cells as well as on the differentiation of CD4$^+$ T cells into Treg and Th17 cells. Finally, we also tested the effect of PF on the cytotoxic activity of the peripheral blood natural killer (NK) cells.

2. Results

2.1. Concentrations of Cytokines and Chemokines in PF

Concentrations of IL-2, IFN-γ, IL-17A, TNF, IL-4, IL-10 and IL-6 in the peritoneal fluid of control women and patients with endometriosis are shown in Table 1. Women with endometriosis had increased concentrations of IL-6 and IL-10. There were no differences between the control and endometriosis groups in concentrations of IL-2, IFN-γ, IL-17A, TNF, and IL-4.

Table 1. Immunoregulatory cytokine concentrations in peritoneal fluid from patients with endometriosis and control women.

Cytokine	Control (n = 14)	Endometriosis (n = 16)	p-Value *
IL-2	0.3 (0.1–0.6)	0.4 (0.1–0.9)	ns
IFN-γ	0.3 (0–1.0)	0.1 (0–0.9)	ns
IL-17A	2.0 (0–8.1)	3.5 (0–28.4)	ns
TNF	1.2 (0.4–1.4)	0.9 (0.4–2.2)	ns
IL-4	0 (0–1.4)	0 (0–0.6)	ns
IL-10	1.5 (0–9.7)	8.0 (1.5–96.9)	0.0107
IL-6	35.8 (1.7–312.8)	313 (26.2–6436)	0.0435

Values are expressed in pg/mL and are shown as medians (range). * p-values were calculated by Mann–Whitney U test. ns, non-significant.

Concentrations of CCL2, CCL5, CXCL8 and CXCL9 in PF of control women and patients with endometriosis are shown in Table 2. PF from the women with endometriosis displayed significantly increased concentrations of CCL2, CXCL8 and CXCL9 as compared with the control subjects.

Table 2. Chemokine concentrations in peritoneal fluid from patients with endometriosis and control women.

Chemokine	Control (n = 14)	Endometriosis (n = 16)	p-Value *
CCL2	64.7 (16.6–198.7)	316.8 (10.1–10,333)	0.0232
CCL5	14.2 (5.8–227.2)	8.0 (5.3–33.9)	ns
CXCL8	7.7 (1.4–62.0)	72.2 (8.7–9027)	0.0015
CXCL9	16.6 (5.2–50.8)	46.2 (24.1–628.3)	0.0030

Values are expressed in pg/mL and are shown as medians and a range. * p-values were calculated by Mann–Whitney U test. ns, non-significant.

2.2. Effect of PF on Cytokine and Chemokine Production by $CD4^+$ T Cells

To reveal whether the PF from the patients with endometriosis and the control subjects may affect the cytokine and chemokine production by $CD4^+$ T cells, we evaluated cytokine and chemokine production following the 5-day culture of unstimulated and CD3/CD28/IL-2-stimulated $CD4^+$ T cells, where stimulation with CD3/CD28 beads mimics antigen stimulation conditions [27,28]. The results of IL-2, IFN-γ, IL-17A, TNF, IL-4, IL-10 and IL-6 concentrations in $CD4^+$ T cell culture supernatants are shown in Figure 1. As can be seen, $CD4^+$ T cell stimulation with CD3/CD28 beads and IL-2 resulted in the very high upregulation of production of all tested cytokines as compared to unstimulated cells. The addition of the endometriotic PF to the culture of $CD4^+$ T cells revealed its suppressive effect on the production of IL-2 (Figure 1A), IFN-γ (Figure 1B), IL-17A (Figure 1C) and TNF (Figure 1D), particularly by stimulated cells. Control PF also displayed some inhibitory activity toward the production of these cytokines; however, a statistically significant inhibition was seen only in the case of IL-2 production (Figure 1A). On the other hand, endometriotic PF significantly upregulated production of IL-4 (Figure 1E) and IL-10 (Figure 1F) by stimulated $CD4^+$ T cells. The production of IL-10 by stimulated $CD4^+$ T cells was also upregulated by the control PF (Figure 1F). The production of IL-6 by unstimulated $CD4^+$ T cells was significantly stimulated by endometriotic PF, whereas the production of this cytokine by stimulated lymphocytes was affected by neither control nor endometriotic

PFs (Figure 1G). There were no significant differences between PF from endometriosis and control group.

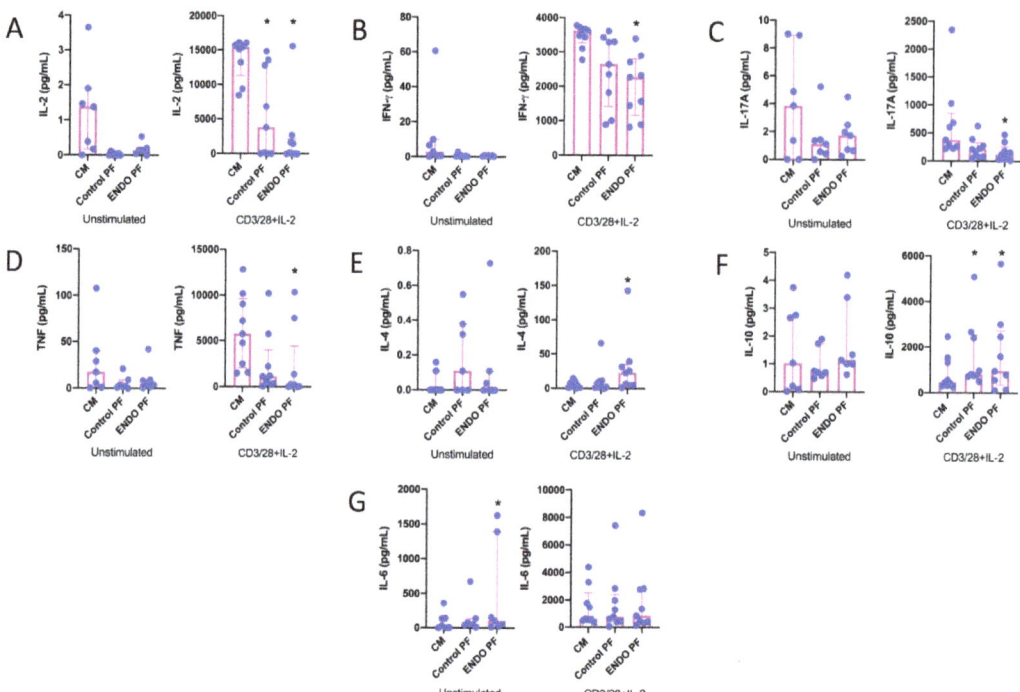

Figure 1. Production of (**A**) IL-2, (**B**) IFN-γ, (**C**) IL-17A, (**D**) TNF, (**E**) IL-4, (**F**) IL-10 and (**G**) IL-6 by cultured CD4+ T cells unstimulated or stimulated with CD3/CD28 beads and IL-2 in the presence of the culture medium alone (CM), peritoneal fluid from control woman (Control PF) or peritoneal fluid from woman with endometriosis (ENDO PF). The results are shown as scatter dot plots with a median and interquartile range. Statistical significance was computed by paired non-parametric ANOVA (Friedman's test) followed by a post hoc test. * Statistically significant from the control group at least at $p < 0.05$. Baseline concentration ranges of the tested cytokines (pg/mL), respectively, in Control PF and ENDO PF used for the experiments were as follows. IL-2, 0.13–0.56 and 0.13–0.88; IFN-γ, 0–0.82 and 0–0.95; IL-17A, 0–8.10 and 0–8.70; TNF, 0.43–1.32 and 0.38–2.24; IL-4, 0–0.70 and 0–0.59; IL-10, 0.59–9.65 and 1.46–11.2; IL-6, 16.4–312.8 and 47.1–492.

The results of the evaluation of the effects of PF on chemokine (CCL2, CCL5, CXCL8 and CXCL9) production by CD4+ T cells are shown in Figure 2. As seen, CD3/CD28/IL-2 stimulation of CD4+ T cells significantly affected the production of all chemokines except CXCL8. It should be stressed, however, that production of the latter was extremely relatively high even in unstimulated CD4+ T cells. The production of CCL2 was significantly upregulated in both unstimulated and stimulated CD4+ T cells by the control as well as endometriotic PF (Figure 2A). The stimulation of CXCL8 production was seen only with endometriotic PF in unstimulated CD4+ T cells (Figure 2C). On the other hand, both control and endometriotic PF significantly inhibited the production of CCL5 (Figure 2B) and CXCL9 (Figure 2D) by stimulated CD4+ T cells. There were no significant differences between PF from endometriosis and control group.

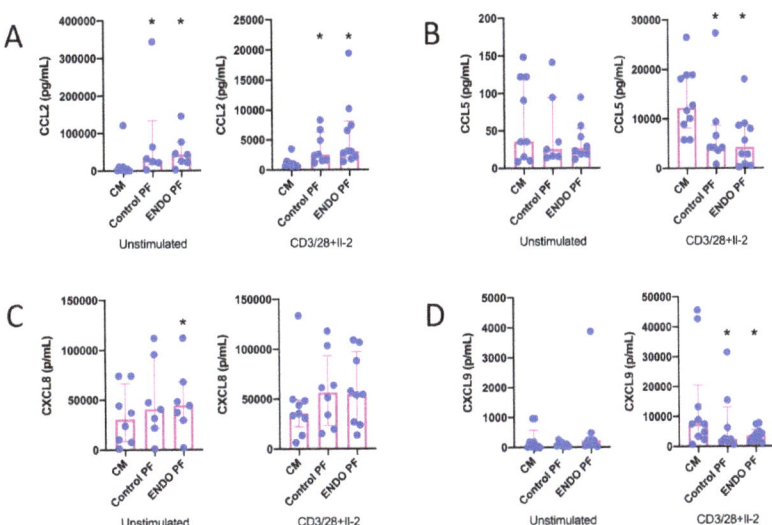

Figure 2. Production of (**A**) CCL2, (**B**) CCL5, (**C**) CXCL8 and (**D**) CXC9 by cultured CD4$^+$ T cells unstimulated or stimulated with CD3/CD28 beads and IL-2 in the presence of the culture medium alone (CM), peritoneal fluid from control woman (Control PF) or peritoneal fluid from woman with endometriosis (ENDO PF). The results are shown as scatter dot plots with a median and interquartile range. Statistical significance was computed by paired non-parametric ANOVA (Friedman's test) followed by a post hoc test. * Statistically significant from the control group at least at $p < 0.05$. Baseline concentration ranges of the tested chemokines (pg/mL), respectively, in Control PF and ENDO PF used for the experiments were as follows. CCL2, 16.6–198.7 and 10.12–393.2; CCL5, 2.5–9.6 and 6.0–33.9; CXCL8, 7.08–61.98 and 15.4–400.0; CXC9, 12.1–50.8 and 39.2–72.6.

2.3. Effect of PF on Generation of Treg and Th17 Cells

To see whether the PF from the patients with endometriosis and the control subjects may affect in vitro generation of Treg and Th17 cells we evaluated specific phenotype changes of the unstimulated and CD3/CD28/IL-2-stimulated CD4$^+$ T cells following their 5-day culture. As seen in Figure 3, stimulation of CD4$^+$ T cells with CD3/CD28 beads and IL-2 resulted in significant generation of CD25^{high} and CD25^{high} FOXP3$^+$ Treg cells. The addition of the endometriotic PF significantly enhanced generation of the CD25^{high} T cells as compared to culture medium control and PF from women without endometriosis. A similar effect of the endometriotic PF on the generation of CD25^{high} FOXP3$^+$ cells was also seen in cultures of unstimulated CD4$^+$ T cells (Figure 3B), whereas there were no differences in the generation of CD25^{high} FOXP3$^+$ cells in CD3/CD28/IL-2-stimulated cultures. Control PF did not affect generation of CD25^{high} and CD25^{high} FOXP3$^+$ T cells in either unstimulated or stimulated CD4$^+$ T cell cultures.

Figure 4 shows that stimulation with CD3/CD28/IL-2 significantly increased the generation of CD161$^+$ T cells while having no significant effect on the generation of the CD161$^+$ RORγ$^+$ cells. Endometriotic PF had a significant suppressive effect on generation of CD161$^+$, both in unstimulated and stimulated CD4$^+$ T cell populations (Figure 4A). Neither PF affected the generation of CD161$^+$ RORγ$^+$ cells (Figure 4B). There were no significant differences between PF from endometriosis and control group.

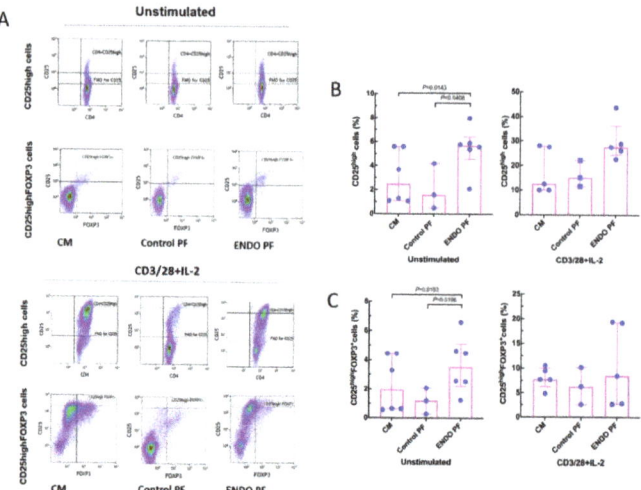

Figure 3. Effect of culture medium alone (CM), peritoneal fluid from control woman (Control PF) or peritoneal fluid from woman with endometriosis (ENDO PF) on generation of CD25^{high} and CD25^{high} FOXP3$^+$ Treg cells in cultures of CD4$^+$ T cells unstimulated or stimulated with CD3/CD28 beads and IL-2. (**A**) Gating strategy and a representative flow cytometry analysis showing identification of the respective CD25^{high} and CD25^{high} FOXP3$^+$ T cell subpopulations in CD4$^+$ T cells under different culture conditions. (**B**) Proportions of CD25^{high} T cells and (**C**) CD25^{high} FOXP3$^+$ Treg cells in population of unstimulated or CD3/CD28 beads+IL-2-stimulated CD4$^+$ T cells. The results are shown as scatter dot plots with a median and interquartile range. Statistical significance was computed by paired (Friedman's test) or unpaired (Kruskal–Wallis test) non-parametric ANOVA followed by a post hoc test.

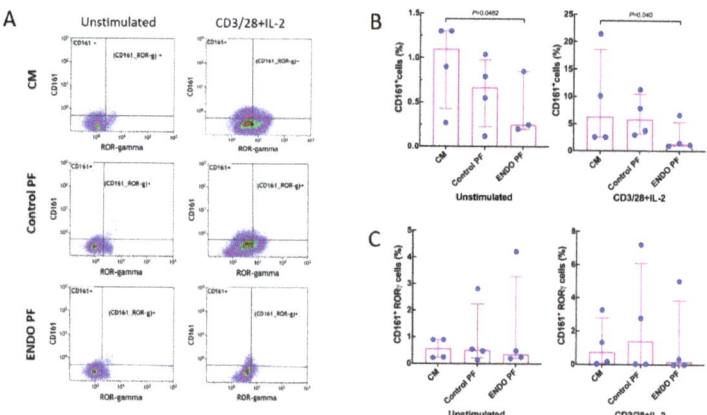

Figure 4. Effect of culture medium alone (CM), peritoneal fluid from control woman (Control PF) or peritoneal fluid from woman with endometriosis (ENDO PF) on generation of CD161$^+$ and CD161$^+$ RORγ$^+$ Th17 cells in cultures of CD4$^+$ T cells unstimulated or stimulated with CD3/CD28 beads and IL-2. (**A**) Gating strategy and a representative flow cytometry analysis showing identification of the respective CD161$^+$ and CD161$^+$ RORγ$^+$ T cell subpopulations in CD4$^+$ T cells under different culture conditions. (**B**) Proportions of CD161$^+$ T cells and (**C**) CD161$^+$ RORγ$^+$ Th17 cells in population of unstimulated or CD3/CD28 beads+IL-2-stimulated CD4$^+$ T cells. The results are shown as scatter dot plots with a median and interquartile range. Statistical significance was computed by paired (Friedman's test) or unpaired (Kruskal–Wallis test) non-parametric ANOVA followed by a post hoc test.

2.4. Effect of PF on NK Cell Cytotoxicity

To reveal an effect of the PF from the patients with endometriosis and the control subjects on the NK cells, we evaluated the cytotoxic activity of the cultured PBMC against K562 erythroleukemia cells. As seen in Figure 5, a one day culture of PBMC with endometriotic PF resulted in a significant decrease in their cytotoxic activity. The control PF also displayed some inhibitory effect; this, however, was not statistically significant. There was also no significant difference between PF from endometriosis and control group.

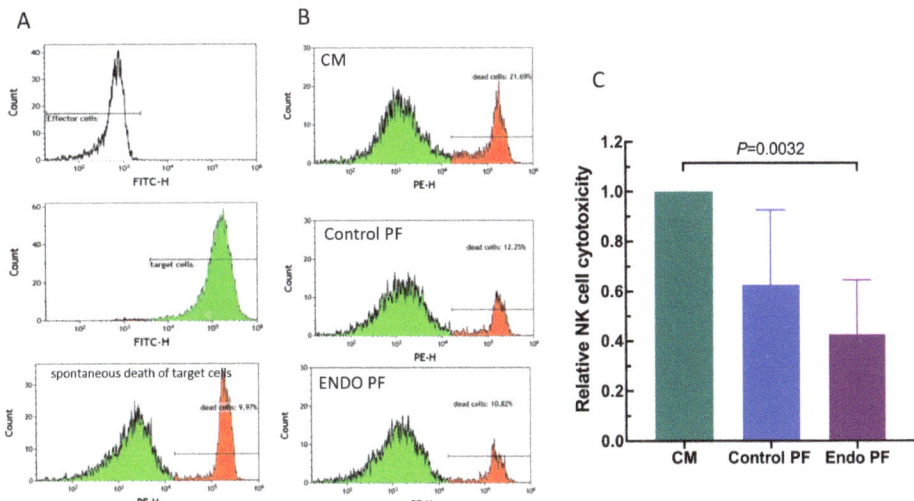

Figure 5. Effect of culture medium alone (CM), peritoneal fluid from control woman (Control PF) or peritoneal fluid from woman with endometriosis (ENDO PF) on the NK cell cytotoxic activity of cultured PBMC. (**A**) The representative flow cytometry analysis showing the controls for the NK assay. Shown are the fluorescence-negative effector cells (PBMC), green fluorescence (FITC) labeled K562 target cells and spontaneously dying K562 cells (red fluorescence, PE). Spontaneous death of target cells was determined in cultures without effector cells. (**B**) An example of identification of target K562 cells killed by NK cells from the PBMC population (red fluorescence). (**C**) Relative cell mediated cytotoxicity of untreated and peritoneal fluid-treated PBMC against K562 cells. The results are expressed as an index of specific cytotoxicity of peritoneal fluid-treated PBMC relative to untreated control PBMC. Each bar represents mean ± SD from 4 independent experiments. Statistical significance was computed by paired non-parametric ANOVA (Friedman's test) followed by a post hoc test.

3. Discussion

The results of the present study show for the first time that PF from women with advanced endometriosis displays immunomodulatory activity toward both unstimulated and CD3/CD28/IL-2-stimulated CD4$^+$ T cells. We chose the stimulation of CD4$^+$ T cells with CD3/CD28 beads and IL-2 as this method is considered to be a good model for assessment of T cell receptor-dependent T cell activation and expansion [27,28]. We found that endometriotic PF inhibited the production of IL-2, IFN-γ, IL-17A and TNF by CD4$^+$ T cells. On the other hand, it stimulated the production of IL-4 and IL-10. The production of IL-2, IFN-γ and TNF is a feature of the Th1 subpopulation of CD4$^+$ T cells, which is responsible for inflammatory and cell-mediated immunity, whereas the production of IL-4 and IL-10 is an attribute of Th2 cells, which are involved in the regulation of antibody production and the downregulation of cell-mediated responses [29,30]. Thus, our results may suggest that endometriotic PF displays an ability to shift CD4$^+$ T cell differentiation into the Th2 phenotype. This observation is in line with the previous suggestions that the Th1/Th2 balance is abrogated in the endometriosis patients and that Th2 cells may favor development of the disease [31,32]. It should be stressed, however, that our observations were limited to cytokine evaluations and further studies on the shifting of the Th1/Th2 balance to Th2 phenotype are required.

We also found that the PF from women with endometriosis modulates the production of some T cell-derived chemokines. The treatment of CD4$^+$ T cells with endometriotic PF resulted in stimulation of CCL2 (also known as MCP-1) release. This is consistent with our observation that CCL2 concentrations are elevated in the PF from endometriosis patients as compared to healthy women (Table 2) as well as previous observations of many other investigators [33]. CCL2 is a key chemokine responsible for chemotaxis/infiltration and activation of monocytes/macrophages [34], thus, our present results strongly argue for the role of the PF milieu in generation of pelvic inflammation in the course of endometriosis. Interestingly, we also found that endometriotic PF inhibited the production of CCL5 (RANTES) and CXCL9 (MIG) by the CD4$^+$ T cells. CCL5 is responsible for the chemotaxis of T cells and some other leukocyte populations [35] and is considered to play a part in the pathogenesis of endometriosis [33]. CXCL9 is also responsible for T and NK cell infiltration, and, in particular, Th1 cells [36,37]. The expression of CXCL9 is upregulated by IFN-γ, thus, its downregulated production in endometriotic PF may reflect the inhibition of this cytokine release. These results seem to be in line with and extend the previous observations of Na et al. that endometriotic PF modulated production of CCL2, CCL3 (MIP-1α) and CCL5 by monocytes, neutrophils and T cells [38]. These findings strongly suggest that the PF from women with endometriosis displays immunosuppressive properties which may affect local infiltration and differentiation of T cells.

In addition to the observation that the PF from women with endometriosis affects cytokine/chemokine production by CD4$^+$ T cells. We also found that it stimulates differentiation/expansion of CD25^{high} FOXP3$^+$ Treg cells. Increased numbers of Treg cells were repeatedly reported in the peritoneum of patients with endometriosis, thus suggesting their role in the suppression of the local immune responses [17,23,25,39,40]. Our present result suggests that the mechanism responsible for the increased numbers of Treg cells in the endometriotic PF may be at least partially due to their local activation by the peritoneal milieu.

A stimulatory effect of the endometriotic PF on generation of Treg cells was accompanied by an inhibition of expansion of CD161$^+$ Th17 cells. However, it should be noted that we did not observe any effect on the CD161$^+$ RORg$^+$ cells. It has been claimed that Th17 cells may play a part in the immunopathogenesis of endometriosis by exacerbation of the inflammatory response [41–43]. Nevertheless, our present observation suggests that the activity of Th17 cells may be suppressed by the factors present in the PF. Our observation might also explain the differential levels of Treg and Th17 cells in patients with different stage of the endometriosis [25].

Finally, we also confirmed the previous observations that the peritoneal fluid form women with endometriosis may also inhibit the cytotoxic activity of the NK cells [44,45].

Interestingly, the suppressive/modulatory effects of the PF of women with endometriosis were also reported on monocytes/macrophages. Accordingly, PF from the patients with endometriosis was reported to downregulate the expression of the MHC class II molecules as well as CD80 and CD86 costimulatory molecules in monocytes [46]. Furthermore, PF from women with endometriosis was also found to inhibit production of matrix metalloproteinases in the peritoneal macrophages [47].

Taken all together, our present results provide evidence that the PF of patients with endometriosis displays immunomodulatory/immunosuppressive activities toward CD4$^+$ T cells. These activities manifest by inhibition of Th1 and stimulation of Th2 cytokine production, the inhibition of some lymphocyte chemotactic factor production, the shift of the Treg/Th17 balance to Treg phenotype and the inhibition of NK cell cytotoxic activity. The nature of these modulatory/suppressive properties of the endometriotic PF remains a subject of speculations. It should be stressed, however, that unlike in comparison to culture medium control, there were no significant differences in immunomodulatory/immunosuppressive activities between endometriotic PF and PF from control women without the disease. Furthermore, some inhibition of IL-2 and stimulation of IL-10 production by CD4$^+$ T cells was also seen in the case of PF from the control women. The control PF also stimulated CCL2 and inhibited CCL5 and CXCL9 production. This strongly suggests that PF from control women with ovarian dermoid cysts also displays some immunoregulatory activity. We included patients with ovarian dermoid cysts as control since this is a benign ovarian teratoma that typically does not manifest with local inflammatory response or systemic immune deviations [48]. Considering that the immunology of ovarian dermoid cysts remains elusive, the significance our present observation and the nature of this phenomenon remains to be elucidated.

The levels of some investigated cytokines and chemokines, such as IL-6, IL-10, CCL2, CXCL8, and CXCL9, were significantly increased in PF from patients with endometriosis as compared to control. This observation is consistent with a variety of previous reports [20,21,49,50] and argues for the role of endometriotic peritoneal milieu in the regulation of local inflammatory responses. It is tempting to speculate that the modulatory/suppressive activity of the endometriotic PF is at least partially attributable to the increased local production of some regulatory cytokines such as TGF-β and IL-10 [20]. Both cytokines exert strong anti-inflammatory activity and were found to be produced by and to facilitate the induction of Treg cells [51–54]. TGF-β may be also responsible for local inhibition of the NK cell activity [45]. It should be stressed, however, that the regulation of the Treg/Th17 balance cannot simply be explained by an excessive stimulation with TGF-β [55] and this issue requires further investigations. Similarly, it is also difficult to speculate about the possible mechanisms responsible for the change of the Th1/Th2 balance. The differentiation of both subpopulations of Th cells appears to be a complicated phenomenon depending on a bulk of immunoregulatory cytokines and accessory cells [56] and also deserves further study.

It should be stressed that due to difficulties in obtaining the sufficient amounts of PF for the research purposes, the present study was performed on a limited number of PF samples. Nevertheless, the present results suggest that the peritoneal milieu of women with endometriosis shows immunosuppressive properties and shifts the Th1/Th2 balance toward the Th2 phenotype. These properties may help us to understand how the endometrioid tissue may escape from under local immune surveillance. The shift of the Th1/Th2 balance may also account for the dysregulated control of antibody production and may explain the origin of endometriosis-associated autoimmune phenomena. This may strongly support the view that the peritoneal milieu plays an important part in the pathogenesis of endometriosis and may be a target for specific clinical interventions.

4. Materials and Methods

4.1. Patients

The study included 16 women (mean age 35.8 years, range 25–46) with laparoscopically and histopathologically confirmed endometriosis. All patients had ovarian endometriotic cysts and the disease was classified as moderate/severe (III/IV) stage according to the revised criteria of the American Society for Reproductive Medicine [57]. The control group comprised 14 women (mean age 31.8 years, range 19–46) without visible endometriosis foci, pelvic inflammation or related pathology who underwent laparoscopic excision of ovarian dermoid cysts. All women had regular menses and none of them had a history of previous pelvic surgery or chronic systemic disease. The patients were not subjected to any hormonal or immunomodulatory therapy for at least six months prior to the study.

All participants gave a written informed consent to the study. The procedures were approved by the Institutional Bioethical Review Board of the Medical University of Warsaw, Poland and were conducted according to the Helsinki Declaration ethical principles.

4.2. PF Sample Collection

PF samples were collected on the same day at the mid-follicular phase (8–10 day) of the menstrual cycle. The mid-follicular menstrual cycle phase was additionally confirmed by the ultrasound examination.

PF was aspirated from the cul de sac at the beginning of the standard laparoscopic procedure under general anesthesia. Samples of the peritoneal fluid contaminated with blood were excluded from the study. PF samples were centrifuged at 400g at 4 °C for 10 min and the cell-free supernatants were collected, aliquoted, and stored frozen at −80 °C until used for further evaluations and experiments. The mean yield of PF obtained from the endometriosis patients and the control subjects was 6.2 (range 2–12.5) and 4.6 (range 0.5–13) mL, respectively.

4.3. Isolation, Stimulation and Culture of $CD4^+$ T Cells

Peripheral blood mononuclear cells (PBMC) were isolated from the buffy coat from healthy volunteers from the local blood drive by Histopaque®-1077 (Sigma-Aldrich, St. Louis, MO, USA) density gradient centrifugation. Then, $CD4^+$ T cells were isolated using $CD4^+$ Cell Isolation Kit (Miltenyi Biotec, Bergisch Gladbach, Germany) according to the detailed protocol provided by the manufacturer. The purity of isolated cells was >90% as evaluated by flow cytometry analysis (see below). A representative flow cytometry analysis of $CD4^+$ T cell purity is shown in Supplementary Figure S1.

Isolated $CD4^+$ T cells were resuspended in RPMI 1640 culture medium supplemented with 10% Fetal Bovine Serum, 1% HEPES buffer and 1% Pen-Strep (all from Invitrogen, ThermoFisher Scientific, Waltham, MA, USA) and subjected or not to stimulation with Dynabeads™ Human T-Activator CD3/CD28 [27,28] at bead-to-cell ratio 1:1 and 30 U/mL rIL-2 (all from Invitrogen, TermoFisher Scientific) according to the protocol provided by the manufacturer. Then, 1×10^6 of unstimulated or stimulated cells were cultured for 5 days in the medium alone or in the medium with control or endometriotic PF at 1:1 ratio without medium refreshment in the wells of 12-well plates (Corning Inc., Corning, NY, USA) at 37 °C and 5% CO_2 atmosphere.

The following culture cell-free supernatants were collected and stored frozen at −70 °C until used for cytokine and chemokine quantification. The cells were also harvested, and their phenotype was evaluated by flow cytometry as described below.

Peritoneal fluids containing particular cytokines or chemokines at concentrations far exceeding interquartile range values were not used in the experiments. Baseline concentration ranges of each tested cytokines and chemokines present in control and endometriotic PF used in the experiments are given in the legends to Figures 2 and 3. As seen, these baseline concentrations of cytokines and chemokines were relatively very low compared to those found in the cell-free supernatants following $CD4^+$ T cell cultures and therefore may be considered as negligible.

4.4. Cytokine Evaluations

Concentrations of cytokines (IL-2, IL-4, IL-6, IL-10, IL-17A, IFN-γ, and TNF) and chemokines (CCL2, CCL5, CXCL8, and CXCL9) in peritoneal fluids and culture media were measured using the BD™ Cytometric Bead Array (CBA) Human Th1/Th2/Th17 Cytokine and Human Chemokine kits (BD Bioscience, USA), respectively. The samples were evaluated using a FACSVerse flow cytometry with BD Suite software (BD Bioscience) according to the protocol provided by the manufacturer. The results were analyzed with FCAP Array software (BD Bioscience). The advertised theoretical limit of detection defined as the corresponding concentration at two standard deviations above the median fluorescence of 20–30 replicates of the negative control (0 pg/mL) for IL-2, IL-4, IL-6, IL-10, IL-17A, IFN-γ, and TNF was 2.6, 4.9, 2.4, 4.5, 18.9, 3.7, and 3.8 pg/mL, respectively. The respective theoretical limit of detection for CCL2, CCL5, CXCL8, and CXCL9 was 2.7, 1.0, 0.2, and 2.5 pg/mL. The measurements were always within the respective standard curve. Raw data of standard curves for all assays are shown in a supplementary file.

4.5. Flow Cytometry Analysis

For flow cytometry analysis 0.5×10^6 cells were labelled with 1 mg/mL of a respective antibody for 30 min at 4 °C, as described in detail elsewhere [23,58]. In brief, for evaluation of the purity of isolated CD4$^+$ T cells the cells were labelled with FITC-conjugated anti-CD4 monoclonal antibodies (BD Biosciences, San Jose, CA, USA). For evaluation of Treg cells in CD4$^+$ T cell cultures the harvested cells were labelled with PerCP-conjugated anti-CD4 and APC-conjugated anti-CD25 monoclonal antibodies (both from BD Biosciences) followed by a permeabilization-fixation procedure and intracellular staining with Phycoerythrin (PE) Anti-Human Foxp3 Staining Set (eBioscience Inc., San Diego, CA, USA) according to the detailed protocol provided by the manufacturer. For identification and evaluation of Th17 cells cultured CD4$^+$ T cells were labelled with FITC-conjugated anti-CD161 monoclonal antibody (BD Biosciences) followed by intracellular staining with Phycoerythrin (PE)-conjugated Anti-Human ROR-γ antibody (eBioscience Inc.). As a negative control served nonspecific isotype IgG antibodies conjugated with the respective fluorochrome.

Cell samples were analyzed on the FACSCalibur using CellQuest / BD FACS Diva™ software (BD Biosciences). The cells were specifically analyzed by selective gating, based on the parameters of forward and side scatter as described elsewhere [23,58]. The results were based on analysis of at least 100,000 cells and were shown as the percentage of positively labelled cells. The gating strategy for identification and evaluation of Treg and Th17 cells is shown in Supplementary Figures S2 and S3, respectively.

4.6. NK Cell Cytotoxicity Assay

PBMC were isolated from the buffy coat by Histopaque®-1077 (Sigma-Aldrich) density gradient centrifugation, washed and cultured in RPMI 1640 + GlutaMAX medium supplemented with 10% FBS and 1% antibiotic–antimycotic solution (all from Invitrogen, TermoFisher Scientific) with or without addition of PF (1:1) from patients with endometriosis or control subjects at a density of 2×10^6/mL in 12-well plates at 37 °C in 5% CO_2 atmosphere. Following 24 h of culture natural cytotoxic activity of PBMC was evaluated by means of NKTEST™ (Glycotope Biotechnology, Heidelberg, Germany) according to the detailed description provided by the manufacturer. In brief, cultured effector PBMC and K562 target cells prestained with a green fluorescent membrane dye were mixed at 50:1, 25:1 and 12.5:1 effector-to-target (E:T) ratio in a test medium and incubated for 3 h at 37 °C in 5% CO_2 atmosphere. Following incubation, the cells were stained with DNA staining solution for 5 min at 4 °C and the cytotoxicity was measured using CytoFLEX (Beckman Coulter) and CytExpert 2.0 software. Specific cytotoxicity was calculated on the basis of analysis of 5000 target cells and shown as percentage of positively stained cells. The results of cytotoxicity of PF-preincubated effector cells were presented in relation to control effector cells preincubated in medium alone.

4.7. Statistical Analyses

All statistical analyses and graphical presentations were performed using GraphPad Prism 8.2.0 (GraphPad Software, San Diego, CA, USA). Statistical differences between groups were calculated using the Mann–Whitney U-test or non-parametric analysis of variance (ANOVA) for paired or unpaired samples followed by post hoc multiple comparison test where applied. Differences were considered significant at least at $p < 0.05$.

Supplementary Materials: The following are available online at https://www.mdpi.com/article/10.3390/ijms22158134/s1.

Author Contributions: J.O.-T.: design of the project, sample collection, experiment conduction, data analysis, interpretation of data, writing of the manuscript, critical revision and final approval of the manuscript. A.B.: design of the project, experiment conduction, data analysis, interpretation of data, critical revision and final approval of the manuscript. A.Z.: design of the project, patients enrolment, sample collection, clinical data acquisition, data analysis, interpretation of data, critical revision and final approval of the manuscript. A.S.-I.: design of the project, sample collection, data analysis, interpretation of data, critical revision and final approval of the manuscript. I.J.: design of the project, sample collection, data analysis, interpretation of data, critical revision and final approval of the manuscript. F.D.: design of the project, patients enrolment, sample collection, clinical data acquisition, data analysis, interpretation of data, critical revision and final approval of the manuscript and of the project, experiment conduction, data analysis, interpretation of data, critical revision and final approval of the manuscript. G.K.-K.: conceptualization, investigation, methodology, writing-review & editing. E.B.: design of the project, patients enrolment, sample collection, clinical data acquisition, data analysis, interpretation of data, critical revision and final approval of the manuscript. K.B.: design of the project, experiment conduction, data analysis, interpretation of data, writing of the manuscript, critical revision and final approval of the manuscript. J.M.: design of the project, data analysis, interpretation of data, writing of the manuscript, critical revision and final approval of the manuscript. All authors have read and agreed to the published version of the manuscript.

Funding: The study was supported by the Polish National Science Centre grant no. 2014/13/B/NZ6/00806 and the 1st Faculty of Medicine, Warsaw Medical University grants 1M15/18 and 1M15/19.

Institutional Review Board Statement: The study was conducted according to the guidelines of the Declaration of Helsinki and approved by the Institutional Review Board of the Medical University of Warsaw. Informed consent was obtained from all subjects involved in the study.

Data Availability Statement: Raw data can be obtained from the corresponding author upon request.

Conflicts of Interest: The authors declare no conflict of the interest.

References

1. Zondervan, K.T.; Becker, C.M.; Missmer, S.A. Endometriosis. *N. Engl. J. Med.* **2020**, *382*, 1244–1256. [CrossRef] [PubMed]
2. Koninckx, P.R.; Ussia, A.; Adamyan, L.; Wattiez, A.; Gomel, V.; Martin, D.C. Pathogenesis of endometriosis: The genetic/epigenetic theory. *Fertil. Steril.* **2019**, *111*, 327–340. [CrossRef] [PubMed]
3. Giudice, L.C.; Kao, L.C. Endometriosis. *Lancet* **2004**, *364*, 1789–1799. [CrossRef]
4. Tomassetti, C.; D'Hooghe, T. Endometriosis and infertility: Insights into the causal link and management strategies. *Best Pract. Res. Clin. Obstet. Gynaecol.* **2018**, *51*, 25–33. [CrossRef] [PubMed]
5. Nisolle, M.; Donnez, J. Peritoneal endometriosis, ovarian endometriosis, and adenomyotic nodules of the rectovaginal septum are three different entities. *Fertil. Steril.* **1997**, *68*, 585–596. [CrossRef]
6. Garcia-Velasco, J.A.; Arici, A. Apoptosis and the pathogenesis of endometriosis. *Semin. Reprod Med.* **2003**, *21*, 165–172. [CrossRef]
7. Balkowiec, M.; Maksym, R.B.; Wlodarski, P.K. The bimodal role of matrix metalloproteinases and their inhibitors in etiology and pathogenesis of endometriosis (Review). *Mol. Med. Rep.* **2018**, *18*, 3123–3136. [CrossRef]
8. Witz, C.A. Cell adhesion molecules and endometriosis. *Semin. Reprod. Med.* **2003**, *21*, 173–182. [CrossRef]
9. Reis, F.M.; Petraglia, F.; Taylor, R.N. Endometriosis: Hormone regulation and clinical consequences of chemotaxis and apoptosis. *Hum. Reprod Update* **2013**, *19*, 406–418. [CrossRef]
10. Sciezynska, A.; Komorowski, M.; Soszynska, M.; Malejczyk, J. NK Cells as Potential Targets for Immunotherapy in Endometriosis. *J. Clin. Med.* **2019**, *8*, 1468. [CrossRef]
11. Matarese, G.; De Placido, G.; Nikas, Y.; Alviggi, C. Pathogenesis of endometriosis: Natural immunity dysfunction or autoimmune disease? *Trends Mol. Med.* **2003**, *9*, 223–228. [CrossRef]
12. Zhang, T.; De Carolis, C.; Man, G.C.W.; Wang, C.C. The link between immunity, autoimmunity and endometriosis: A literature update. *Autoimmun. Rev.* **2018**, *17*, 945–955. [CrossRef] [PubMed]
13. Riccio, L.; Santulli, P.; Marcellin, L.; Abrao, M.S.; Batteux, F.; Chapron, C. Immunology of endometriosis. *Best Pract. Res. Clin. Obstet Gynaecol.* **2018**, *50*, 39–49. [CrossRef]
14. Eisenberg, V.H.; Zolti, M.; Soriano, D. Is there an association between autoimmunity and endometriosis? *Autoimmun. Rev.* **2012**, *11*, 806–814. [CrossRef] [PubMed]
15. Berbic, M.; Fraser, I.S. Regulatory T cells and other leukocytes in the pathogenesis of endometriosis. *J. Reprod. Immunol.* **2011**, *88*, 149–155. [CrossRef]
16. Ulukus, M.; Arici, A. Immunology of endometriosis. *Minerva Ginecol.* **2005**, *57*, 237–248.
17. de Barros, I.B.L.; Malvezzi, H.; Gueuvoghlanian-Silva, B.Y.; Piccinato, C.A.; Rizzo, L.V.; Podgaec, S. What do we know about regulatory T cells and endometriosis? A systematic review. *J. Reprod. Immunol.* **2017**, *120*, 48–55. [CrossRef] [PubMed]
18. Vallve-Juanico, J.; Houshdaran, S.; Giudice, L.C. The endometrial immune environment of women with endometriosis. *Hum. Reprod Update* **2019**, *25*, 564–591. [CrossRef] [PubMed]
19. Izumi, G.; Koga, K.; Takamura, M.; Makabe, T.; Satake, E.; Takeuchi, A.; Taguchi, A.; Urata, Y.; Fujii, T.; Osuga, Y. Involvement of immune cells in the pathogenesis of endometriosis. *J. Obstet. Gynaecol. Res.* **2018**, *44*, 191–198. [CrossRef]
20. Zhou, W.J.; Yang, H.L.; Shao, J.; Mei, J.; Chang, K.K.; Zhu, R.; Li, M.Q. Anti-inflammatory cytokines in endometriosis. *Cell Mol. Life Sci.* **2019**, *76*, 2111–2132. [CrossRef]

21. Gazvani, R.; Templeton, A. Peritoneal environment, cytokines and angiogenesis in the pathophysiology of endometriosis. *Reproduction* **2002**, *123*, 217–226. [CrossRef]
22. Basta, P.; Majka, M.; Jozwicki, W.; Lukaszewska, E.; Knafel, A.; Grabiec, M.; Stasienko, E.; Wicherek, L. The frequency of CD25+CD4+ and FOXP3+ regulatory T cells in ectopic endometrium and ectopic decidua. *Reprod. Biol. Endocrinol.* **2010**, *8*, 116. [CrossRef]
23. Olkowska-Truchanowicz, J.; Bocian, K.; Maksym, R.B.; Bialoszewska, A.; Wlodarczyk, D.; Baranowski, W.; Zabek, J.; Korczak-Kowalska, G.; Malejczyk, J. CD4(+) CD25(+) FOXP3(+) regulatory T cells in peripheral blood and peritoneal fluid of patients with endometriosis. *Hum. Reprod.* **2013**, *28*, 119–124. [CrossRef]
24. Podgaec, S.; Rizzo, L.V.; Fernandes, L.F.; Baracat, E.C.; Abrao, M.S. CD4(+) CD25(high) Foxp3(+) cells increased in the peritoneal fluid of patients with endometriosis. *Am. J. Reprod. Immunol.* **2012**, *68*, 301–308. [CrossRef]
25. Khan, K.N.; Yamamoto, K.; Fujishita, A.; Muto, H.; Koshiba, A.; Kuroboshi, H.; Saito, S.; Teramukai, S.; Nakashima, M.; Kitawaki, J. Differential levels of regulatory T-cells and T-helper-17 cells in women with early and advanced endometriosis. *J. Clin. Endocrinol. Metab.* **2019**, *104*, 4715–4729. [CrossRef]
26. Sikora, J.; Smycz-Kubanska, M.; Mielczarek-Palacz, A.; Bednarek, I.; Kondera-Anasz, Z. The involvement of multifunctional TGF-beta and related cytokines in pathogenesis of endometriosis. *Immunol. Lett.* **2018**, *201*, 31–37. [CrossRef]
27. Trickett, A.; Kwan, Y.L. T cell stimulation and expansion using anti-CD3/CD28 beads. *J. Immunol. Methods* **2003**, *275*, 251–255. [CrossRef]
28. Martkamchan, S.; Onlamoon, N.; Wang, S.; Pattanapanyasat, K.; Ammaranond, P. The Effects of Anti-CD3/CD28 Coated Beads and IL-2 on Expanded T Cell for Immunotherapy. *Adv. Clin. Exp. Med.* **2016**, *25*, 821–828. [CrossRef] [PubMed]
29. Romagnani, S. T-cell subsets (Th1 versus Th2). *Ann. Allergy Asthma Immunol.* **2000**, *85*, 9–18. [CrossRef]
30. Hirahara, K.; Nakayama, T. CD4+ T-cell subsets in inflammatory diseases: Beyond the Th1/Th2 paradigm. *Int. Immunol.* **2016**, *28*, 163–171. [CrossRef] [PubMed]
31. Antsiferova, Y.S.; Sotnikova, N.Y.; Posiseeva, L.V.; Shor, A.L. Changes in the T-helper cytokine profile and in lymphocyte activation at the systemic and local levels in women with endometriosis. *Fertil. Steril.* **2005**, *84*, 1705–1711. [CrossRef]
32. Podgaec, S.; Abrao, M.S.; Dias, J.A., Jr.; Rizzo, L.V.; de Oliveira, R.M.; Baracat, E.C. Endometriosis: An inflammatory disease with a Th2 immune response component. *Hum. Reprod.* **2007**, *22*, 1373–1379. [CrossRef]
33. Borrelli, G.M.; Carvalho, K.I.; Kallas, E.G.; Mechsner, S.; Baracat, E.C.; Abrao, M.S. Chemokines in the pathogenesis of endometriosis and infertility. *J. Reprod. Immunol.* **2013**, *98*, 1–9. [CrossRef] [PubMed]
34. Deshmane, S.L.; Kremlev, S.; Amini, S.; Sawaya, B.E. Monocyte chemoattractant protein-1 (MCP-1): An overview. *J. Interferon Cytokine Res.* **2009**, *29*, 313–326. [CrossRef] [PubMed]
35. Marques, R.E.; Guabiraba, R.; Russo, R.C.; Teixeira, M.M. Targeting CCL5 in inflammation. *Expert Opin. Ther. Targets* **2013**, *17*, 1439–1460. [CrossRef] [PubMed]
36. Tokunaga, R.; Zhang, W.; Naseem, M.; Puccini, A.; Berger, M.D.; Soni, S.; McSkane, M.; Baba, H.; Lenz, H.J. CXCL9, CXCL10, CXCL11/CXCR3 axis for immune activation—A target for novel cancer therapy. *Cancer Treat Rev.* **2018**, *63*, 40–47. [CrossRef]
37. Neo, S.Y.; Lundqvist, A. The Multifaceted Roles of CXCL9 Within the Tumor Microenvironment. *Adv. Exp. Med. Biol.* **2020**, *1231*, 45–51. [CrossRef]
38. Na, Y.J.; Lee, D.H.; Kim, S.C.; Joo, J.K.; Wang, J.W.; Jin, J.O.; Kwak, J.Y.; Lee, K.S. Effects of peritoneal fluid from endometriosis patients on the release of monocyte-specific chemokines by leukocytes. *Arch. Gynecol. Obstet.* **2011**, *283*, 1333–1341. [CrossRef]
39. Berbic, M.; Hey-Cunningham, A.J.; Ng, C.; Tokushige, N.; Ganewatta, S.; Markham, R.; Russell, P.; Fraser, I.S. The role of Foxp3+ regulatory T-cells in endometriosis: A potential controlling mechanism for a complex, chronic immunological condition. *Hum. Reprod.* **2010**, *25*, 900–907. [CrossRef]
40. Braundmeier, A.; Jackson, K.; Hastings, J.; Koehler, J.; Nowak, R.; Fazleabas, A. Induction of endometriosis alters the peripheral and endometrial regulatory T cell population in the non-human primate. *Hum. Reprod.* **2012**, *27*, 1712–1722. [CrossRef]
41. Chang, K.K.; Liu, L.B.; Jin, L.P.; Zhang, B.; Mei, J.; Li, H.; Wei, C.Y.; Zhou, W.J.; Zhu, X.Y.; Shao, J.; et al. IL-27 triggers IL-10 production in Th17 cells via a c-Maf/RORgammat/Blimp-1 signal to promote the progression of endometriosis. *Cell Death Dis.* **2017**, *8*, e2666. [CrossRef]
42. Gogacz, M.; Winkler, I.; Bojarska-Junak, A.; Tabarkiewicz, J.; Semczuk, A.; Rechberger, T.; Adamiak, A. Increased percentage of Th17 cells in peritoneal fluid is associated with severity of endometriosis. *J. Reprod. Immunol.* **2016**, *117*, 39–44. [CrossRef]
43. Hirata, T.; Osuga, Y.; Hamasaki, K.; Yoshino, O.; Ito, M.; Hasegawa, A.; Takemura, Y.; Hirota, Y.; Nose, E.; Morimoto, C.; et al. Interleukin (IL)-17A stimulates IL-8 secretion, cyclooxygenase-2 expression, and cell proliferation of endometriotic stromal cells. *Endocrinology* **2008**, *149*, 1260–1267. [CrossRef] [PubMed]
44. Oosterlynck, D.J.; Meuleman, C.; Waer, M.; Koninckx, P.R.; Vandeputte, M. Immunosuppressive activity of peritoneal fluid in women with endometriosis. *Obstet. Gynecol.* **1993**, *82*, 206–212. [PubMed]
45. Guo, S.W.; Du, Y.; Liu, X. Platelet-derived TGF-beta1 mediates the down-modulation of NKG2D expression and may be responsible for impaired natural killer (NK) cytotoxicity in women with endometriosis. *Hum. Reprod.* **2016**, *31*, 1462–1474. [CrossRef]
46. Lee, K.S.; Baek, D.W.; Kim, K.H.; Shin, B.S.; Lee, D.H.; Kim, J.W.; Hong, Y.S.; Bae, Y.S.; Kwak, J.Y. IL-10-dependent down-regulation of MHC class II expression level on monocytes by peritoneal fluid from endometriosis patients. *Int. Immunopharmacol.* **2005**, *5*, 1699–1712. [CrossRef] [PubMed]

47. Wu, M.H.; Shoji, Y.; Wu, M.C.; Chuang, P.C.; Lin, C.C.; Huang, M.F.; Tsai, S.J. Suppression of matrix metalloproteinase-9 by prostaglandin E(2) in peritoneal macrophage is associated with severity of endometriosis. *Am. J. Pathol.* **2005**, *167*, 1061–1069. [CrossRef]
48. Ahmed, A.; Lotfollahzadeh, S. Cystic Teratoma. In *Treasure Island*; StatPearls Publishing (Internet Publisher): Treasure Island, FL, USA, 2021.
49. Barcz, E.; Milewski, L.; Dziunycz, P.; Kaminski, P.; Ploski, R.; Malejczyk, J. Peritoneal cytokines and adhesion formation in endometriosis: An inverse association with vascular endothelial growth factor concentration. *Fertil. Steril.* **2012**, *97*, 1380–1386.e1381. [CrossRef]
50. Milewski, L.; Dziunycz, P.; Barcz, E.; Radomski, D.; Roszkowski, P.I.; Korczak-Kowalska, G.; Kaminski, P.; Malejczyk, J. Increased levels of human neutrophil peptides 1, 2, and 3 in peritoneal fluid of patients with endometriosis: Association with neutrophils, T cells and IL-8. *J. Reprod. Immunol.* **2011**, *91*, 64–70. [CrossRef]
51. Kanamori, M.; Nakatsukasa, H.; Okada, M.; Lu, Q.; Yoshimura, A. Induced Regulatory T Cells: Their Development, Stability, and Applications. *Trends Immunol.* **2016**, *37*, 803–811. [CrossRef]
52. Sanjabi, S.; Zenewicz, L.A.; Kamanaka, M.; Flavell, R.A. Anti-inflammatory and pro-inflammatory roles of TGF-beta, IL-10, and IL-22 in immunity and autoimmunity. *Curr. Opin. Pharmacol.* **2009**, *9*, 447–453. [CrossRef]
53. Li, M.O.; Flavell, R.A. TGF-beta: A master of all T cell trades. *Cell* **2008**, *134*, 392–404. [CrossRef]
54. Li, M.O.; Flavell, R.A. Contextual regulation of inflammation: A duet by transforming growth factor-beta and interleukin-10. *Immunity* **2008**, *28*, 468–476. [CrossRef] [PubMed]
55. Lee, G.R. The Balance of Th17 versus Treg Cells in Autoimmunity. *Int. J. Mol. Sci.* **2018**, *19*, 730. [CrossRef] [PubMed]
56. Zhang, Y.; Zhang, Y.; Gu, W.; Sun, B. TH1/TH2 cell differentiation and molecular signals. *Adv. Exp. Med. Biol.* **2014**, *841*, 15–44. [CrossRef]
57. ASRM. Revised American Society for Reproductive Medicine classification of endometriosis: 1996. *Fertil. Steril.* **1997**, *67*, 817–821. [CrossRef]
58. Bocian, K.; Borysowski, J.; Wierzbicki, P.; Wyzgal, J.; Klosowska, D.; Bialoszewska, A.; Paczek, L.; Gorski, A.; Korczak-Kowalska, G. Rapamycin, unlike cyclosporine A, enhances suppressive functions of in vitro-induced CD4+CD25+ Tregs. *Nephrol. Dial. Transplant* **2010**, *25*, 710–717. [CrossRef]

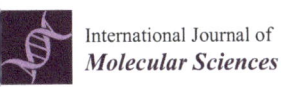

Article

BMI-1 Expression Heterogeneity in Endometriosis-Related and Non-Endometriotic Ovarian Carcinoma

Ludmila Lozneanu [1,2,†], Raluca Anca Balan [1,3,†], Ioana Păvăleanu [4], Simona Eliza Giuşcă [1,5], Irina-Draga Căruntu [1,5,*] and Cornelia Amalinei [1,6]

1. Department of Morpho-Functional Sciences I–Histology, Pathology,
"Grigore T. Popa" University of Medicine and Pharmacy, 700115 Iasi, Romania;
ludmila.lozneanu@umfiasi.ro (L.L.); raluca.balan@umfiasi.ro (R.A.B.); simonaelizagiusca@gmail.com (S.E.G.); cornelia.amalinei@umfiasi.ro (C.A.)
2. Department of Pathology, "Sf. Spiridon" County Clinical Emergency Hospital, 700111 Iasi, Romania
3. Department of Pathology, "Elena Doamna" Obstetrics and Gynecological Hospital, 700398 Iasi, Romania
4. Department of Mother and Child Medicine, "Grigore T. Popa" University of Medicine and Pharmacy, 700115 Iaşi, Romania; ipavaleanu@gmail.com
5. Department of Pathology, "Dr. C. I. Parhon" University Hospital, 700503 Iasi, Romania
6. Department of Histopathology, Institute of Legal Medicine, 700455 Iasi, Romania
* Correspondence: irinadragacaruntu@gmail.com
† These authors contributed equally to this work.

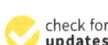

Citation: Lozneanu, L.; Balan, R.A.; Păvăleanu, I.; Giuşcă, S.E.; Căruntu, I.-D.; Amalinei, C. BMI-1 Expression Heterogeneity in Endometriosis-Related and Non-Endometriotic Ovarian Carcinoma. *Int. J. Mol. Sci.* **2021**, *22*, 6082. https://doi.org/10.3390/ijms22116082

Academic Editor: Antonio Simone Laganà

Received: 26 April 2021
Accepted: 30 May 2021
Published: 4 June 2021

Publisher's Note: MDPI stays neutral with regard to jurisdictional claims in published maps and institutional affiliations.

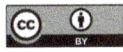

Copyright: © 2021 by the authors. Licensee MDPI, Basel, Switzerland. This article is an open access article distributed under the terms and conditions of the Creative Commons Attribution (CC BY) license (https://creativecommons.org/licenses/by/4.0/).

Abstract: BMI-1 is a key component of stem cells, which are essential for normal organ development and cell phenotype maintenance. BMI-1 expression is deregulated in cancer, resulting in the alteration of chromatin and gene transcription repression. The cellular signaling pathway that governs BMI-1 action in the ovarian carcinogenesis sequences is incompletely deciphered. In this study, we set out to analyze the immunohistochemical (IHC) BMI-1 expression in two different groups: endometriosis-related ovarian carcinoma (EOC) and non-endometriotic ovarian carcinoma (NEOC), aiming to identify the differences in its tissue profile. Methods: BMI-1 IHC expression has been individually quantified in epithelial and in stromal components by using adapted scores systems. Statistical analysis was performed to analyze the relationship between BMI-1 epithelial and stromal profile in each group and between groups and its correlation with classical clinicopathological characteristics. Results: BMI-1 expression in epithelial tumor cells was mostly low or negative in the EOC group, and predominantly positive in the NEOC group. Moreover, the stromal BMI-1 expression was variable in the EOC group, whereas in the NEOC group, stromal BMI-1 expression was mainly strong. We noted statistically significant differences between the epithelial and stromal BMI-1 profiles in each group and between the two ovarian carcinoma (OC) groups. Conclusions: Our study provides solid evidence for a different BMI-1 expression in EOC and NEOC, corresponding to the differences in their etiopathogeny. The reported differences in the BMI-1 expression of EOC and NEOC need to be further validated in a larger and homogenous cohort of study.

Keywords: ovarian cancer; endometriosis; BMI-1; epithelial tumor cells; stroma

1. Introduction

Ovarian cancer (OC) is a gynecological malignancy that commonly originates from the ovaries, fallopian tubes, and peritoneum [1] and is considered as the most lethal malignancy with a high rate of chemoresistance and relapses. Regarding their histology, 90% of ovarian tumors are of the epithelial type [2].

Endometriosis represents a precursor lesion for certain types of epithelial OC, being related to microenvironment changes (such as estrogen production and dependency, progesterone resistance, and inflammation), which lead to genetic alterations and/or genetic susceptibilities that favour endometriosis-associated ovarian carcinogenesis [2–4]. It has been demonstrated that ovarian endometriosis, ovarian atypical endometriosis, and endometriosis-related OC (EOC) share the same genetic alterations and express clonality, while the ovarian malignant endometriosis-associated phenotype is promoted by chronic inflammation, which provides permanent mutations and nonpermanent cytokine production [2]. The different clinicopathological features and distinct mutational statuses justify the classification of OC into EOC, represented mainly by clear cell and endometrioid subtypes, and non-endometriotic OC (NEOC) [5].

OC is commonly diagnosed in advanced stages III and IV when the tumor has a high potential of metastasis [6]. Therefore, the early detection of OC by using different biomarkers is an important clinical desideration. Concomitantly, the researchers' interest is directed towards a deep insight into the genetic and molecular substrate of ovarian carcinogenesis, aiming not only to understand the sequence of carcinogenic events, but also to identify new potential prognostic factors and therapeutic targets. The exclusive recent list of potential candidate biomarkers includes molecules expressed by the cancer stem and stem-like cells [7], BMI-1 protein being one of them [8,9]. BMI-1 protein, a stem-like marker, represents a homologue of the *Drosophila polycomb* group of proteins, and its role is the regulation of homeotic genes expression by transcription repression [10]. The BMI-1 gene has been initially isolated as an oncogene, which cooperates with c-Myc in lymphoma experimental models [11]. It belongs to the Polycomb-group (PcG) of proteins, which are involved in axial pattern establishment, hematopoiesis, cementogenesis, and senescence [11].

Considering BMI-1's involvement in cellular proliferation and tumor progression, this gene has been identified, as expected, in a large variety of human tumors, such as: lymphoma [12–14], brain [15], prostate [16], oropharynx and nasopharynx [10,17,18], breast [19,20], bladder [11], gastric [21], pancreas [22], esophagus [23], lungs [24,25], head and neck cancers [26], malignant melanoma [27], pleomorphic adenoma [28], and also displaying a prognosis value in mielodysplastic syndromes [29] and in gallbladder cancer [30]. Although its action has been initially thought to be achieved by p16 suppressor gene repression, subsequent studies have demonstrated another specific mechanism of action by intercellular adhesion pathway modulation [31].

Limited information is available about BMI-1 in OC, as few studies address this topic, mainly providing experimental evidences [10,32–41]. BMI-1 increased expression mirrors an early and maybe reversible event in carcinogenesis [10], suggestive for an invasive and aggressive phenotype during tumor development [10,42]. It is demonstrated that BMI-1 regulates cell cycle and promotes cell proliferation, which has self-renewal and differentiation potential [9], acts as a potential modulator of cellular adhesion in endometriotic tumor cells, and alters endometrial stromal cells by changing microenvironment interactions in OC [43]. Several results support its potential value as an independent predictor for poor outcomes [39] and as a possible new therapeutic target in chemoresistant OC [7,9,33,40,41].

Currently, there is a high interest in a better understanding and characterization of EOC, in an attempt to provide a different clinical and therapeutic management compared to that of NEOC. In this regard, the purpose of our study was to evaluate the immunohistochemical (IHC) BMI-1 expression in two different groups of OC (associated or not with endometriosis), aiming to identify the differences in its tissue profile. The novelty of this research consisted in a double assessment of BMI-1, in tumor epithelial cells and stromal cells, following the potentiation relationship of these two cell types in tumor progression. Nevertheless, the BMI-1 expression was correlated with clinicopathological data that offer a solid functional image of the tumor progression.

2. Results

2.1. BMI-1 Expression—Qualitative Assessment

The qualitative evaluation showed, at a glance, a heterogeneous expression in both groups, without a specific pattern for each group.

A double BMI-1 staining was found: a nuclear and cytoplasmic/membrane immunoexpression in EOC group. Strong expression of epithelial cells was observed in cases with poor prognosis, such as high-grade serous and endometrioid carcinomas (HGSCs and HGECs), as well in clear cell ovarian carcinomas (COCs). A negative BMI-1 stroma expression in the endometrioid phenotype of EOC group was found, while positive stroma was dominant in the serous phenotype, clear cell and mixed subtypes. Relevant aspects of BMI-1 expression in EOC are presented in Figure 1.

In the NEOC group, the intensity of BMI-1 was predominantly moderate or strong in epithelial (nuclear or cytoplasmic/membrane immunoexpression) and stromal cells. Moderate and strong nuclear expression and weaker cytoplasmic expression was observed in cases with a serous phenotype and a more aggressive course, such as HGSC, while the endometrioid phenotype preserved a strong, diffuse, membrane BMI-1 staining. In undifferentiated carcinomas, BMI-1 expression was heterogeneous, displaying a weak cytoplasmic staining. Differences between BMI-1 expression in variable types of NEOC are illustrated in Figure 2.

We also noted the lack of BMI-1 expression in normal ovary or ovarian surface, and its positivity in the normal tubal surface epithelium.

2.2. BMI Expression—Semi-Quantitative Assessment

In the whole group of study, without division into EOC and NEOC categories, the BMI-1 semi-quantitative assessment showed the following: a high expression in 31 cases (65.96%) and a low expression in 16 cases (34.04%), in tumor cells, along with immunopositivity in 34 cases (72.34%), and immunonegativity in 13 cases (27.65%) in tumor stroma. The statistical analysis revealed significant correlations between BMI-1 expression in epithelial tumor cells (low/high) versus tumor stroma (negative/positive) ($p = 0.01$).

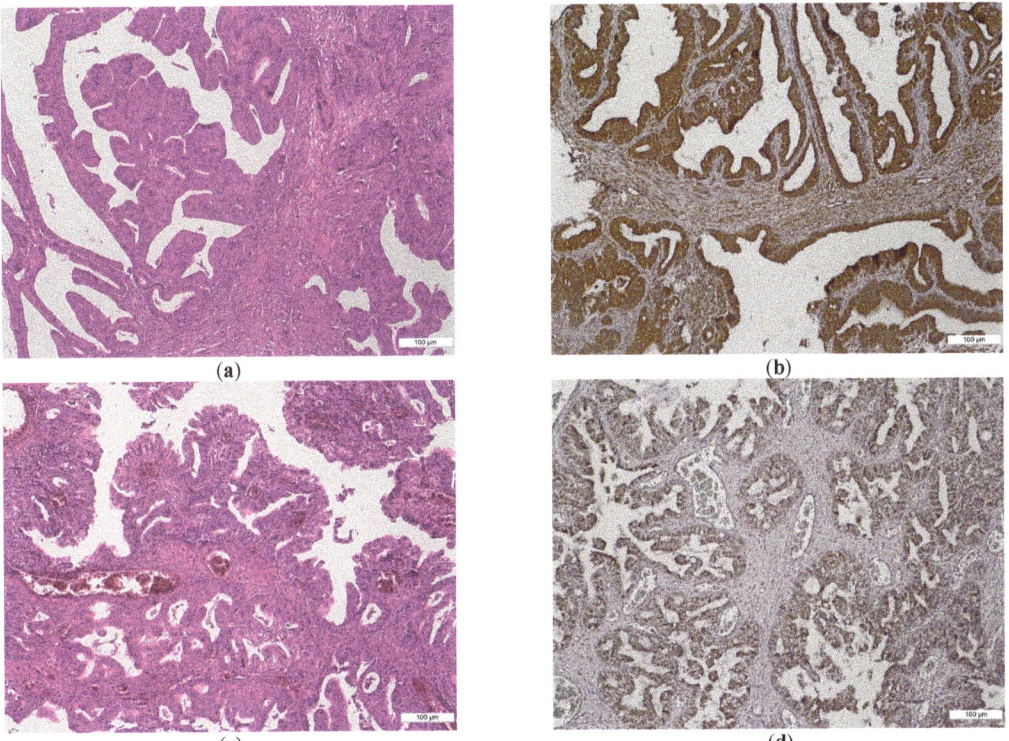

Figure 1. Cont.

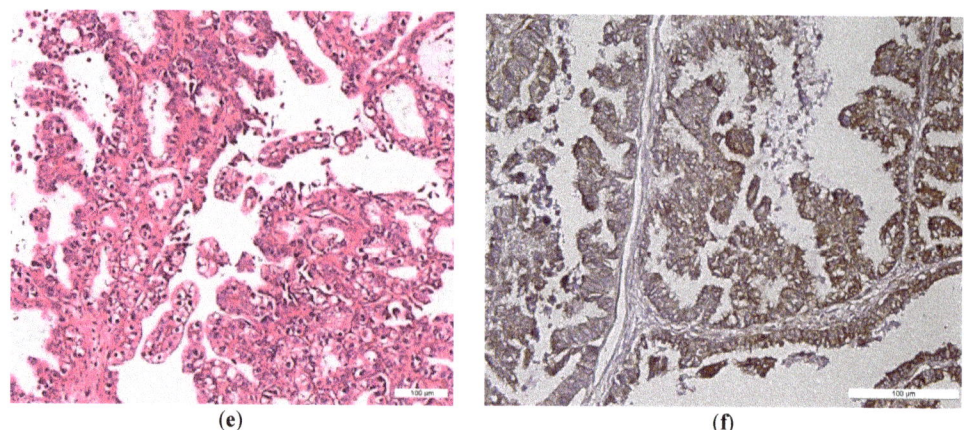

Figure 1. (**a**–**f**) Histologic features and BMI-1 expression in EOC group in different ovarian tumor subtypes: (**a**,**b**) HGSC: (**a**) papillary growth, enlarged and irregular nuclei, prominent nucleoli, high cellular size and shape (hematoxylin and eosin–H&E, magnification 10×), (**b**) strong BMI-1 nuclear staining in epithelial tumor cells of HGSC (magnification 10×); (**c**,**d**) HGEC: (**c**) crowded back-to-back glands, lined by atypical columnar epithelium, and smooth luminal borders (H&E, magnification 10×), (**d**) weak BMI-1 cytoplasmic staining in epithelial tumor cells of HGEC (magnification 10×); (**e**,**f**) COC: (**e**) papillary and tubulocystic pattern, combined with clear and eosinophilic cells and stromal hyalinization (H&E, magnification 10×), (**f**) strong BMI-1 cytoplasmic staining of tumor cells and stroma in COC (magnification 10×).

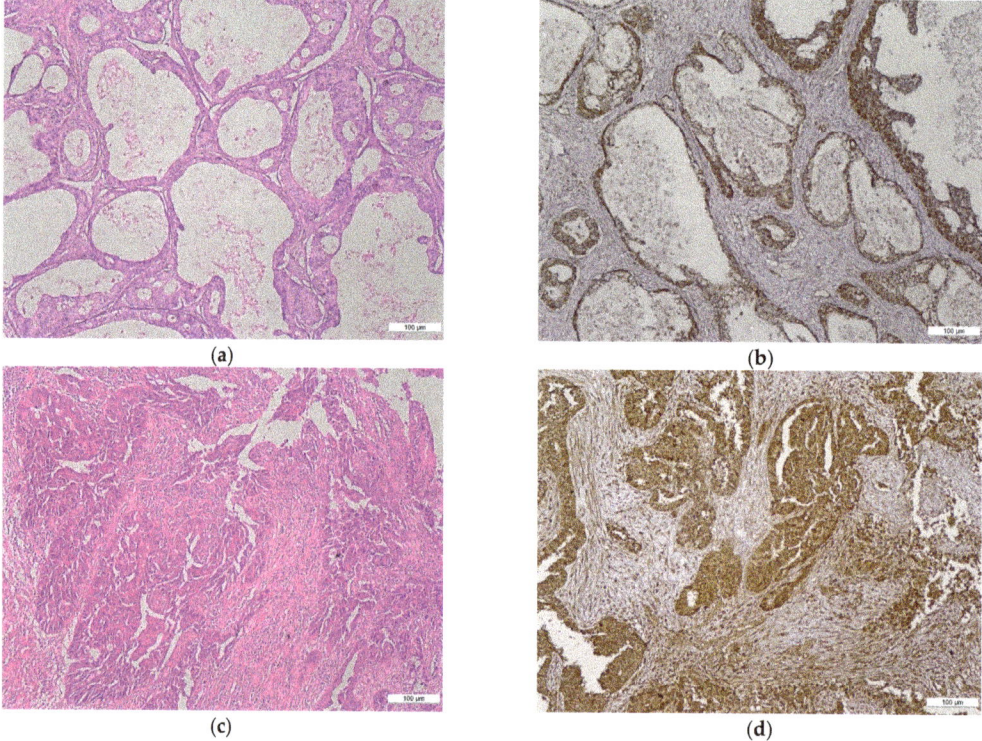

Figure 2. *Cont.*

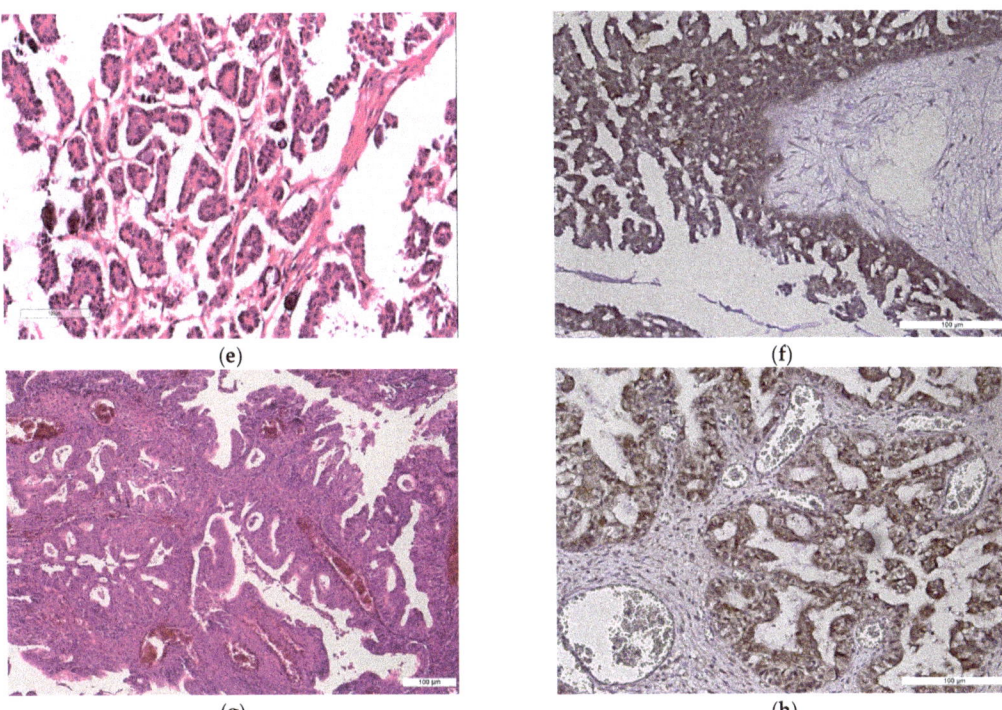

Figure 2. (**a–h**) Histologic features and BMI-1 expression in NEOC group in different ovarian tumor subtypes: (**a,b**) MOC: (**a**) atypical mucin-producing tumor cells with an infiltrative pattern of invasion (H&E, magnification 10×), (**b**) negative BMI-1 staining in tumor stroma of MOC (magnification 10x); (**c,d**) HGSC: (**c**) variation in cellular size and shape, marked nuclear atypia, dense fibrous stroma, and inflammation around the tumor nests (H&E, magnification 10×), (**d**) strong BMI-1 cytoplasmic staining of tumor stroma in HGSC (magnification 10×); (**e,f**) LGSC: (**e**) micropapillary growth with minimal nuclear atypia in LGSC (H&E, magnification 10×), (**f**) moderate BMI-1 cytoplasmic staining of tumor cells and stroma in LGSC (magnification 10×); (**g,h**) LGEC: (**g**) papillary and glandular differentiation in LGEC (H&E, magnification 10×), (**h**) strong BMI-1 cytoplasmic staining of tumor cells and stroma in LGEC (magnification 10×).

The semi-quantitative expression of BMI-1 showed a different profile in the two analyzed groups.

BMI-1 expression in epithelial tumor cells was mostly low or negative in the EOC group and predominantly positive in NEOC group. On the other hand, the cases of the EOC group expressed positive and negative stromal BMI-1 immunoreactions approximately equally, whereas the stromal BMI-1 expression was mainly strong in the NEOC group (Table 1). We noted statistically significant differences between the BMI-1 epithelial and stromal profiles in each group (Table 1).

Comparing the epithelial and stromal BMI-1 expressions between the EOC and NEOC groups, we obtained statistically significant differences only for the epithelial component ($p = 0.0002$), not for the stromal one ($p = 0.06$).

2.3. Relationship between BMI-1 Epithelial and Stromal Expression, and Clinicopathological Parameters in EOC

The results of the statistical analysis revealed a significant relationship between BMI-1 expression in tumor cells (low/high) and tumor grade (well and moderately differentiated versus poorly differentiated) ($p = 0.04$). On the other hand, stromal BMI-1 expression was significantly correlated with the median value of cancer antigen 125 (CA 125) ($p = 0.03$). No other significant differences were registered (Table 2).

Table 1. Correlations between the epithelial and stromal BMI-1 expression in the EOC and the NEOC groups.

BMI-1	EOC			NEOC		
	High Score/ Positive Reaction	Low Score/ Negative Reaction	p Value	High Score/ Positive Reaction	Low Score/ Negative Reaction	p Value
Epithelial tumor cells	5 (26.31%)	14 (73.68%)	0.04	26 (92.85%)	2 (7.14%)	0.001
Stromal cells	11 (57.89%)	8 (42.10%)		23 (82.14%)	5 (17.85%)	

Table 2. Correlations between BMI-1 expression in tumoral cells and clinicopathological parameters—EOC group.

Clinicopathological Characteristics	#	Tumor Cells BMI-1				p Value	Stromal BMI-1				p Value
		Low Score		High Score			Negative Reaction		Positive Reaction		
		#	%	#	%		#	%	#	%	
Age											
<55 age	8	5	62.5	3	37.5	0.34	4	50	4	50	0.55
≥55 age	11	9	81.82	2	18.18		4	36.36	7	63.64	
Tumor stage											
1	4	4	100	0	0	0.48	1	25	3	75	0.55
2	6	4	66.66	2	33.33		3	50	3	50	
3	8	5	62.50	3	37.50		3	37.50	5	62.50	
4	1	1	100	0	0		1	100	0	0	
Tumor grade											
I/II	7	7	100	0	0	0.04	4	57.14	3	42.85	0.31
III	12	7	58.33	5	41.66		4	33.33	8	66.66	
Histological subtype											
LGSC	0	0	0	0	0	0.78	0	0	0	0	0.93
LGEC	0	0	0	0	0		0	0	0	0	
COC	4	3	75	1	25		1	25	3	75	
MOC	0	0	0	0	0		0	0	0	0	
HGSC	3	1	33.33	2	66.66		1	33.33	2	66.66	
HGEC	8	6	75	2	25		5	62.50	3	37.50	
Undifferentiated	0	0	0	0	0		0	0	0	0	
Mixed	4	4	100	0	0		1	25	3	75	
Type											
Type I	4	3	75	1	25	0.94	1	25	3	75	0.57
Type II	15	11	73.33	4	26.67		7	46.67	8	53.33	
Residual disease											
NED/<1 cm	6	5	83.33	1	16.67	0.51	2	33.33	4	66.67	0.59
≥1 cm	13	9	69.23	4	30.77		6	46.15	7	53.85	
CA 125—median value											
<1201.5 U/mL	10	8	80	2	20	0.51	2	20	8	80	0.03
≥1201.5 U/mL	9	6	66.67	3	33.33		6	66.67	3	33.33	

LGSC (low-grade serous carcinoma); LGEC (low-grade endometrioid carcinoma); COC (clear cell ovarian carcinoma); MOC (mucinous ovarian carcinoma); HGSC (high-grade serous carcinoma); HGEC (high-grade endometrioid carcinoma); NED (no evident data about residual tumor).

2.4. Relationship between BMI-1 Epithelial and Stromal Expression and Clinicopathological Parameters in NEOC

The statistical analysis showed significant correlations between BMI-1 expression in the tumor cells (low/high), the stroma (negative/positive), and the tumor histological subtypes ($p = 0.002$ and $p = 0.04$, respectively) (Table 3). No associations were found for the other clinical clinicopathological parameters.

Table 3. Correlations between BMI-1 expression in tumor stroma and clinicopathological parameters—NEOC group.

Clinicopathological Characteristics	#	Tumor Cells BMI-1				p Value	Stromal BMI-1				p Value
		Low Score		High Score			Negative Reaction		Positive Reaction		
		#	%	#	%		#	%	#	%	
Age											
<55 age	14	1	7.14	13	92.86	0.30	2	14.29	12	85.71	0.62
≥55 age	14	1	7.14	13	92.86		3	21.43	11	78.57	
Tumor stage											
1	13	1	7.69	12	92.30	0.91	3	23.07	10	76.92	0.71
2	5	0	0	5	100		0	0	5	100	
3	10	1	10	9	90		2	20	8	80	
4	0	0	0	0	0		0	0	0	0	
Tumor grade											
I/II	15	0	0	15	100	0.11	3	20	12	80	0.75
III	13	2	15.38	11	84.61		2	15.38	11	84.61	
Histological subtype											
LGSC	4	0	0	4	100	0.002	0	0	4	100	0.04
LGEC	5	0	0	5	100		3	60	2	40	
COC	5	0	0	5	100		0	0	5	100	
MOC	5	1	20	4	80		1	20	4	80	
HGSC	5	0	0	5	100		0	0	5	100	
HGEC	3	0	0	3	100		0	0	3	100	
Undifferentiated	1	1	100	0	0		1	100	0	0	
Mixed	0	0	0	0	0		0	0	0	0	
Type											
Type I	19	1	5.26	18	94.74	0.57	4	21.05	15	78.95	0.43
Type II	9	1	11.11	8	88.89		0	0	9	100	
Residual disease											
NED/<1 cm	16	1	6.25	15	93.75	0.83	2	12.5	14	87.5	0.72
≥1 cm	12	1	8.33	11	91.67		1	8.33	11	91.67	
CA 125—median value											
<101	14	1	7.14	13	92.86	1	4	28.57	10	71.43	0.13
≥101	14	1	7.14	13	92.30		1	7.14	13	92.86	

LGSC (low-grade serous carcinoma); LGEC (low-grade endometrioid carcinoma); COC (clear cell ovarian carcinoma); MOC (mucinous ovarian carcinoma); HGSC (high-grade serous carcinoma); HGEC (high-grade endometrioid carcinoma); NED (no evident data about residual tumor).

3. Discussion

Numerous hypotheses regarding the mechanisms involved in OC etiopathogenesis have been proposed over time as attempts to explain the multiple tumor phenotypes, poor prognosis, and chemoresistance. Endometriosis represents a precursor lesion for certain types of epithelial OC, since the identification of the same genetic alterations in both diseases are demonstrated [3,4,31]. Accordingly, the corroboration of specific clinicopathological findings with specific mutations led to the EOC and NEOC categories distinction [44].

The BMI-1 protein, involved in homeotic genes regulation by transcription inhibition [10], represents a survival factor of malignant stem cells [10], and is correlated to hormonal receptor expression, and is considered as a prognosis factor surrogate [44,45].

BMI-1 has been identified in experimental studies of OC (cell lines, clone derivation, and animal experiments) [32–38], both in protein and the protein-coding gene [39], and in human ovarian tumors or ascites fluid samples [10,32,34,36,39,46,47]. Despite these reported results, BMI-1 expression is not fully established in OC. The review of the literature shows that less than 10 studies have addressed BMI-1's involvement in OC, most of them highlighting the molecular action and potential therapeutic value of this protein. A positive correlation between BMI-1 positive expression in human epithelial OC and elevated telomerase activity was demonstrated [46,47]. Another study, based on human specimens and ovarian cancer cells, showed that BMI-1 expression is downregulated by MiR-15a or MiR-16 underexpression, with subsequent significant decreases in cell proliferation and clonal growth [40]. Therefore, BMI-1 seems to be a potential target in OC therapy. Eloquent evidences in this direction are provided in recent papers that have demonstrated the therapeutic activity of PTC-028 as a novel inhibitor of BMI-1 function in OC [37] and the role of MiR-132 in cisplatin resistance and OC metastasis by the targeted regulation of BMI-1 [41]. In terms of the number of human OC samples, the studies on BMI-1 have been generally performed on small groups, with a median number of research sample of 41 (range 5–179) [10,32,34,36,40,46,47]. These samples were collected from tumor tissue [10,32,34,36,39,40,46,47], fresh ascites [34], and frozen ovarian tissues [47].

The reported data target only BMI-1 in epithelial tumor cells, showing a high expression in 80.9% of OC and its relationship with tumor aggressiveness [46]. Moreover, a positive correlation between BMI-1 expression and advanced International Federation of Gynecology and Obstetrics (FIGO) stages, bilaterality, higher tumor grades, and serous morphology [42,47], and a progressive incremental number of BMI-1-positive cases in accordance with the increase of tumor grade and stage were demonstrated, while increased BMI-1 expression was associated with reduced patient survival [39].

This short review of data concerning the correlation between BMI-1 and OC shows that the current knowledge is predominantly based on experimental data as the first level of evidence regarding its role in carcinogenesis, while the results obtained by the investigation of BMI-1 in human tissues is very scarce. Within this general context, our study complements the knowledge on BMI-1 in OC by doing research that translates the evidences level from the experimental area to the clinical domain by reference to the clinicopathological characteristics of OC with different parameters for EOC and NEOC.

Our work has demonstrated high BMI-1 expression levels in the epithelial tumor cells in 66% of OC (26% in EOC and 93% in NEOC). Moreover, our study provides valuable data on BMI-1 profile in OC, bringing to the foreground the relationship of OC with endometriosis, and the differences between the epithelial and stromal expression. This endeavor was possible by consistent differences in the design of the patient's cohort, comprising 47 cases of OC separated in two different tumor groups: EOC and NEOC. Thus, we have demonstrated, for the first time, the possible correlations between epithelial and stromal BMI-1 profiles in EOC and NEOC and several classical clinicopathological parameters.

The segregation into EOC and NEOC has been justified by the findings that certain histological types of EOC, mainly endometrioid and clear cell carcinomas, have different clinical features, such as younger age at diagnosis, unilaterality, identification at an earlier stage, and a better survival rate, compared to the counterpart entities of NEOC [5]. Our study supports the hypothesis of EOC development within endometriosis, showing mostly an endometrioid (42% in EOC versus 28.57% in NEOC) or clear cell phenotype (21% in EOC versus 18% in NEOC), and, implicitly, the quality of precursor lesion of ovarian endometriosis. Endometriosis and EOC represent two entities with the same target organ (ovary), the same tissue of origin (endometrial-like), and the same pathogenic mechanism which progresses from benign to atypical and malignant phenotypes. Having these in mind, tubal ligature or salpingectomy may be used as preventative maneuvers which may be applied within a screening and early therapy algorithm.

An original finding in our research is the dual staining pattern, nuclear and cytoplasmic/membrane in both study groups, although only a nuclear staining is reported in literature [27,41,42,48]. This immunostaining pattern may indicate a possible relocation of protein during the transition to tumor phenotype. Moreover, it may suggest the involvement of additional factors as a possible reflection of adhesion molecules interrelationship in the context of epithelial mesenchymal transition (EMT) [27,48] or of the involvement of variable ovarian microenvironmental factors in both EOC and NEOC.

Our study confirms the relationship between BMI-1 in epithelial tumor cells and stroma in three instances: (i) in the general OC group ($p = 0.01$), (ii) in the NEOC group ($p = 0.001$), and (iii) in the EOC group ($p = 0.04$). In parallel, the comparative analysis of BMI-1 expression in EOC and NEOC showed a statistically significant higher expression of BMI-1 in the epithelial tumor component than in the stroma ($p = 0.0002$). Our results clearly show EOC's association with BMI-1 low expression in epithelial tumor cells without a dominant expression profile in stromal cells, while NEOC is characterized by high BMI-1 expression in both the epithelial and stromal types of cells. However, stromal BMI-1 expression is reflecting EMT involvement in tumor progression and the interrelationship between the two cellular components, which result in BMI-1 synthesis as a stromal-dependent mechanism. Therefore, if present, stromal BMI-1 could be considered as a valuable marker for poor survival.

To the best of our knowledge, our study provides for the first time evidence for BMI-1 expression in human EOC. Differently from NEOC group findings, a progressive gain of BMI-1 expression in epithelial tumor cells has been noticed in the EOC group along with tumor grade, with statistically significant differences when we compared well and moderately differentiated with poorly differentiated tumors. This finding indicates a relationship between BMI-1 epithelial overexpression and a poorer prognosis in the selected EOC cases. Currently, CA125, expressed in the embryonic development of ovaries and re-expressed in endometriosis and ovarian neoplasms, can be used as a prognostic and predictive biomarker related to patient survival, independent of OC treatment [48].

CA 125 shows significant different values in the two major types of OC, suggesting that they occur as a result of different factors, following specific pathway initiations and progressions [49]. Many studies have shown that the CA125 profiles of HGSC and HGEC are different from other subtypes [50]. We also found a statistically significant correlation between stromal BMI-1 and CA 125 level, suggesting that EOC may be influenced by a microenvironment modulation specific for endometriosis-based ovarian carcinomas, supporting the rapid growth pattern and the unfavorable prognosis in a subcategory of cases. Thus, we may conclude that the interrelationship and reciprocal stimulation between a tumor's epithelial and stromal components occurs latter during the endometriosis-related carcinogenic process, with a subsequent uptake of BMI-1 expression by stromal component, which may be reflected in an increased CA-125 level. The aggressive behavior of these EOC cases has a different significance from that of aggressive type I OC, probably originating from fallopian tube epithelium. It is worth mentioning that BMI-1 was absent in the normal ovaries or ovarian surface in the study groups, while BMI-1 expression has been identified in the normal tubal surface epithelium; this finding comports with the hypothesis of some OCs development from the fallopian tube, providing another support for this pathogenic mechanism.

On the other hand, in the NEOC group, we have shown statistically significant differences between BMI-1 immunopositivity in the tumor's epithelial cells, stromal cells, and histological subtypes. In our opinion, these results may be considered as solid evidence for the association of BMI-1 with high grade OC phenotypes and, consequently, with tumor aggressiveness.

Overall, our study reveals a different BMI-1 profile in the EOC an NEOC groups, thus underlying the differences in their etiopathogeny. We are aware of the limitations of our study due to the small size of the study groups and their heterogeneity in histological types, as the selection criteria have been strictly applied. Despite these limitations, our results open promising perspectives for differentiation of EOC from NEOC that need to be further validated in a larger and homogenous cohort of study. An interesting research item can be directed to the high-grade serous phenotype of OC that may be further subdivided into subcategories according to their affiliation to the EOC or to NEOC groups.

4. Materials and Methods

4.1. Patients

Our study group included 47 cases of OC, diagnosed between 2006 and 2017 and treated in several hospitals of Iasi, Romania: "Sf. Spiridon" County Clinical Emergency Hospital, "Cuza Vodă" and "Elena Doamna" Obstetrics and Gynecological Hospitals, and Oncology Regional Institute. All cases were histopathologically reassessed by two pathologists to ascertain the OC histological subtype and then divided into two groups: EOC and NEOC. The study has been approved by the Ethics Committee of "Grigore T. Popa" University of Medicine and Pharmacy, Iași, based on the patients' informed consent (12378/June 2015). All subjects who provided ovarian tissue had given written and informed consent prior the surgery.

4.1.1. Clinicopathological and Tumor Serum Marker Profile of the Study Cohort

At the time of the diagnosis, the age of the patients ranged between 37 and 76 years old: 22 patients were younger (<55 years old) and 25 patients were older ($\geq$55 years old).

Based on the standards of the FIGO staging, 17 cases were staged as FIGO stage I, 11 cases as FIGO stage II, 18 cases as FIGO stage III, and 1 case FIGO stage IV. According to tumor grade, 13 cases were graded as G1 (well differentiated), 9 cases as G2 (moderately differentiated), and 25 cases as G3 (poorly differentiated or undifferentiated). The distribution of OC histological variants was as follows: LGSC—4 cases; LGEC—5 cases; COC—9 cases; MOC—5 cases; HGSC—8 cases; HGEC—11 cases; undifferentiated—1 case; and mixed tumor (serous, endometrioid, and clear cells phenotypes)—4 cases. According to the pathogenic classification, the cases have been divided in low-grade (type I; 23 cases) and high-grade (type II; 24 cases). The histopathological exam revealed the tumor extension (residual tumor after primary surgery) in 25 cases (residual tumor $\geq$ 1 cm), with 13 patients diagnosed with a residual tumor < 1 cm and 9 cases without evident data about a residual tumor. Preoperatory CA125 levels higher than 35 U/mL were found in all cases comprised in the study group, ranging between 46–4163 U/mL.

4.1.2. Clinicopathological and Tumor Serum Marker Profile of the EOC and NEOC Groups

In the whole group, 19 of 47 (40%) patients belonged to the EOC group and 28 patients (60%) belonged to the NEOC group.

Cases included in the EOC group were characterized by the presence of associate endometriotic lesions consisting of the endometriosis area in the form of an endometriotic cyst lined with endometrial epithelium and endometrial stroma, as well as evidence of hemosiderin deposits and chronic hemorrhage or proliferative endometriosis foci with a well-developed glandular profile.

The mean age of patients was 59.10 $\pm$ 8.66 years in the EOC group and 56.57 $\pm$ 2.64 years in the NEOC group. The EOC group comprised the following histological types: COC—4 cases; HGSC—3 cases; HGEC—8 cases; mixed tumors—4 cases; and none of LGSC, LGEC, MOC, or undifferentiated carcinoma cases were classified as EOC. The histological types in NEOC group were: LGSC—4 cases; LGEC—5 cases; COC—5 cases; HGEC—3 cases; MOC—5 cases; HGSC—5 cases; and undifferentiated—1 case. The median value of the preoperatory CA 125 level in the EOC group was 1201.5 U/mL, while a median value of 101 U/mL was found in the NEOC group.

4.2. Immunohistochemistry (IHC)

The immunohistochemical staining for the identification of Antigens has been achieved using BenchMark XT automatic system (Ventana Medical System, Inc., Tucson, AZ, USA), according to protocols that needed standardization for different types of antibodies. The sections obtained from the selected paraffin-embedded blocks were dewaxed in xylene, rehydrated in ethanol, and rinsed in distilled water. The antigen retrieval was made by using the Heat-Induced Epitope Retrieval (HIER) procedure, with an antigen retrieval solution of pH 9 using CC1 solution (Ventana Medical System, Tucson, AZ, USA), consisting of a combination of ethylenediaminetetraacetic and boric acid diluted in Tris buffer for 30—60 minutes. After the endogenous peroxidase blocking with 3% hydrogen peroxide and treatment with normal goat serum 10%, used to block the non-specific protein bonds, the sections were incubated with the primary antibody BMI-1 (clone F6/ABCAM, 1/50 dilution, Abcam, Cambridge, MA, USA). Consequently, the incubation with Ultra-Vision Quanto Detection System Horseradish peroxidase (HRP) (Igs; Ventana Medical Systems) has been performed. Antigen-antibody reaction has been visualized using 3,3'-Diaminobenzidine as a chromogen (UltraView, Ventana Medical Systems, Tucson, AZ, USA). The counterstaining of the sections was done with Mayer's Hematoxylin. After counterstaining, the slides have been washed with liquid soap in order to eliminate the oily film, they have been rinsed with taping water and have been also bathed twice in distilled water. Negative controls have been used for results interpretation, in which primary antibodies have been skipped and replaced with distilled water and positive controls have been considered as endothelial cells and stromal fibroblasts immunostaining.

4.3. Semi-Quantitative Assessment

BMI-1 expression has been individually quantified in the epithelial and in the stromal components. The semi-quantitative assessment of the BMI-1 in tumor cells was done by using adapted scores based on literature reports [27,51] that took into account the staining intensity (I) and the percentage of positive cells (P). BMI-1 showed a double immunostaining, nuclear, and cytoplasmic/membrane [27,51]. The intensity of BMI-1 immunoreaction was scored as: 0—absent, 1—weak, 2—moderate, and 3—strong. The percentage of BMI-1 positive cells was scored as follows: 1—< 10%, 2—10–50%, 3—> 50%. The final BMI-1 score was obtained by multiplying P by I. BMI-1 score values < 3 were considered as a low score, and score values ≥ 3 were considered as a high score.

For the semi-quantitative assessment of stromal BMI-1, we used a standard 2-point scale scoring system. The immunoreaction was considered negative when $\leq 10\%$ of the tumor stromal area had a positive immunostaining of BMI-1, and positive when > 10% of the stromal area showed BMI-1 immunostaining, regardless of the level of staining intensity.

BMI-1 expression has been independently evaluated and scored by three histopathologists with experience in immunohistochemistry interpretation and scoring differences have been revised in the evaluation panel in order to reach a consensus.

4.4. Statistical Analysis

Statistical analysis was carried out with Statistical Package for the Social Sciences (SPSS) v. 19 program (SPSS Inc., IBM Corporation, Chicago, IL, USA). A Chi-square (χ^2) test was performed to analyze the differences in BMI-1 epithelial and stromal profile in each group and between groups, and its relationship with classical clinicopathological characteristics (age, tumor stage, grade, histological subtype, tumorigenic dualistic tumor types, residual disease, and preoperatory CA 125 level). Yates' correction was applied when the number of cases in a subgroup was lower than five. Statistical significance was considered when $p < 0.05$.

5. Conclusions

Our study provides solid evidence for a different BMI-1 expression in EOC and NEOC, corresponding to the differences in their etiopathogeny. The EOCs were largely characterized by a low BMI-1 expression in epithelial tumor cells, without a dominant expression profile in stromal cells. Epithelial BMI-1 is progressively increased alongside the tumor grade and strong stromal BMI-1 may be correlated to microenvironment modulation, supporting the rapid growth pattern and the recognized poor prognosis in a subcategory of EOC cases. The NEOCs were characterized by high BMI-1 expression in both the epithelial and stromal types of cells; therefore, BMI-1 expression could be regarded as an indicator of aggressiveness of this type of malignancies in general, and for HGSC in particular. Additionally, BMI-1 expression limited to the normal tubal surface epithelium and its lack in normal germinal/surface ovarian epithelium may support the hypothesis that many OCs are originating from the fallopian tube epithelium.

Nevertheless, the reported differences in BMI-1 expression in EOC and NEOC need to be further validated in a larger and homogenous cohort of study.

Author Contributions: Conceptualization, L.L., C.A. and I.-D.C.; methodology, L.L., R.A.B. and S.E.G.; software, R.A.B.; validation, L.L., C.A., S.E.G. and R.A.B.; investigation, L.L., R.A.B. and I.P.; writing—original draft preparation, L.L. and R.A.B.; writing—review and editing, C.A.; supervision, I.-D.C. All authors have read and agreed to the published version of the manuscript.

Funding: No funding was received for this study.

Institutional Review Board Statement: The study was conducted according to the guidelines of the Declaration of Helsinki, and approved by the Ethics Committee of the "Grigore T. Popa" University of Medicine and Pharmacy, Iași (12378/June 2015).

Informed Consent Statement: Informed consent was obtained from all subjects involved in the study.

Data Availability Statement: The data used to support the findings of this study are available upon request to the authors.

Conflicts of Interest: The authors declare no conflict of interest.

References

1. Bray, F.; Ferlay, J.; Soerjomataram, I.; Siegel, R.L.; Torre, L.A.; Jemal, A. Global Cancer Statistics 2018: GLOBOCAN Estimates of Incidence and Mortality Worldwide for 36 Cancers in 185 Countries. *CA Cancer J. Clin.* **2018**, *68*, 394–424. [CrossRef]
2. Wei, J.-J.; William, J.; Bulun, S. Endometriosis and Ovarian Cancer: A Review of Clinical, Pathologic, and Molecular Aspects. *Int. J. Gynecol. Pathol.* **2011**, *30*, 553–568. [CrossRef] [PubMed]
3. Laganà, A.S.; Vitale, S.G.; Salmeri, F.M.; Triolo, O.; Ban Frangež, H.; Vrtačnik-Bokal, E.; Stojanovska, L.; Apostolopoulos, V.; Granese, R.; Sofo, V. Unus pro Omnibus, Omnes pro Uno: A Novel, Evidence-Based, Unifying Theory for the Pathogenesis of Endometriosis. *Med. Hypotheses* **2017**, *103*, 10–20. [CrossRef]
4. Herreros-Villanueva, M.; Chen, C.-C.; Tsai, E.-M.; Er, T.-K. Endometriosis-Associated Ovarian Cancer: What Have We Learned so Far? *Clin. Chim. Acta* **2019**, *493*, 63–72. [CrossRef] [PubMed]
5. Brilhante, A.; Augusto, K.; Portela, M.; Sucupira, L.C.; Oliveira, L.A.; Pouchaim, A.J.; Mesquita Nóbrega, L.R.; de Magalhães, T.F.; Sobreira, L.R. Endometriosis and Ovarian Cancer: An Integrative Review (Endometriosis and Ovarian Cancer). *APJCP* **2017**, *18*. [CrossRef]
6. Vargas, A.N. Natural History of Ovarian Cancer. *Ecancermedicalscience* **2014**, *8*, 465. [CrossRef] [PubMed]
7. Motohara, T.; Yoshida, G.J.; Katabuchi, H. The Hallmarks of Ovarian Cancer Stem Cells and Niches: Exploring Their Harmonious Interplay in Therapy Resistance. *Semin. Cancer Biol.* **2021**, S1044579X21000997. [CrossRef]
8. Pieterse, Z.; Amaya-Padilla, M.A.; Singomat, T.; Binju, M.; Madjid, B.D.; Yu, Y.; Kaur, P. Ovarian Cancer Stem Cells and Their Role in Drug Resistance. *Int. J. Biochem. Cell Biol.* **2019**, *106*, 117–126. [CrossRef]
9. Muinao, T.; Deka Boruah, H.P.; Pal, M. Diagnostic and Prognostic Biomarkers in Ovarian Cancer and the Potential Roles of Cancer Stem Cells—An Updated Review. *Exp. Cell Res.* **2018**, *362*, 1–10. [CrossRef]
10. Honig, A.; Weidler, C.; Häusler, S.; Krockenberger, M.; Buchholz, S.; Köster, F.; Segerer, S.E.; Dietl, J.; Engel, J.B. Overexpression of Polycomb Protein BMI-1 in Human Specimens of Breast, Ovarian, Endometrial and Cervical Cancer. *Anticancer Res.* **2010**, *30*, 1559–1564.

11. Qin, Z.-K.; Yang, J.-A.; Ye, Y.-L.; Zhang, X.; Xu, L.-H.; Zhou, F.-J.; Han, H.; Liu, Z.-W.; Song, L.-B.; Zeng, M.-S. Expression of Bmi-1 Is a Prognostic Marker in Bladder Cancer. *BMC Cancer* **2009**, *9*, 61. [CrossRef] [PubMed]
12. Beà, S.; Tort, F.; Pinyol, M.; Puig, X.; Hernández, L.; Hernández, S.; Fernandez, P.L.; van Lohuizen, M.; Colomer, D.; Campo, E. BMI-1 Gene Amplification and Overexpression in Hematological Malignancies Occur Mainly in Mantle Cell Lymphomas. *Cancer Res.* **2001**, *61*, 2409–2412. [PubMed]
13. van Kemenade, F.J.; Raaphorst, F.M.; Blokzijl, T.; Fieret, E.; Hamer, K.M.; Satijn, D.P.; Otte, A.P.; Meijer, C.J. Coexpression of BMI-1 and EZH2 Polycomb-Group Proteins Is Associated with Cycling Cells and Degree of Malignancy in B-Cell Non-Hodgkin Lymphoma. *Blood* **2001**, *97*, 3896–3901. [CrossRef] [PubMed]
14. Raaphorst, F.M. Deregulated Expression of Polycomb-Group Oncogenes in Human Malignant Lymphomas and Epithelial Tumors. *Hum. Mol. Genet.* **2005**, *14* (Suppl. 1), R93–R100. [CrossRef] [PubMed]
15. Cui, H.; Hu, B.; Li, T.; Ma, J.; Alam, G.; Gunning, W.T.; Ding, H.-F. Bmi-1 Is Essential for the Tumorigenicity of Neuroblastoma Cells. *Am. J. Pathol.* **2007**, *170*, 1370–1378. [CrossRef]
16. Crea, F.; Duhagon Serrat, M.A.; Hurt, E.M.; Thomas, S.B.; Danesi, R.; Farrar, W.L. BMI1 Silencing Enhances Docetaxel Activity and Impairs Antioxidant Response in Prostate Cancer. *Int. J. Cancer* **2011**, *128*, 1946–1954. [CrossRef] [PubMed]
17. Huber, G.F.; Albinger-Hegyi, A.; Soltermann, A.; Roessle, M.; Graf, N.; Haerle, S.K.; Holzmann, D.; Moch, H.; Hegyi, I. Expression Patterns of Bmi-1 and P16 Significantly Correlate with Overall, Disease-Specific, and Recurrence-Free Survival in Oropharyngeal Squamous Cell Carcinoma. *Cancer* **2011**, *117*, 4659–4670. [CrossRef]
18. Song, L.-B.; Zeng, M.-S.; Liao, W.-T.; Zhang, L.; Mo, H.-Y.; Liu, W.-L.; Shao, J.-Y.; Wu, Q.-L.; Li, M.-Z.; Xia, Y.-F.; et al. Bmi-1 Is a Novel Molecular Marker of Nasopharyngeal Carcinoma Progression and Immortalizes Primary Human Nasopharyngeal Epithelial Cells. *Cancer Res.* **2006**, *66*, 6225–6232. [CrossRef]
19. Kim, J.H.; Yoon, S.Y.; Jeong, S.-H.; Kim, S.Y.; Moon, S.K.; Joo, J.H.; Lee, Y.; Choe, I.S.; Kim, J.W. Overexpression of Bmi-1 Oncoprotein Correlates with Axillary Lymph Node Metastases in Invasive Ductal Breast Cancer. *Breast* **2004**, *13*, 383–388. [CrossRef]
20. Guo, B.-H.; Feng, Y.; Zhang, R.; Xu, L.-H.; Li, M.-Z.; Kung, H.-F.; Song, L.-B.; Zeng, M.-S. Bmi-1 Promotes Invasion and Metastasis, and Its Elevated Expression Is Correlated with an Advanced Stage of Breast Cancer. *Mol. Cancer* **2011**, *10*, 10. [CrossRef]
21. Lu, Y.-W.; Li, J.; Guo, W.-J. Expression and Clinicopathological Significance of Mel-18 and Bmi-1 MRNA in Gastric Carcinoma. *J. Exp. Clin. Cancer Res.* **2010**, *29*, 143. [CrossRef]
22. Proctor, E.; Waghray, M.; Lee, C.J.; Heidt, D.G.; Yalamanchili, M.; Li, C.; Bednar, F.; Simeone, D.M. Bmi1 Enhances Tumorigenicity and Cancer Stem Cell Function in Pancreatic Adenocarcinoma. *PLoS ONE* **2013**, *8*, e55820. [CrossRef]
23. Yoshikawa, R.; Tsujimura, T.; Tao, L.; Kamikonya, N.; Fujiwara, Y. The Oncoprotein and Stem Cell Renewal Factor BMI1 Associates with Poor Clinical Outcome in Oesophageal Cancer Patients Undergoing Preoperative Chemoradiotherapy. *BMC Cancer* **2012**, *12*, 461. [CrossRef] [PubMed]
24. Vonlanthen, S.; Heighway, J.; Altermatt, H.J.; Gugger, M.; Kappeler, A.; Borner, M.M.; van Lohuizen, M.; Betticher, D.C. The Bmi-1 Oncoprotein Is Differentially Expressed in Non-Small Cell Lung Cancer and Correlates with INK4A-ARF Locus Expression. *Br. J. Cancer* **2001**, *84*, 1372–1376. [CrossRef]
25. Breuer, R.H.J.; Snijders, P.J.F.; Sutedja, G.T.; Sewalt, R.G.A.B.; Otte, A.P.; Postmus, P.E.; Meijer, C.J.L.M.; Raaphorst, F.M.; Smit, E.F. Expression of the P16(INK4a) Gene Product, Methylation of the P16(INK4a) Promoter Region and Expression of the Polycomb-Group Gene BMI-1 in Squamous Cell Lung Carcinoma and Premalignant Endobronchial Lesions. *Lung Cancer* **2005**, *48*, 299–306. [CrossRef] [PubMed]
26. Elkashty, O.A.; Ashry, R.; Tran, S.D. Head and Neck Cancer Management and Cancer Stem Cells Implication. *Saudi Dent. J.* **2019**, *31*, 395–416. [CrossRef] [PubMed]
27. Bachmann, I.M.; Puntervoll, H.E.; Otte, A.P.; Akslen, L.A. Loss of BMI-1 Expression Is Associated with Clinical Progress of Malignant Melanoma. *Mod. Pathol.* **2008**, *21*, 583–590. [CrossRef]
28. Sedassari, B.T.; Rodrigues, M.F.S.D.; Mariano, F.V.; Altemani, A.; Nunes, F.D.; Sousa, S. The Stem Cell Marker Bmi-1 Is Sensitive in Identifying Early Lesions of Carcinoma Ex Pleomorphic Adenoma. *Medicine* **2015**, *94*, e1035. [CrossRef]
29. Mihara, K.; Chowdhury, M.; Nakaju, N.; Hidani, S.; Ihara, A.; Hyodo, H.; Yasunaga, S.; Takihara, Y.; Kimura, A. Bmi-1 Is Useful as a Novel Molecular Marker for Predicting Progression of Myelodysplastic Syndrome and Patient Prognosis. *Blood* **2006**, *107*, 305–308. [CrossRef]
30. Jiao, K.; Jiang, W.; Zhao, C.; Su, D.; Zhang, H. Bmi-1 in Gallbladder Carcinoma: Clinicopathology and Mechanism of Regulation of Human Gallbladder Carcinoma Proliferation. *Oncol. Lett.* **2019**, *18*, 1365–1371. [CrossRef]
31. Douglas, D.; Hsu, J.H.-R.; Hung, L.; Cooper, A.; Abdueva, D.; van Doorninck, J.; Peng, G.; Shimada, H.; Triche, T.J.; Lawlor, E.R. BMI-1 Promotes Ewing Sarcoma Tumorigenicity Independent of CDKN2A Repression. *Cancer Res.* **2008**, *68*, 6507–6515. [CrossRef]
32. Zhang, S.; Balch, C.; Chan, M.W.; Lai, H.-C.; Matei, D.; Schilder, J.M.; Yan, P.S.; Huang, T.H.-M.; Nephew, K.P. Identification and Characterization of Ovarian Cancer-Initiating Cells from Primary Human Tumors. *Cancer Res.* **2008**, *68*, 4311–4320. [CrossRef] [PubMed]
33. Wang, E.; Bhattacharyya, S.; Szabolcs, A.; Rodriguez-Aguayo, C.; Jennings, N.B.; Lopez-Berestein, G.; Mukherjee, P.; Sood, A.K.; Bhattacharya, R. Enhancing Chemotherapy Response with Bmi-1 Silencing in Ovarian Cancer. *PLoS ONE* **2011**, *6*, e17918. [CrossRef] [PubMed]

34. Vathipadiekal, V.; Saxena, D.; Mok, S.C.; Hauschka, P.V.; Ozbun, L.; Birrer, M.J. Identification of a Potential Ovarian Cancer Stem Cell Gene Expression Profile from Advanced Stage Papillary Serous Ovarian Cancer. *PLoS ONE* **2012**, *7*, e29079. [CrossRef] [PubMed]
35. Xin, T.; Zhang, F.B.; Sui, G.J.; Jin, X.M. Bmi-1 SiRNA Inhibited Ovarian Cancer Cell Line Growth and Decreased Telomerase Activity. *Br. J. Biomed. Sci.* **2012**, *69*, 62–66. [CrossRef] [PubMed]
36. He, Q.-Z.; Luo, X.-Z.; Wang, K.; Zhou, Q.; Ao, H.; Yang, Y.; Li, S.-X.; Li, Y.; Zhu, H.-T.; Duan, T. Isolation and Characterization of Cancer Stem Cells from High-Grade Serous Ovarian Carcinomas. *Cell Physiol. Biochem.* **2014**, *33*, 173–184. [CrossRef]
37. Dey, A.; Xiong, X.; Crim, A.; Dwivedi, S.K.D.; Mustafi, S.B.; Mukherjee, P.; Cao, L.; Sydorenko, N.; Baiazitov, R.; Moon, Y.-C.; et al. Evaluating the Mechanism and Therapeutic Potential of PTC-028, a Novel Inhibitor of BMI-1 Function in Ovarian Cancer. *Mol. Cancer Ther.* **2018**, *17*, 39–49. [CrossRef]
38. Shishido, A.; Mori, S.; Yokoyama, Y.; Hamada, Y.; Minami, K.; Qian, Y.; Wang, J.; Hirose, H.; Wu, X.; Kawaguchi, N.; et al. Mesothelial Cells Facilitate Cancer Stem-like Properties in Spheroids of Ovarian Cancer Cells. *Oncol. Rep.* **2018**, *40*, 2105–2114. [CrossRef] [PubMed]
39. Yang, G.-F.; He, W.-P.; Cai, M.-Y.; He, L.-R.; Luo, J.-H.; Deng, H.-X.; Guan, X.-Y.; Zeng, M.-S.; Zeng, Y.-X.; Xie, D. Intensive Expression of Bmi-1 Is a New Independent Predictor of Poor Outcome in Patients with Ovarian Carcinoma. *BMC Cancer* **2010**, *10*, 133. [CrossRef]
40. Bhattacharya, R.; Nicoloso, M.; Arvizo, R.; Wang, E.; Cortez, A.; Rossi, S.; Calin, G.A.; Mukherjee, P. MiR-15a and MiR-16 Control Bmi-1 Expression in Ovarian Cancer. *Cancer Res.* **2009**, *69*, 9090–9095. [CrossRef]
41. Zhang, X.-L.; Sun, B.-L.; Tian, S.-X.; Li, L.; Zhao, Y.-C.; Shi, P.-P. MicroRNA-132 Reverses Cisplatin Resistance and Metastasis in Ovarian Cancer by the Targeted Regulation on Bmi-1. *Eur. Rev. Med. Pharmacol. Sci.* **2019**, *23*, 3635–3644. [CrossRef] [PubMed]
42. Abd El hafez, A.; El-Hadaad, H.A. Immunohistochemical Expression and Prognostic Relevance of Bmi-1, a Stem Cell Factor, in Epithelial Ovarian Cancer. *Ann. Diagn. Pathol.* **2014**, *18*, 58–62. [CrossRef] [PubMed]
43. Horie, K.; Iseki, C.; Kikuchi, M.; Miyakawa, K.; Yoshizaki, M.; Yoshioka, H.; Watanabe, J. Bmi-1 Immunohistochemical Expression in Endometrial Carcinoma Is Correlated with Prognostic Activity. *Medicina* **2020**, *56*, 72. [CrossRef]
44. Silva, J.; García, V.; García, J.M.; Peña, C.; Domínguez, G.; Díaz, R.; Lorenzo, Y.; Hurtado, A.; Sánchez, A.; Bonilla, F. Circulating Bmi-1 MRNA as a Possible Prognostic Factor for Advanced Breast Cancer Patients. *Breast Cancer Res.* **2007**, *9*, R55. [CrossRef]
45. Choi, Y.J.; Choi, Y.L.; Cho, E.Y.; Shin, Y.K.; Sung, K.W.; Hwang, Y.K.; Lee, S.J.; Kong, G.; Lee, J.E.; Kim, J.S.; et al. Expression of Bmi-1 Protein in Tumor Tissues Is Associated with Favorable Prognosis in Breast Cancer Patients. *Breast Cancer Res. Treat.* **2009**, *113*, 83–93. [CrossRef]
46. Zhang, F.; Sui, L.; Xin, T. Correlations of BMI-1 Expression and Telomerase Activity in Ovarian Cancer Tissues. *Exp. Oncol.* **2008**, *30*, 70–74.
47. Zhang, F.B.; Sui, L.H.; Xin, T. Correlation of Bmi-1 Expression and Telomerase Activity in Human Ovarian Cancer. *Br. J. Biomed. Sci.* **2008**, *65*, 172–177. [CrossRef]
48. Zhang, H.; Yang, Y.; Wang, Y.; Gao, X.; Wang, W.; Liu, H.; He, H.; Liang, Y.; Pan, K.; Wu, H.; et al. Relationship of Tumor Marker CA125 and Ovarian Tumor Stem Cells: Preliminary Identification. *J. Ovarian Res.* **2015**, *8*, 19. [CrossRef]
49. Charkhchi, P.; Cybulski, C.; Gronwald, J.; Wong, F.O.; Narod, S.A.; Akbari, M.R. CA125 and Ovarian Cancer: A Comprehensive Review. *Cancers* **2020**, *12*, 3730. [CrossRef] [PubMed]
50. Köbel, M.; Kalloger, S.E.; Boyd, N.; McKinney, S.; Mehl, E.; Palmer, C.; Leung, S.; Bowen, N.J.; Ionescu, D.N.; Rajput, A.; et al. Ovarian Carcinoma Subtypes Are Different Diseases: Implications for Biomarker Studies. *PLoS Med.* **2008**, *5*, e232. [CrossRef] [PubMed]
51. Bachmann, I.M.; Halvorsen, O.J.; Collett, K.; Stefansson, I.M.; Straume, O.; Haukaas, S.A.; Salvesen, H.B.; Otte, A.P.; Akslen, L.A. EZH2 Expression Is Associated with High Proliferation Rate and Aggressive Tumor Subgroups in Cutaneous Melanoma and Cancers of the Endometrium, Prostate, and Breast. *J. Clin. Oncol.* **2006**, *24*, 268–273. [CrossRef] [PubMed]

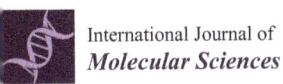

Review

The Inflammatory Role of Pro-Resolving Mediators in Endometriosis: An Integrative Review

Cássia de Fáveri [1], Paula M. Poeta Fermino [2], Anna P. Piovezan [3] and Lia K. Volpato [3,4,*]

1. Medical Residency Program in Ginecology and Obstetric, Hospital Regional Dr. Homero Miranda Gomes, São José 88103-901, Brazil; cassia_faveri@hotmail.com
2. Department Curso de Medicina, Campus Pedra Branca, Undergraduate Medical School, Universidade Sul de Santa Catarina—UNISUL, Palhoça 88137-272, Brazil; paulampf@icloud.com
3. Postgraduate Studies in Health Science Program, Universidade do Sul de Santa Catarina—UNISUL, Palhoça 88137-272, Brazil; Anna.Piovezan@unisul.br
4. Ginecology and Obstetric Department, Hospital Regional Dr. Homero Miranda Gomes, São José 88103-901, Brazil
* Correspondence: liakarina@hotmail.com

Abstract: The pathogenesis of endometriosis is still controversial, although it is known that the inflammatory immune response plays a critical role in this process. The resolution of inflammation is an active process where the activation of endogenous factors allows the host tissue to maintain homeostasis. The mechanisms by which pro-resolving mediators (PRM) act in endometriosis are still little explored. Thus, this integrative review aims to synthesize the available content regarding the role of PRM in endometriosis. Experimental and in vitro studies with Lipoxin A4 demonstrate a potential inhibitory effect on endometrial lesions' progression, attenuating pro-inflammatory and angiogenic signals, inhibiting proliferative and invasive action suppressing intracellular signaling induced by cytokines and estradiol, mainly through the FPR2/ALX. Investigations with Resolvin D1 demonstrated the inhibition of endometrial lesions and decreased pro-inflammatory factors. Annexin A1 is expressed in the endometrium and is specifically present in women with endometriosis, although the available studies are still inconsistent. Thus, we believe there is a gap in knowledge regarding the PRM pathways in patients with endometriosis. It is important to note that these substances' therapeutic potential is evident since the immune and abnormal inflammatory responses play an essential role in endometriosis development and progression.

Keywords: endometriosis; inflammation mediators; annexin A1; Lipoxin A4; receptors; Lipoxin; Resolvin; review

1. Introduction

Endometriosis is a chronic, inflammatory and estrogen-dependent disease characterized by endometrial tissue outside the uterine cavity. It affects approximately 10% of women of reproductive age and is associated with chronic pelvic pain and infertility [1]. The pathophysiology of endometriosis is controversial. Sampson's (1927) retrograde menstruation theory is still the most accepted, describing that the reflux of endometrial fragments would allow the implantation of these cells outside the uterus, especially in the pelvic cavity [2]. However, genetic, neuronal, hormonal and immunological variations may facilitate the adhesion and development of endometrial implants [3].

It is known that 17-β-estradiol (E2) plays a strong influence on the development and progression of endometriosis, acting via estrogen receptors (ER) that are abundant in reproductive tissues, in addition to activating several intracellular signaling cascades in the inflammatory process [4].

Several studies demonstrate that the immune response plays an essential role in the genesis of endometriosis. Many active immune cells, especially peritoneal macrophages, are involved in the development, maintenance and progression of endometrial lesions [1]. High concentrations of cytokines, growth factors and angiogenic factors are observed in the peritoneal fluid of subjects with endometriosis [5]. Interleukins, tumor necrosis factors (TNF) and other chemotactic cytokines act as recruiting macrophages and T lymphocytes to the peritoneum, modulating the inflammatory response associated with endometriosis [6]. Among the factors that support the invasive and proliferative activity of endometrial implants, the epithelial-mesenchymal transition (EMT) is characterized as a biological process in which cells lose cell polarity cell-cell adhesion, and gain migratory and invasive properties to become mesenchymal stem cells [7]. Additionally, matrix metalloproteinases (MMPs) act out as cell-matrix remodeling enzymes that induce the release of growth factors and pro-inflammatory cytokines, favoring the progression of inflammation angiogenesis, tissue remodeling and, therefore, contributing to the implantation and increase of endometriotic lesions [8].

Furthermore, cellular signaling proteins such as p38 MAPK (p38 mitogen-activated protein kinases) and ERK (extracellular signal-regulated kinase) are critical in the inflammatory response. They are characterized as intracellular signal transduction molecules activated by phosphorylation via membrane receptors, increasing levels of cytokines such as interleukins, and TNF, in addition to increasing MMP activity. In addition, several studies show its influence on the pathogenesis of endometriosis [9]. The multidrug resistance-associated protein 4 (MRP4) can transport several endogenous molecules, playing a critical role in cellular communication and signaling. Among these molecules, there is a strong affinity with Prostaglandin E2 (PGE2), consequently potentiating the inflammatory process [10].

Several inflammatory response events can limit their magnitude and duration [5]. The resolution of inflammation is an active process where the activation of endogenous factors allows the host tissue to maintain homeostasis [11]. This process occurs differently concerning the known anti-inflammatory pathways since the pro-resolving molecules act in a multifactorial way at the inflammatory site. In addition to producing powerful signals to reduce neutrophils and eosinophils' infiltration, they also promote the uptake and elimination of apoptotic cells and microorganisms by macrophages at the inflamed tissue. At the beginning of the inflammatory process, classic lipid mediators such as prostaglandins and leukotrienes are released, activating and amplifying the inflammatory process. After the acute phase, some of these molecules start to produce substances that synthesize endogenous mediators with anti-inflammatory and pro-resolving activity, such as lipoxins, resolvins, protectins and maresines [12–14].

The pro-resolving mediators (PRM) are lipids or proteins. Lipid mediators are generated through lipoxygenases (LOX) and cyclooxygenases (COX) by the metabolism of arachidonic acid (AA), such as lipoxins, or originated from omega-3 polyunsaturated fatty acids (omega-3 PUFAS), represented by the acid eicosapentaenoic (EPA)-derived resolvin E (RvE) and docosahexaenoic acid (DHEA)-derived resolvin D (RvD), protectins and maresines. These mediators promote the sequestration of pro-inflammatory cytokines, in addition to removing polymorphonuclear cells (PMN) from the epithelial surface, phagocyting apoptotic PMNs, removing inflammatory residues through the lymphatic vessels and reducing inflammatory pain [15–17].

In endometriosis, the signaling pathways for Lipoxin A4 (LXA4) are the most studied. Its cascades are mediated by several membrane receptors [18] with higher affinity for the formyl peptide 2/"aspirin-triggered lipoxin" receptor (FPR2/ALX); therefore, most studies show how LXA4 acts through this receptor [19], allowing it to act in a double, anti-inflammatory and pro-resolutive manner [12]. Some works have already shown that LXA4 presents a high structural similarity with estriol, a weak agonist of the ER-α in the endometrium's epithelial cells. For this reason, LXA4 can also occupy these receptors and decrease E2-mediated signaling, triggering anti-inflammatory and pro-resolving effects, in addition to modulating the expression of ERs [4,18,20].

The PRM proteins are Annexin A1 (ANXA1), galectins and melanocortins. These mediators have a crucial modulating function in neutrophil trafficking. They can reduce infiltration, activate apoptosis at the inflammatory site, stimulate phagocytosis and the elimination of apoptotic neutrophils, in addition to inducing the phenotypic change from inflammatory M1 macrophages to M2 anti-inflammatory macrophages, which causes a reparative response [17,21,22]. ANXA1 is a calcium-dependent phospholipid-binding protein and has been observed as an anti-inflammatory mediator, regulating physiological and pathological cellular processes. Additionally, ANXA1 is expressed in several tissues, including the endometrium, where it acts via the FPR2/ALX and other mediators [23].

The FPR2/ALX regulates the action of PRM, such as ANXA1 and LXA4, belonging to the superfamily of formyl peptide receptors. These receptors are critical in endometriosis since the expression of FPR2/ALX proved to be more significant in the cells of endometriotic lesions compared to the normal endometrium. In addition, these receptors are regulated by estrogen and other cytokines and mediate specific cellular pathways to suppress inflammation [18,23].

Failures in these pro-resolving pathways can predispose the host to chronic inflammatory diseases [12]. In this process, cellular mechanisms and their biochemical pathways open new strategies for potential therapeutic interventions [24]. Evidence that PRM are promising targets for the development of pharmacological treatments for chronic inflammatory diseases is pointed out by Serhan (2017); in this, the author demonstrates examples of conditions for which drugs like PRM have been successfully studied in clinical trials in humans (phase I and phase II), including periodontal diseases, inflammation associated with dry eye and childhood eczema [25].

The mediators that act as PRM in endometriosis are still little explored. Thus, this review aims to synthesize the information available in the literature regarding the inflammatory role of PRM in endometriosis.

2. Methods

2.1. Search Strategy

For this integrative review, a survey of all articles published and indexed in the main known databases was conducted: MEDLINE (PubMed), Bireme (LILACS, ADOLEC, IBECS and BDENF), EMBASE (Elsevier) and DOAJ. The search was carried out between June and August 2020, without restrictions regarding the date limit of publication or language. The terms "endometriosis", "pro-resolution mediators", "lipoxin", "maresin", "resolvin", "protectin", "FPR", "Annexin A1", "galectin" and "melanocortin" were used, and additionally the Boolean operators "AND" and "OR" applied for "endometriosis" and the other terms, respectively.

2.2. Articles Eligibility Criteria

The eligibility criteria were applied to the selected articles with support of the reference manager software Mendeley© Version 1.19.4 (Mendeley Ltd., London, UK), by which duplicates were identified and excluded. Two independent researchers screened the articles by reading the title and abstract. Full-length original articles whose theme covered the role of PRM in endometriosis by experimental models, cell culture or in humans were included. Articles written in an alphabet other than the Roman alphabet and review articles were excluded.

2.3. Data Processing

After the screening, two independent researchers performed the data extraction by filling out a clinical form in a previously established spreadsheet. Finally, the findings were analyzed and the written data descriptively synthesized.

3. Results and Discussions

In the initial search, 336 articles were identified, 90 of which were duplicates, resulting in 246 articles. The studies were screened by reading the title and abstract, with 19 articles selected and one excluded since the full-length text was only available in the Mandarin language (Figure 1). The distribution of the captured articles and the related terms are shown in Table 1. No research was found addressing the terms "protectin", "galectin" or "melanocortin" associated with "endometriosis". The included studies and their main findings are shown in Table 2.

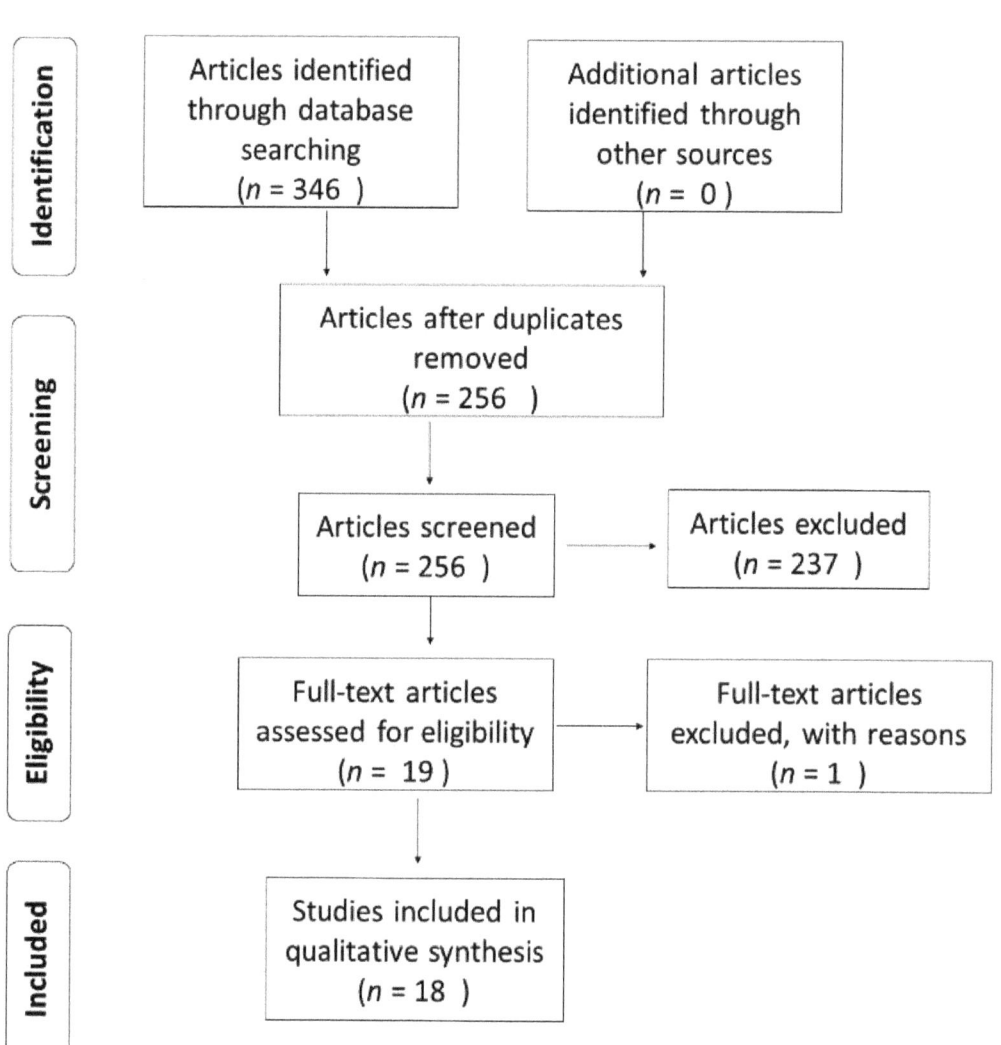

Figure 1. Flowchart of article selection. São José-SC—Brazil, 2021.

Table 1. Articles captured in the database and grouped according to the main observed mediators. São José, SC—Brazil, 2021.

Database	PRM	Lipoxin	Resolvin	Maresin	ANXA1	FPR
DOAJ	-	2	-	-	3	-
EMBASE	2	92	25	9	81	25
PUBMED	-	20	2	-	4	3
BIREME/LILACS	2	20	2	-	32	3
Total	4	134	39	18	120	31

PRM: pro-resolving mediators; ANXA1: Annexin A1; FPR: formyl peptide receptors.

Table 2. Categorization of articles selected by the main authors, journal, design and study target. São José-SC—Brazil, 2021.

Authors	Journal/Year	Study Design	Study Target
Motohashi et al. [26]	Biomed Pharmacother, 2005	Experimental—treatment with LXA4	FPR2/ALX
		Cross-sectional	
Chen et al. [27]	Eur J Obstet Gynecol Reprod Biol, 2009	In vitro: ESC culture—treatment with LXA4 and IL-β	LXA4
Chen et al. [28]	Fertil Steril, 2010	Experimental—treatment with LXA4	LXA4
Xu et al. [29]	Am J Reprod Immunol, 2012	Experimental—treatment with LXA4	LXA4
Gori et al. [30]	Fertil Steril, 2013	Cross-sectional	LXA4
		In vitro: ESC culture—treatment with LXA4	
Wu et al. [19]	British J Pharmacol, 2014	Experimental—treatment with LXA4	LXA4
		In vitro: Endometrioma culture—treatment with LXA4, Boc-2 and IL-1β	LXA4 and FPR2/ALX
		Cross-sectional	
Chen et al. [31]	Fertil Steril, 2014	In vitro: ESC culture—treatment with LXA4	LXA4
		Cross-sectional	
Kumar et al. [32]	PloS ONE, 2014	Experimental—treatment with LXA4	LXA4 and FPR2/ALX
Sobel et al. [33]	Front Endocrinol, 2016	In vitro: ESC culture—treatment with LXA4 and E2	LXA4
Wu et al. [34]	J Obst Gynaecol Res, 2017	In vitro: ESC culture—treatment with LXA4 and IL-1β	LXA4
Wu et al. [6]	Reprod Sci, 2017	Experimental—treatment with LXA4 and Boc-2	LXA4 and FPR2/ALX
		In vitro: Endometrioma culture—treatment with LXA4, Boc-2 and E2	
Dai et al. [35]	Reprod Sci, 2019	Experimental—treatment with LXA4 and Boc-2	LXA4 and FPR2/ALX
		In vitro: Endometrioma culture—treatment with LXA4, MAPK inhibitor and IL-1β	
Li et al. [36]	Chin Med J, 2008	Cross-sectional	ANXA1
Rasheed et al. [37]	J Stem Cel Regen Med, 2010	In vitro: stem cell culture	ANXA1
Paula Jr et al. [38]	J Mol Hist, 2015	Cross-sectional	ANXA1 and FPR1
Volpato et al. [39]	J Reprod Immunol, 2018	Cross-sectional	ANXA1 and FPR2/ALX
Tomio et al. [40]	PloS ONE, 2013	Experimental	RvE2
Dmitrieva et al. [41]	Fertil Steril, 2014	Experimental	RvD1

3.1. Methods Used in the Studies Reviewed

3.1.1. Experimental Studies: Methods to Induce and Evaluate Endometriosis

In experimental studies, endometriosis is induced in mice with transplantation of endometrial fragments in the peritoneal cavity by autologous or heterologous transplantation of the uterine horns. The endometrium-rich fragments are obtained by removing the uterine corn from the donor or through minor surgery to collect endometrial tissue and transplant it in the same animal. The fragments are injected or implanted in the recipient animals' peritoneal cavity. The animals have randomly grouped accordingly: those submitted to endometriosis that received treatment, those submitted to endometriosis without treatment and a control group not submitted to experimental endometriosis. Following the treatment with the respective mediator, the mice are sacrificed or re-operated to assess the lesions and collect the tissue to measure the intervention effects [7,19,26,28,29,32,35,40,41].

Some studies have also carried out hormonal stimulation of endometrial lesions with estrogen administration [29] or estrogen and 17-OH-progesterone [26]. In Tomio et al. investigation, donor and recipient were oophorectomized and stimulated with estrogen [31]. In addition, researchers have used vaginal cytology in mice to define its estrous cycle stage [27–29,41]. Further, Dmitrieva et al. injected Evans Blue dye to assess leakage in endometrial lesions and implant a telemetric probe to analyze vaginal nociception in mice [30].

3.1.2. In Vitro Studies

In vitro studies were carried out using primary endometriotic stromal cells (ESCs) collected and isolated from endometriotic lesions or cells from patients' eutopic endometrium endometriosis diagnosed by surgery and histological process. The disease stage was established according to the American Society for Reproductive Medicine (ASRM). Control group patients were confirmed with the absence of endometriosis; tissue cells from the peritoneal cavity were collected when operated due to other reasons. In these studies, patients were at least 3–6 months without hormonal or anti-inflammatory treatment. ESCs were treated in cell culture with the mediator under investigation, and the evaluation was carried out through several types of laboratory analysis [7,19,30,31,33–35]. Rasheed et al. analyzed in vitro halogenic stem cells by adding serum from patients diagnosed with endometriosis to evaluate cell differentiation and the expression of ANXA1 [37].

3.1.3. Cross-Sectional Studies in Humans

Cross-sectional studies evaluated biopsies of endometrial lesions and peritoneal fluid in patients with endometriosis who underwent surgery. The disease stage was classified according to criteria established by the ASRM. Additionally, patients in the control group were confirmed with the absence of endometriosis and tissue cells from the peritoneal cavity collected when operated on due to other reasons. Then, the study was conducted based on an analysis of different types of laboratory exams [26,31,36–39].

3.2. PRM and Endometriosis

3.2.1. Lipoxin A4

LXA4 Inhibits the Progression of Endometrial Lesions in Experimental Studies

According to the studies evaluated here, treatment with LXA4 or the analog 15-epi-LXA4 performed according to the experimental model previously mentioned does not alter the mice's estrous cycle or ovarian function. Therefore, it does not prevent the development of endometriosis [27–29]. However, it inhibits established lesions' progression by significantly reducing endometriotic lesions' size and weight that histologically present a rudimentary architecture, with less glandular and stromal development [7,19,27–29,32,35].

LXA4 Attenuates Pro-Inflammatory and Angiogenic Effects Associated with Endometriosis

Evidence shows that LXA4 attenuates pro-inflammatory and angiogenic effects associated with endometriosis. In an experimental study, LXA4 reduced the expression of COX-2 [32,35] and PGE2 levels in endometriotic lesions and peritoneal fluid cells [32]. LXA4 reduced pro-inflammatory cytokines in lesions, ESCs and peritoneal fluid cells during in vivo and in vitro experiments. Among the studied cytokines, treatment with LXA4 reduced the expression of interleukine 1β (IL-1β), interleukin 6 (IL-6), interleukin 10 (IL-10), interleukin 16 (IL-16), vascular endothelial growth factor (VEGF), TNF, transforming growth factor (TGF)-β1 and TGF-β2 [19,27,29,31–33].

LXA4 Suppresses MMP Activity, Proliferative Action and Cell Cycle Progression

In experimental models of endometriosis, evidence has shown that LXA4 suppresses the activity of MMPs (MMP-9 and MMP-2) in endometrial lesions via the FPR2/ALX in mice [7,28,29,32]. Treatment with LXA4 in vitro also inhibited the cell cycle's progression in ESCs, consequently attenuating the invasive and proliferative activity associated with endometriotic lesions [19].

LXA4 Modulates the Expression of Estrogen Receptors

A cross-sectional study of ESCs has shown that treatment with LXA4 and E2 triggered a higher ER-β expression and decreased pro-inflammatory signals. The authors suggest that LXA4 may selectively modulate ER-β in ESCs. In addition, the human endometrium analysis showed a strong positive correlation between the expression of LXA4 and ER-α. In contrast, a negative correlation with ER-β was observed in an in vitro analysis. Further, there was no association between LXA4 and the progesterone receptor (RP). Despite the divergence, it is evident that LXA4 regulates ERs by attenuating E2-induced inflammatory signaling pathways in addition to acting as an E2 receptor agonist [31].

LXA4 Suppresses Cell Signaling, p38 MAPK and ERK Phosphorylation Induced by Estrogen in ESCs

Another in vitro effect elicited by LXA4 in ESCs is reducing E2-induced p38 MAPK and ERK phosphorylation. Important, estradiol is known to stimulate the activity of these enzymes. Additionally, E2-induced p38 MAPK phosphorylation is significantly reduced in cells treated with E2 and LXA4, suggesting that LXA4 may inhibit endometriosis development by this route, probably through ERs [31]. Further, the inhibition of E2-induced p38 MAPK and ERK phosphorylation is mediated by the FPR2/ALX in vitro [7]. In a proteomic analysis, the combined treatment with E2 and LXA4 resulted in reduced regulated proteins, with LXA4 mediating a suppressive effect on E2-mediated inflammatory cell signaling [33].

LXA4 Suppresses E2-Induced Epithelial-Mesenchymal Transition

LXA4 suppressed E2-induced EMT of ESCs in vitro, reversing in a dose-dependent manner the reduced expression of epithelial markers (E-cadherin) and the increased expression of mesenchymal markers (Vimentin, N-cadherin and Zinc Finger E-box-binding homeobox 1 (ZEB1)) induced by E2, thus preventing the progress, migration and invasion promoted by endometriosis [7].

LXA4 Reduces p38 MAPK Phosphorylation, Cytokine Release and COX-2 Expression Induced by Interleukin-1β in ESCs via FPR2/ALX

IL-1β is an important pro-inflammatory cytokine that stimulates other cytokines and angiogenic factors. Important to note, LXA4 inhibited IL-1β-induced cytokine release, additionally also inhibited IL-1β-induced p38 MAPK phosphorylation via FPR2/ALX in an in vitro assay [19,35]. Further, LXA4 inhibited COX-2 expression induced by IL-1β in ESCs through the FPR2/ALX modulation. According to Wu et al. in proteomic analysis, LXA4 can suppress proteins that facilitate IL-1β-induced migration and invasion in ESC [34].

LXA4 Attenuates MRP4 Expression in ESCs

Gori et al. first described the expression of MRP4 in the human endometrium, showing increased peritoneal endometriotic lesions associated with high levels of PGE2 in the peritoneal fluid. The same study showed that LXA4 significantly attenuated the expression of MRP4 in vitro, thus disabling intracellular signals associated with inflammation in endometriosis [30].

3.2.2. Resolvins

Resolvin D1 (RvD1) Decreases Inflammatory Signs Associated with Endometriosis

The treatment with RvD1 and the analog 17(R)-RvD1 decreased the inflammatory signs of vascular permeability and neurogenic activity as reflected by the significant reduction of Evans Blue dye leakage in ectopic lesions in mice submitted to the experimental model previously mentioned. Moreover, RvD1 effectively reduced vaginal hyperalgesia in mice, proving its potential to relieve abnormal endometriosis-related pelvic pain [41].

Resolvin E3 (RvE3) Inhibits the Progression of Endometriosis

In an experimental study, 15/12-LOX-KO mice (animals with 15/12 lipoxygenase enzyme deficiency) and wild mice submitted to endometriosis received oral EPA to investigate the effects of 12/15-LOX-related mediators in endometriotic lesions and compared with wild mice subjected to endometriosis which did not receive oral EPA. The administration of EPA significantly decreased the number of endometriotic lesions in wild mice, although the suppressive effect of EPA on the development of endometriotic lesions was not observed in 12/15-LOX-KO mice. In addition, the number of endometriotic lesions was similar in 12/15-LOX-KO mice treated or not with EPA. Interestingly, the EPA-derived bioactive mediator 18S/R-RvE3, which was biosynthesized from 18-HEPE (hydroxyicosapentaenoic acid) by 15/12-LOX was increased in the peritoneal fluid of wild mice following the administration of EPA. However, this increase was not observed in 12/15-LOX-KO mice, suggesting that RvE3 may be involved in modulating endometriotic lesions [40].

3.2.3. Annexin A1

Expression of ANXA1 Protein in Endometriosis

Cross-sectional studies have assessed the role of ANXA1 in the pathogenesis of endometriosis in humans. It was shown that its expression is more significant in the endometrium of women with endometriosis [36] and higher in endometriotic lesions (abdominal wall endometrioma). Furthermore, the high levels correlate with morphological changes in this tissue, suggesting that ANXA1 may be involved in cell differentiation and proliferation [38]. However, these data are inconsistent since another study showed a reduced expression of ANXA1 in patients with endometriosis, suggesting that this decrease can facilitate the inflammatory process [39]. In this sense, the lack of studies to better assess the role of ANXA1 and its pathways in endometriosis is evidenced.

ANXA1 as Endometriosis Inducing Factors

The involvement of predisposing factors in endometriosis was investigated by adding the serum of patients with endometriosis into halogenic stem cells. Most of these cells showed morphological changes that resembled endometrial cells and glands, and this differentiation was more intense and faster, the more significant the severity of endometriosis. In addition, differentiated cells expressed ANXA1. These data reveal that there may be inducing factors in women's blood with endometriosis, highlighting a new theory in endometriosis's pathogenesis. However, further studies are needed to ratify this and help decipher this substance's nature and its molecular composition [37].

3.2.4. FPR2/ALX Receptor

Expression of FPR2/ALX in Endometriosis

According to the literature, in experimental endometriosis, the expression of FPR2/ALX is more significant in the endometrium and uterus than in the ovary. In addition, this expression is increased in the proestral phase (which corresponds to the ovarian follicular phase) and decreased in the estrous phase (corresponding to the ovulatory stage). In parallel, progesterone administration as 17-OH-progesterone also reduced the expression of FPR2/ALX. Furthermore, in both cross-sectional analysis of endometriosis in humans and experimental endometriosis induced in mice, the FPR2/ALX expression was more significant in endometrial lesions than topical endometrium. These data suggest that this receptor is more expressed in women with endometriosis and even more critical in endometriotic lesions, in addition to being regulated by estrogen and progesterone [26].

4. Conclusions

The pro-resolving mediators of inflammation represent potent endogenous factors, allowing the host tissue to maintain homeostasis and prevent chronic inflammatory diseases. Currently, the treatment of endometriosis includes hormonal and anti-inflammatory therapies. However, these therapies are limited due to the high cost, side effects and recurrence of the disease after discontinuing treatment. Among the mediators, LXA4 is the most studied, acting positively in several aspects related to endometriosis progression and maintenance.

According to the reviewed literature, we believe that there is still a knowledge gap regarding the PRM pathways in patients with endometriosis. It is important to note that these substances' therapeutic potential is evident since the immune response and abnormal inflammatory responses play an essential role in developing, maintaining and progressing this chronic disease.

Author Contributions: All authors whose names appear in this article made substantial contributions to the conception and interpretation of data; A.P.P. had the idea for the article, L.K.V. and P.M.P.F. performed the literature search, L.K.V. and C.d.F. performed data analysis. All authors drafted the work or revised it critically for important intellectual content; approved the version to be published; and agree to be accountable for all aspects of the work in ensuring that questions related to the accuracy or integrity of any part of the work are appropriately investigated and resolved. All authors have read and agreed to the published version of the manuscript.

Funding: This research received no external funding.

Acknowledgments: The authors thank the Coordenação de Aperfeiçoamento de Pessoal de Nível Superior—Brasil (CAPES) for the partial financing of this study.

Conflicts of Interest: The authors have no conflict of interest to declare relevant to this article's content.

References

1. Giudice, L.C.; Kao, L.C. Endometriosis. *Lancet* **2004**. [CrossRef]
2. Lebovic, D.I.; Mueller, M.D.; Taylor, R.N. Immunobiology of endometriosis. *Fertil. Steril.* **2001**. [CrossRef]
3. Rakhila, H.; Al-Akoum, M.; Bergeron, M.E.; Leboeuf, M.; Lemyre, M.; Akoum, A.; Pouliot, M. Promotion of angiogenesis and proliferation cytokines patterns in peritoneal fluid from women with endometriosis. *J. Reprod. Immunol.* **2016**. [CrossRef]
4. Clark, J.H.; Markaverich, B.M. The agonistic and antagonistic actions of estriol. *J. Steroid. Biochem.* **1984**. [CrossRef]
5. Gazvani, R.; Templeton, A. Peritoneal environment, cytokines and angiogenesis in the pathophysiology of endometriosis. *Reproduction* **2002**. [CrossRef]
6. Kralickova, M.; Vetvicka, V. Immunological aspects of endometriosis: A review. *Ann. Transl. Med.* **2015**. [CrossRef]
7. Wu, R.F.; Huang, Z.X.; Ran, J.; Dai, S.J.; Lin, D.C.; Ng, T.W.; Chen, Q.X.; Chen, Q.H.; Lipoxin, A. Lipoxin A_4 suppresses estrogen-induced epithelial-mesenchymal transition via ALXR-dependent manner in endometriosis. *Reprod. Sci.* **2017**. [CrossRef]
8. Mott, J.D.; Werb, Z. Regulation of matrix biology by matrix metalloproteinases. *Curr. Opin. Cell Biol.* **2004**. [CrossRef]
9. Levy, B.D.; Clish, C.B.; Schmidt, B.; Gronert, K.; Serhan, C.N. Lipid mediator class switching during acute inflammation: Signals in resolution. *Nat. Immunol.* **2001**. [CrossRef] [PubMed]
10. Reid, G.; Wielinga, P.; Zelcer, N.; van der Heijden, I.; Kuil, A.; de Haas, M.; Wijnholds, J.; Borst, P. The human multidrug resistance protein MRP4 functions as a prostaglandin efflux transporter and is inhibited by nonsteroidal anti-inflammatory drugs. *Proc. Natl. Acad. Sci. USA* **2003**. [CrossRef] [PubMed]
11. Serhan, C.N.; Brain, S.D.; Buckley, C.D.; Gilroy, D.W.; Haslett, C.; O'Neill, L.A.; Perretti, M.; Rossi, A.G.; Wallace, J.L. Resolution of inflammation: State of the art, definitions, and terms. *FASEB J.* **2007**. [CrossRef] [PubMed]
12. Serhan, C.N.; Chiang, N.; Van Dyke, T.E. Resolving inflammation: Dual anti-inflammatory and pro-resolution lipid mediators. *Nat. Rev. Immunol.* **2008**. [CrossRef]
13. Gilroy, D.W.; Lawrence, T.; Perretti, M.; Rossi, A.G. Inflammatory resolution: New opportunities for drug discovery. *Nat. Rev. Drug. Discov.* **2004**. [CrossRef] [PubMed]
14. Campbell, E.L.; Louis, N.A.; Tomassetti, S.E.; Canny, G.O.; Arita, M.; Serhan, C.N.; Colgan, S.P. Resolvin E1 promotes mucosal surface clearance of neutrophils: A new paradigm for inflammatory resolution. *FASEB J.* **2007**. [CrossRef] [PubMed]

15. Recchiuti, A.; Serhan, C.N. Pro-resolving lipid mediators (SPMs) and their actions in regulating miRNA in novel resolution circuits in inflammation. *Front. Immunol.* **2012**. [CrossRef] [PubMed]
16. Seki, H.; Sasaki, T.; Ueda, T.; Arita, M. Resolvins as regulators of the immune system. *Sci. World J.* **2010**. [CrossRef]
17. Serhan, C.N. Novel pro-resolving lipid mediators in inflammation are leads for resolution. *Nature* **2014**. [CrossRef]
18. Russell, R.; Gori, I.; Pellegrini, C.; Kumar, R.; Achtari, C.; Canny, G.O. Lipoxin A$_4$ is a novel estrogen receptor modulator. *FASEB J.* **2011**. [CrossRef]
19. Wu, R.; Zhou, W.; Chen, S.; Shi, Y.; Su, L.; Zhu, M.; Chen, Q.; Chen, Q. Lipoxin A$_4$ suppresses the development of endometriosis in an ALX receptor-dependent manner via the p38 MAPK pathway. *Br. J. Pharmacol.* **2014**. [CrossRef]
20. Bulun, S.E. Endometriosis. *N. Engl. J. Med.* **2009**. [CrossRef] [PubMed]
21. Kamal, A.M.; Flower, R.J.; Perretti, M. An overview of the effects of Annexin 1 on cells involved in the inflammatory process. *Mem. Inst. Oswaldo Cruz.* **2005**. [CrossRef] [PubMed]
22. Lim, L.H.; Pervaiz, S. Annexin 1: The new face of an old molecule. *FASEB J.* **2007**. [CrossRef] [PubMed]
23. Bena, S.; Brancaleone, V.; Wang, J.M.; Perretti, M.; Flower, R.J. Annexin A1 interaction with the FPR2/ALX receptor: Identification of distinct domains and downstream associated signaling. *J. Biol. Chem.* **2012**. [CrossRef] [PubMed]
24. Bannenberg, G.L.; Chiang, N.; Ariel, A.; Arita, M.; Tjonahen, E.; Gotlinger, K.H.; Hong, S.; Serhan, C.N. Molecular circuits of resolution: Formation and actions of resolvins and protectins. *J. Immunol.* **2005**. [CrossRef] [PubMed]
25. Serhan, C.N. Treating inflammation and infection in the 21st century: New hints from decoding resolution mediators and mechanisms. *FASEB J.* **2017**. [CrossRef]
26. Motohashi, E.; Kawauchi, H.; Endo, H.; Kondo, H.; Kitasato, H.; Kuramoto, H.; Majima, M.; Unno, N.; Hayashi, I. Regulatory expression of lipoxin A$_4$ receptor in physiologically estrus cycle and pathologically endometriosis. *Biomed. Pharmacother.* **2005**. [CrossRef]
27. Chen, Q.H.; Zhou, W.D.; Pu, D.M.; Huang, Q.S.; Li, T.; Chen, Q.X. 15-Epi-lipoxin A$_4$ inhibits the progression of endometriosis in a murine model. *Fertil. Steril.* **2010**. [CrossRef]
28. Chen, Q.; Zhou, W.; Pu, D.; Li, Z.; Huang, Q.; Chen, Q. The inhibitory effect of 15-R-LXA$_4$ on experimental endometriosis. *Eur. J. Obstet. Gynecol. Reprod. Biol.* **2009**. [CrossRef]
29. Xu, Z.; Zhao, F.; Lin, F.; Chen, J.; Huang, Y. Lipoxin A4 inhibits the development of endometriosis in mice: The role of anti-inflammation and antiangiogenesis. *Am. J. Reprod. Immunol.* **2012**. [CrossRef]
30. Gori, I.; Rodriguez, Y.; Pellegrini, C.; Achtari, C.; Hornung, D.; Chardonnens, E.; Wunder, D.; Fiche, M.; Canny, G.O. Augmented epithelial multidrug resistance-associated protein 4 expression in peritoneal endometriosis: Regulation by lipoxin A$_4$. *Fertil. Steril.* **2013**. [CrossRef]
31. Chen, S.; Wu, R.F.; Su, L.; Zhou, W.D.; Zhu, M.B.; Chen, Q.H. Lipoxin A$_4$ regulates expression of the estrogen receptor and inhibits 17β-estradiol-induced p38 mitogen-activated protein kinase phosphorylation in human endometriotic stromal cells. *Fertil. Steril.* **2014**. [CrossRef] [PubMed]
32. Kumar, R.; Clerc, A.C.; Gori, I.; Russell, R.; Pellegrini, C.; Govender, L.; Wyss, J.C.; Golshayan, D.; Canny, G.O. Lipoxin A$_4$ prevents the progression of de novo and established endometriosis in a mouse model by attenuating prostaglandin E$_2$ production and estrogen signaling. *PLoS ONE* **2014**. [CrossRef]
33. Sobel, J.A.; Waridel, P.; Gori, I.; Quadroni, M.; Canny, G.O. Proteome-wide effect of 17-β-estradiol and lipoxin A$_4$ in an endometriotic epithelial cell line. *Front. Endocrinol.* **2006**. [CrossRef] [PubMed]
34. Wu, R.F.; Yang, H.M.; Zhou, W.D.; Zhang, L.R.; Bai, J.B.; Lin, D.C.; Ng, T.W.; Dai, S.J.; Chen, Q.H.; Chen, Q.X. Effect of interleukin-1β and lipoxin A$_4$ in human endometriotic stromal cells: Proteomic analysis. *J. Obstet. Gynaecol. Res.* **2017**. [CrossRef] [PubMed]
35. Dai, S.; Zhu, M.; Wu, R. Lipoxin A$_4$ suppresses IL-1b-induced cyclooxygenase-2 expression through inhibition of p38 MAPK activation in endometriosis. *Reprod. Sci.* **2019**. [CrossRef]
36. Li, C.Y.; Lang, J.H.; Liu, H.Y.; Zhou, H.M. Expression of Annexin-1 in patients with endometriosis. *Chin. Med. J.* **2008**, *121*, 927–931. [CrossRef]
37. Rasheed, K.; Atta, H.; Taha, T.F.; Azmy, O.; Sabry, D.; Selim, M.; El-Sawaf, A.; Bibars, M.; Ramzy, A.; El-Garf, W.; et al. A novel endometriosis inducing factor in women with endometriosis. *J. Stem. Cells Regen. Med.* **2017**. [CrossRef]
38. Paula, J.R.; Oliani, A.H.; Vaz-Oliani, D.C.M.; D'Ávila, S.C.; Oliani, S.M.; Gil, C.D. The intricate role of mast cell proteases and the annexin A1-FPR1 system in abdominal wall endometriosis. *J. Mol. Hist.* **2015**. [CrossRef]
39. Volpato, L.K.; Horewicz, V.V.; Bobinski, F.; Martins, D.F.; Piovezan, A.P. Annexin A1, FPR2/ALX, and inflammatory cytokine expression in peritoneal endometriosis. *J. Reprod. Immunol.* **2018**. [CrossRef]
40. Tomio, K.; Kawana, K.; Taguchi, A.; Isobe, Y.; Iwamoto, R.; Yamashita, A.; Kojima, S.; Mori, M.; Nagamatsu, T.; Arimoto, T.; et al. Omega-3 polyunsaturated fatty acids suppress the cystic lesion formation of peritoneal endometriosis in transgenic mouse models. *PLoS ONE* **2013**. [CrossRef]
41. Dmitrieva, N.; Suess, G.; Russell, S. Resolvins RvD1 and 17(R)-RvD1 alleviate signs of inflammation in a rat model of endometriosis. *Fertil. Steril.* **2014**. [CrossRef] [PubMed]

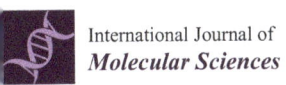

Review

Neurogenic Inflammation in the Context of Endometriosis—What Do We Know?

Renata Voltolini Velho [1], Eliane Taube [2], Jalid Sehouli [1] and Sylvia Mechsner [1,*]

[1] Department of Gynecology Charité with Center of Oncological Surgery, Endometriosis Research Center Charité, Campus Virchow-Klinikum, Augustenburger Platz 1, 13353 Berlin, Germany; renata.voltolini-velho@charite.de (R.V.V.); jalid.sehouli@charite.de (J.S.)

[2] Institute of Pathology, Charité Universitätsmedizin Berlin, Campus Mitte, Charitéplatz 1, 10117 Berlin, Germany; eliane.taube@charite.de

* Correspondence: sylvia.mechsner@charite.de; Tel.: +49-030-450664866

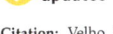

Citation: Velho, R.V.; Taube, E.; Sehouli, J.; Mechsner, S. Neurogenic Inflammation in the Context of Endometriosis—What Do We Know? *Int. J. Mol. Sci.* **2021**, *22*, 13102. https://doi.org/10.3390/ijms222313102

Academic Editors: Antonio Simone Laganà and Kanako Hayashi

Received: 20 October 2021
Accepted: 1 December 2021
Published: 3 December 2021

Publisher's Note: MDPI stays neutral with regard to jurisdictional claims in published maps and institutional affiliations.

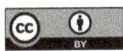

Copyright: © 2021 by the authors. Licensee MDPI, Basel, Switzerland. This article is an open access article distributed under the terms and conditions of the Creative Commons Attribution (CC BY) license (https://creativecommons.org/licenses/by/4.0/).

Abstract: Endometriosis (EM) is an estrogen-dependent disease characterized by the presence of epithelial, stromal, and smooth muscle cells outside the uterine cavity. It is a chronic and debilitating condition affecting ~10% of women. EM is characterized by infertility and pain, such as dysmenorrhea, chronic pelvic pain, dyspareunia, dysuria, and dyschezia. Although EM was first described in 1860, its aetiology and pathogenesis remain uncertain. Recent evidence demonstrates that the peripheral nervous system plays an important role in the pathophysiology of this disease. Sensory nerves, which surround and innervate endometriotic lesions, not only drive the chronic and debilitating pain associated with EM but also contribute to a growth phenotype by secreting neurotrophic factors and interacting with surrounding immune cells. Here we review the role that peripheral nerves play in driving and maintaining endometriotic lesions. A better understanding of the role of this system, as well as its interactions with immune cells, will unearth novel disease-relevant pathways and targets, providing new therapeutics and better-tailored treatment options.

Keywords: endometriosis; neurogenic inflammation; neuroimmune modulation; nerve signalling; peripheral nerve; inflammation; non-hormonal treatment

1. Introduction

Endometriosis (EM) is an estrogen-dependent benign, chronic inflammatory disease affecting up to 10 to 15% of reproductive-aged women [1–3]. It is associated with a significant societal and economic burden that costs the US economy USD 22 billion annually in lost productivity and direct healthcare costs [3–6]. The main symptoms of EM include dysmenorrhea, dyspareunia, dyschezia, dysuria, noncyclic chronic pelvic pain, and primary or secondary fertility problems [7–9].

EM is a disease of the uterine tissues (epithelium, stroma, and smooth muscle cells) that leads to ectopic colonization by detachment/desquamation of basal endometrial stem cells during menstruation or by infiltration into the myometrium [10–12]. Even if the pathogenesis is unclear, over the last 20 years, our understanding of the mechanisms driving EM lesion growth and pain presentation has evolved (Figure 1). Significant advances have been made in understanding how estrogen drives tissue pathology, resulting in aberrant inflammatory and neuronal states, and promoting the invasion of lesions into the surrounding tissues [13].

In this review, we summarize the role of neurogenic inflammation in endometriotic pain. A better understanding of the role of the peripheral nerve system, as well as its interactions with immune cells, will unearth novel disease-relevant pathways and targets, providing new therapeutics and better-tailored treatment options.

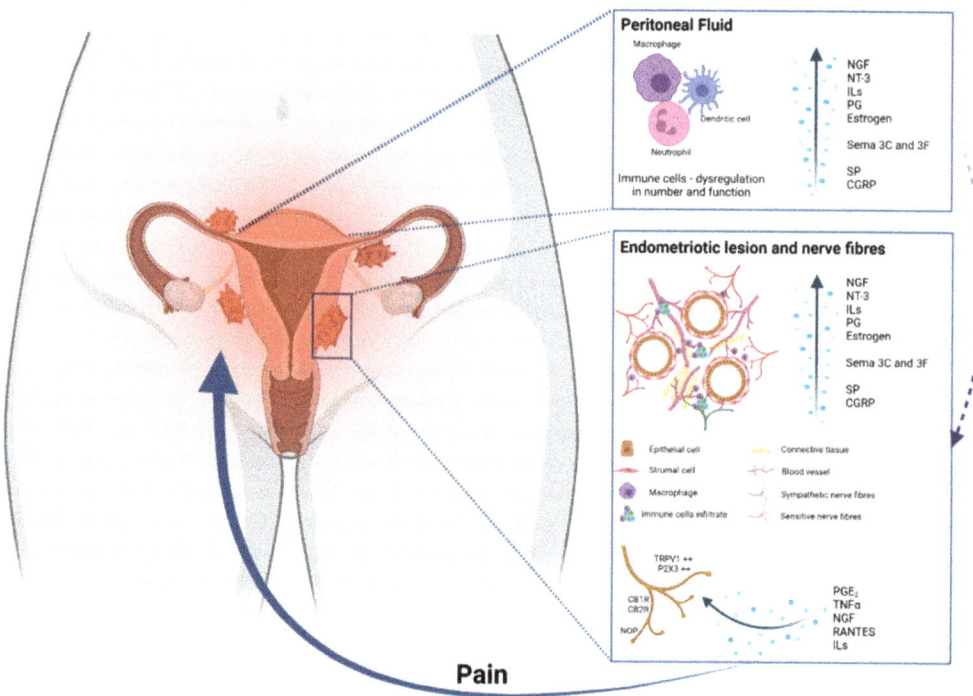

Figure 1. Main pathways involved in the pathogenesis of inflammatory pain in endometriosis. Endometrial fragments in the peritoneum lead to peritoneal inflammation. The same immune response is seen at endometriotic lesions, where the increased production of cytokines, chemokines, growth factors and immune cells also contributes to an enhanced inflammatory environment present in the peritoneal cavity of women with EM. Of these inflammatory mediators, PGE2, tumour necrosis factor-α (TNFα), nerve growth factor (NGF), RANTES and interleukins are also able to stimulate sensory nerve endings and activate a positive feedback loop, further increasing proinflammatory modulator production. The expression of pain receptors is also increased in EM patients' nerve fibres. The enhanced stimulation and activation of peripheral nerve endings in the peritoneal cavity increase the painful stimuli, initiating and maintaining chronic pelvic pain.

2. Patient Presentation, Diagnosis and Current Treatments

There are various symptom patterns and different patient cohorts due to the different kinds of lesions, organs affected, size and diversity of the patient population [14–16]. Additionally, non-specific complaints may lead to consultations of various medical disciplines, delaying the diagnosis. An, on average, 10-year-long delay after the onset of symptoms in diagnosis is common [14,15]. After all, more than 60% of those diagnosed with EM report that their complaints started before the age of 20. Furthermore, there is a clear correlation between the duration, the intensity of the complaints, and the extent of the EM manifestations [14,17].

EM remains a clinically suggested diagnosis and is only definitively diagnosed after surgical exploration yields pathologically confirmed EM. Pathologic examination will demonstrate ectopic endometrial-like tissue outside of the uterus containing endometrial epithelium, glands, or stroma, or hemosiderin-laden macrophages (Mφ) [18]. Imaging techniques such as transvaginal sonography and magnetic resonance imaging may be utilized to aid diagnosis but the methodical limitations should be taken into consideration [19,20]. So far, there are no validated biomarkers for diagnosis or therapy monitoring [21].

After diagnosis, EM patients have three classes of treatments available to them: (i) analgesics to manage symptoms, (ii) hormonal therapies designed to inhibit estrogen-dependent growth of lesions, or (iii) surgical ablation/excision of lesions [14]. Beyond medical treatment, many women also find symptom relief during pregnancy/breastfeeding or after menopause [22].

3. Pathophysiology of Endometriosis Related Pain

Pain has been defined as a "complex constellation of unpleasant sensory, emotional and cognitive experiences provoked by real or perceived tissue damage and manifested by certain autonomic, psychological, and behavioural reactions" [23]. For the perception of pain, a biochemical signal (1) is converted into a neural signal (2) (sensitization of sensory nerve fibres via activation of the nociceptors). At the spinal level, this signal is modulated (3) and referred (attenuated/amplified) to the brain, where the pain perception occurs (4). Steps one and two are called peripheral sensitization and three and four are central sensitizations [14,16].

If severe EM-associated pelvic pain remains untreated, it will recur monthly. Initially, the pain is perceived cyclically (hormonal-dependent pain) reflecting the classical nociceptive inflammatory pain. If this pain occurs repeatedly, such as monthly, the body's warning signals take effect, and it is classified as threatening. At this point, the modulation at the spinal level does not regulate it down but rather increases it (hormonal-independent pain). The release of neurotransmitters is altered and several modulating mechanisms are set in motion: the nociceptive field is expanded and EM symptoms such as dysuria and dyschezia may occur [24].

Increasing pain frightens the person experiencing it and makes pain processing more difficult. Severe cramps, accompanied by vegetative reactions, lead the patient to adopt a pain-relieving posture. However, this leads to a reflex contraction of the pelvic floor muscles and eventually to pelvic floor dysfunction. This increases the experienced pain and is known to lead to dyspareunia [25]. Fear of pain during intercourse can strongly influence the ability to relax and the disorder manifests itself. Changes at the central level develop and the patients have an increased risk of developing complex chronic pain syndromes with bladder dysfunction, irritable bowel syndrome, and vulvodynia [24]. This explains the often severe pain that accompanies patients, even in the absence of pathological findings.

4. Neurogenic Inflammation

The concept of neurogenic inflammation was first postulated by Bayliss (1901) [26] and stated that peripherally located nerve fibres caused vasodilation in the hind limbs of dogs when stimulated by mechanical, chemical or thermal stimuli. This suggests that afferent fibres could also fire in an antidromic direction. These local antidromic currents were termed the "axon reflex" which is responsible for the vascular flare observed following tissue injury. This activation of sensory neurones leads to an inflammatory response called neurogenic inflammation [26]. This phenomenon is very well investigated in other chronic pain conditions, such as asthma, rheumatoid arthritis, and inflammatory bowel disease, for example. Here, we would like to show the increasing evidence of neurogenically derived inflammatory mechanisms occurring in the EM.

In some EM patients, pain characterization shifts from the more cyclical into an acyclical pattern (see Section 3). In this case, the ongoing activation of sensory nerve fibres releases proinflammatory neuropeptides such as substance P (SP) and calcitonin gene-related peptide (CGRP), both of which are found close to endometrial lesions [6,27]. Furthermore, activation of sensory afferent nerves might initiate the recruitment of mast cells and, subsequently, the release of proinflammatory cytokines as TNFα, NGF, PGE2 and a variety of interleukins, such as IL-1β [28,29]. This inflammation encourages further stimulation of locally circulating mast cells and Mφ [30]. Different studies have shown a high number of these cells in endometriotic lesions as well as an increased amount of proinflammatory cytokines in the peritoneal fluid of EM patients [3,20,21,31–34]. This contributes to a chronic state of neurogenic inflammation. Increased levels of TNFα and glycodelin correlate with central hyperexcitability in response to repeated electrical stimulation and altered pain response to nociceptive withdrawal reflex [6]. The nociceptive ion channel TRPV1 showed elevated expression on infiltrating adhesions in EM patients, the increase correlating with pain intensity [35–37].

Taken together, elevated expression and activation of nociceptors and elevated levels of neuropeptides, other proinflammatory chemicals and cytokines imply that neuroinflammatory processes are present in the central nervous system in EM.

5. Neuroimmunomodulation in Endometriosis
5.1. Neuro Fibres and Neurotransmitters

Important work over the past years has been performed to understand the mechanisms by which endometriotic lesions induce pain, the primary symptom of patients. Much of this effort has focused on understanding the extent and type of nerves present in endometriotic lesions compared to surrounding tissues. The presence of nerves in endometriotic lesions has been confirmed. In humans, murine models and rat models, ectopic endometrium implants develop sympathetic, parasympathetic, and sensory nerve fibres [24,25,38]. An imbalance in the distribution of sensitive and sympathetic nerve fibres in peritoneal EM lesions in favour of the sensitive nerve fibres of 4:1 has been observed [38]. In the peritoneum of patients without EM, on the other hand, the ratio of sensitive nerve fibres to sympathetic nerve fibres is 1:5. An inverse ratio of the nerve fibres to one another is evident in EM-aged tissue. In line with these data, similar results were also found in intestinal EM [39]. The sympathetic innervation in the intestinal wall, in particular, speaks for influence on the pathogenesis mechanisms, especially since patients with intestinal infection often complain about functional intestinal disorders. The total nerve fibre density is reduced in the periphery of the peritoneal lesion (an area more than 4 mm away from the actual endometrial lesion), most likely due to a reduced number of sympathetic nerves fibres [38].

The neurotransmitters norepinephrine, adenosine, neuropeptide Y (NPY), substance P (SP), vasoactive intestinal peptide (VIP), and endogenous opioids of the different nerve fibre types exert different effects on inflammatory processes by binding to specific receptors of the immune cells. Furthermore, nerve fibres seem to play an immunomodulatory role [40,41]. The expression of neurotransmitter receptors is not evenly distributed among immune cells but appears to be dependent on the microenvironment [42–44]. Nerve fibres communicate with immune cells in a synapse-like manner and thus modulate immune cell function [45]. Both efferent (sympathetic and parasympathetic) and afferent (sensitive) nerve fibres influence immune cells through the local release of neurotransmitters [40].

A recent study [46] showed that sensory nerve-derived neuropeptides SP and CGRP facilitate epithelial–mesenchymal transition (EMT), fibroblast-to-myofibroblast transdifferentiation (FMT) and further turn stromal cells into smooth muscle cells (SMCs) in EM, yielding increased collagen production, elevated cellular contractility, and eventually fibrosis. Neutralization of their respective receptors, such as NK1R, RAMP-1 and CRLR, however, abrogates these processes. More remarkably, they showed that lesional nerve fibre density correlated with the lesional expression levels of the receptors, with the extent of lesional fibrosis as well as the severity of pain in EM patients [46]. These data provide strong evidence that sensory nerve fibres play a potent facilitatory role in expediting the development and fibrogenesis of endometriotic lesions.

More and more data indicate that the peritoneal EM lesions in particular lead to the release of neurotrophic substances into the peritoneal fluid. Significantly increased NGF and NT-3 levels [47] and also estrogen levels [27] have been detected, especially in patients with peritoneal lesions. In vitro analyses using a neuronal growth assay also demonstrated the neuromodulatory properties of EM at the functional level. Peritoneal fluids from patients with and without EM were incubated with sensitive and sympathetic ganglia. The incubation with peritoneal fluid from patients with peritoneal EM showed a significantly increased sprouting of sensitive nerve fibres, but lower sprouting of sympathetic ones. The peritoneal fluid of patients without EM, however, showed the exact opposite: sympathetic nerve fibres were induced, while sensitive nerve fibres were inhibited. This reflects the results of the changes associated with peritoneal EM and demonstrates serious changes in peritoneal innervation, which are caused by EM, lead to far-reaching changes in the entire peritoneal milieus, and may be the cause of the complex symptoms of the patients [48]. Interactions between endometrial lesions, nerve fibres, and immune cells are considered to be essential factors in these changes.

5.2. Semaphorins and Neuromodulation

The semaphorin family of proteins includes many secreted and membrane-associated proteins. There are approximately 20 distinct members in higher vertebrates, and all contain the family's signature semaphorin domain, a ~500 amino acid N-terminal that is the key extracellular signalling domain of these proteins. Semaphorins act as nerverepulsive factors that become extracellularly effective through a specific repulsive influence on either sympathetic or primary afferent sensitive fibres through various surface receptors, neuropilin-1 (Nrp1), and neuropilin-2 (Nrp2) [49,50].

In normal human endometrial tissue, the expression of many semaphorins is upregulated in the proliferative stage of the menstrual cycle, when estrogen is at its highest [39]. Estrogen has been found to induce the expression of semaphorins in uterine tissue [51]. Semaphorins 3C and 3F (Sema 3C and Sema 3F, respectively), in particular, are known as nerve repellent factors and are upregulated in EM-associated Mφ in rat and mouse models [51,52]. In women with EM, studies revealed an affected innervation and a significant increase of Sema 3C and 3F and their receptors in peritoneal endometriotic tissue. Thereby, the expression of the receptors was identified on the membrane of noradrenergic nerve fibres and vessels. Mφ and activated fibroblasts were found in higher density levels and additionally express semaphorins in peritoneal endometriotic tissue. Inflammation leads to an increased release of immune cells, which secrete a variety of inflammatory factors capable of affecting innervation. Therefore, these data suggest that the chronic inflammatory condition in EM might contribute to the increase of semaphorins, which could affect the innervation in peritoneal EM [53,54].

6. Pain Receptors in Endometriosis-Associated Nerve Fibres

The understanding of pain generation, as this is the main problem in EM patients, is of great importance: the ectopic lesions themselves release pain mediators and activate nociceptors (transduction and transmission). In most cases, this is strongly estrogen-dependent and leads to cyclical nociceptive pain (dysmenorrhoea and cyclical pelvic pain), which is treated by hormones or non-steroidal antiphlogistics (NSAP). However, with ongoing disease, the cyclical pain characterization shifts into an acyclical chronic pain (pain development under hormonal treatment, NSDAP resistant pain, increasing pain severity) [55,56]. We analyzed this phenomenon in nearly 100 patients with acyclical pain under hormonal treatment and found it in 100% of the peritoneal ectopic lesions with extended inflammatory reactions [16]. This phenomenon might especially be due to neurogenic inflammation and activation of peripheral sensory nerve fibres. The peripheral sensitization seems to be stressed and for this, the development of non-hormonal anti-inflammatory compounds is of great interest. So, besides the understanding of the inflammatory reaction, the peripheral sensitization of nerve fibres is also of great importance.

6.1. Purinergic Receptors

In acute and chronic pain models, small- and medium-diameter sensory neurons, which express transient receptor vanilloid-1 (TRPV1) channels and/or adenosine triphosphate (ATP)-gated P2X3 receptors, are the important pain transducers of noxious stimuli [57]. In women with EM, TRPV1 receptor expression has been demonstrated to be elevated in endometriotic lesions and correlated with pain [36,37,57].

Purinergic receptors are ligand-gated ion channels that are expressed in sensory neurons which can be activated by adenosine triphosphate (ATP). P2X3 is one such purinergic receptor. In women with EM, ATP released during retrograde menstruation and due to mechanical stretch from endometriotic adhesions or fibrotic scar tissue could potentially activate P2X3 receptors, leading to neuronal hypersensitivity and pain [58]. Indeed, its expression in the endometrium of women with EM was significantly higher compared to control endometrium and interestingly was also correlated with the severity of pain reported [58,59]. Current interest in targeting P2X3 in EM is high, with multiple pharmaceutical companies having initiated drug programs, one of which has begun to enter Phase IIb clinical trials (NCT04614246).

6.2. Opioid Receptors

The endogenous opioid peptides (EOPs) are derived from proopiomelanocortin (POMC), proenkephalin (PENK), and prodynorphin (PDYN) precursors and exert their effects by binding to the G-protein-coupled receptors δ-opioid receptor (DOR), κ-opioid receptor (KOR), μ-opioid receptor (MOR), and nociceptin/orphanin FQ opioid peptide receptor (NOP) [59,60]. The peripheral opioid system plays a crucial role in inflammatory reactions and neurogenic inflammation since this system is activated and modulated by inflammation. During this process, analgetic factors such as anti-inflammatory cytokines and opioid peptides are released, promoting antinociceptive actions. In chronic inflammation, the release of anti-inflammatory mediators and opioid peptides is decreased, improving the perpetuation of inflammation. Since EM is a chronic inflammatory disease with a disturbing pain mediation and analgesia, disruption in the expression of opioid peptides or opioid receptors might be involved in the inflammatory condition and pain pathogenesis in this disease and alterations in the expression of those receptors and their respective ligands should be urgently investigated. Indeed, the mRNA of three opioid peptide precursors has been described in the endometrium [61]. Finally, DOR and KOR have been described in Ishikawa human endometrial cells, while MOR is absent [62,63]; in fact, MOR has been localized only in the uterine luminal epithelium cells of the pregnant mouse [64] and in EM stromal cells [65–67]. NOP has not been tested. The proven presence of most of the compounds of the opioid system in the endometrium denotes the role of this system in processes occurring in the endometrium, including EM.

6.3. Endocannabinoid Receptors

The first biologically active component of cannabis was identified in the 1960s as delta-9-tetrahydrocannabinol (THC), a potent drug classified as a sedative-hypnotic. This was followed by the discovery of two cannabinoid receptors, cannabinoid receptor 1 (CB1R) and cannabinoid receptor 2 (CB2R), in the early 1990s. Both are G-protein-coupled receptors and serve as the primary sites of action for THC. Together, they are involved in the major neuromodulatory endocannabinoid system (ECS), whose primary goal is to promote homeostasis [68]. The ECS is widespread, and CB1Rs are found throughout the central nervous system and some peripheral tissues, while CB2Rs are primarily found in peripheral tissues and immune cells [69]. Cannabinoids act on receptors other than CB1R and CB1R. They modulate transient receptor potential (TRP) channels, including TRP vanilloid (TRPV) channels, which are involved in neuropathic pain signals in EM [70].

There is a broad range of mechanisms by which cannabinoids modulate pain, and given the high impact of EM on women's quality of life such as the high prevalence of EM, cannabinoid-mediated effects on EM-related pain have become a subject of inquiry [68,69].

Different categories of EM pain may be modulated by cannabinoids [71,72]. There is evidence that a disruption of the normal ECS potentiates pain in EM patients. In women with EM, decreased CB1R expression compared to controls and increased anandamide (AEA) and 2-arachidonoylglycerol (2-AG) expression, both endogenous ligands of the CB1R and CB2R, are consistent with a negative feedback loop that is permissive of inflammation [68].

In vitro studies have shown that exogenous cannabinoids could correct these dysregulations. When endometrial cells were treated with cannabinoid agonist WIN 5512-2, the result was decreased cell proliferation, decreased reactive oxygen species production, and reduction in alpha-smooth muscle actin expression, lending supporting evidence to the anti-inflammatory effects of cannabinoids [73]. Bilgic et al. [74] also found that CB1R and CB2R expressions are decreased in EM tissue compared to control, with concurrently decreased apoptosis indexes. The same study found that exposure of EM tissue to CB1R and CB2 agonists resulted in pro-apoptotic effects. However, animal model studies have shown divergent results. A nude mouse model of transplanted human deep infiltrating EM confirmed the antiproliferative effects of cannabinoids on the growth of deep infiltrating lesions [64]. In contrast, in a mouse analogue of early-stage EM, the activation resulted in an increased disease burden [75]. The complexity of the ECS superimposed on the two different mouse models used may account for the different results [76].

Endocannabinoids have also been shown to trigger endometrial cell migration [77]. Moreover, CB1Rs have been found on the sensory and sympathetic neurons innervating EM lesions [78]. Given the above role of the ECS in the EM modulation, cannabinoids have been proposed as a putative therapy. In fact, an Australian cross-sectional survey showed that self-management strategies were very common in EM patients and that cannabis and cannabis products were among the most effective at pain reduction [79].

7. Endometriosis and Inflammation

Menstruation is an inflammatory process characterized by an increase in a variety of tissue-resident immune cells. A complex interaction between resident immune cells and uterine stromal cells modulates the biosynthesis and release of pro-inflammatory cytokines, chemokines, and prostaglandins (PGs), resulting in local vasoconstriction [3,6]. When retrograde menstruation occurs, endometrial fragments adhere and form lesions within the peritoneum. During this process, inflammatory cells are recruited to the lesions. This immune response is evident at lesion sites, with increased inflammatory cytokines/chemokines, growth factors, neutrophils and PGs found within the peritoneal cavity of EM patients [3,6,20,80,81].

Since EM is considered a chronic inflammatory disorder, the neuromodulatory mechanisms of the EM-associated immune cell infiltrate (EMaICI) need to be considered. In all investigated types of EM, immune cell infiltrates were observed and characterized as a mixture of several immunocompetent cells (T cells, B cells, and Mφ) [31,82,83]. In endometriotic lesions and also in eutopic endometrial tissue of EM patients, the numbers of EMaICI were significantly higher than in control tissue and seem to be associated with a chronic inflammatory process [84]. EMaICI were observed and characterized in all the types of EM by our group as T lymphocytes (CD3+), helper T lymphocytes (CD4+), cytotoxic T lymphocytes (CD8+), antigen-experienced T lymphocytes "memory cells" (CD45RO+), macrophages (CD68+), and B lymphocytes (CD20+) [85]. The characterization of various types of immunocompetent cells in EMaICI demonstrated several distinct immunological reactions within the microenvironment of different endometriotic lesions.

Dendritic cells (DC), Mφ, mast cells (MC) and neutrophils play a central role in chronic inflammatory diseases [32,86,87]. Under normal conditions, immature DCs mature and travel to the lymph nodes in response to foreign antigens or other inflammatory signals, where the antigens are presented to T cells. However, the maturation of DCs declines in EM, with it being hypothesized that immunological components form part of the antigen capture and/or presentation activity. This process might be altered in the endometrium of women with EM. Consequently, EM-circulating anti-endometrial antibodies could mask endometrial antigens. As a result, endometrial antigens might not be effectively recognized, with lost endometrial fragments remaining, potentially leading to ectopic establishment [83,88,89].

Mφ are abundantly recruited to lesions of EM after activation by certain chemokines and cytokines. These cells can release different types of inflammatory substances, creating an inflammatory microenvironment that contributes to the establishment and growth of endometriotic lesions. In turn, these changes can induce the Mφ recruitment and as a result, form a vicious circle during the development of the disease [3]. Mφ are classified as M1 Mφ, which exhibit proinflammatory activity, and M2 Mφ, which provide an anti-inflammatory environment and are capable of remodelling tissue through pro-fibrotic activity. In the context of EM, the differentiation between M1 and M2 Mφ seems to be shifted in favour of M2 in EM and this is particularly important since M2 Mφ are more immunologically tolerant [20,30,90]. It has been reported that endogenous Mφ are involved in tissue remodelling during the development of EM, and the M2 Mφ, in particular, is required for the growth of ectopic lesions in a mouse model [30]. More recently, two independent groups found a decrease in the percentage of M1 and an increase in M2 Mφ in peritoneal washings of EM patients, especially those with advanced disease (stages III–IV) [91,92].

MCs are known to be key players of the immune system, especially during allergic reactions. However, increasing evidence supports the involvement of these cells also in the inflammatory process of EM. High numbers of degranulated MC have been found in endometriotic lesions showing their influence on EM lesions in development, survival, phenotype, and function via the regulation of other immune cells (monocytes/Mφ, granulocytes, DC, and T-B lymphocytes) [31–34,93,94].

Neutrophils are considered simple foot soldiers of the innate immune system and are undoubtedly the major effectors of acute inflammation. Several lines of evidence indicate that they also contribute to chronic inflammatory conditions as well as adaptive immune responses [95]. The infiltration of neutrophils into the peritoneal cavity is significantly increased in EM patients compared with that in healthy women, especially in the early stage of EM [96,97]. In EM, neutrophils in the abdominal cavity can secrete an effective pro-angiogenic factor, VEGF, which is also increased in the PF in the EM. As a result, neutrophils may support the growth of endometriotic lesions by secreting VEGF. Moreover, there may be some other nonclassical factors secreted by neutrophils that can promote inflammation and neovascularization in EM [97].

Aberrant expression of several cytokines by inflammatory cells, such as IL-1, IL-4, IL-6, IL-8, IL-10, IL-33, TNFα and growth factors, e.g., transforming growth factor (TGF-β), insulin-like growth factor (IGF-1), hepatocyte growth factor (HGF), epidermal growth factor (EGF), platelet-derived growth factor (PDGF), and vascular endothelial growth factor (VEGF), have been reported in EM [89,98]. Indeed, cytokines such as IL-8 and TNF-α are known to promote endometrial cell proliferation, endometrial adhesion, and angiogenesis. Furthermore, endometriotic lesions can induce the expression of PGs, MCP1, glycodelin, and other inflammatory mediators [25,99]. Specifically, PGE2, PGF2α, and TNF-α are produced and increased in the early stage; TNF-α, NGF, and IL-17 can cause persistent inflammation; and PGE2, PGF2α, transforming growth factor-β (TGF-β), glycodelin, and TNF-α can induce the sensation of pain [3,25,100]. A recent study showed that cytokine analysis of PFs could differentiate women diagnosed and stratified laparoscopically with ovarian endometrioma, peritoneal, or deep infiltrating EM. This suggests that certain cytokine signatures could be driving different biological signalling events and immune responses in these patients [101]. These inflammation-associated substances act on inflammatory cells in turn. These retroactions lead to more inflammatory cell recruitment in lesions with a subsequent alteration in the original peritoneal and pelvic environments and the formation of a new inflammatory microenvironment. The growth, implantation, infiltration, and migration of EM lesions occur subsequently and retroact on inflammatory cells and substances. This vicious cycle contributes to the aggregation of EM-associated inflammation [3].

8. Conclusions

Even if the pathophysiology of EM is not completely understood, it is well established that the immune system plays a key role in this disease. Moreover, the peripheral and central nervous systems are intimately involved in EM disease and symptomatology. Nociceptor neurons possess many of the same molecular recognition pathways for danger as immune cells and in response to danger, the peripheral nervous system directly communicates with the immune system, forming an integrated protective mechanism. The dense innervation network of sensory and autonomic fibres in peripheral tissues and high speed of neural transduction allows for rapid local and systemic neurogenic modulation of immunity. Peripheral neurons also appear to play a significant role in immune dysfunction in autoimmune and allergic diseases. The literature provides evidence for an overall heterogeneity in EM, rather than a standard approach. This strongly suggests a personalized treatment approach based on aetiology and symptomatology. Current treatments, both pharmacological and surgical, are addressed at providing symptom relief and are mainly focused on complex pain management, without effective results for all patients. Several studies are attempting to overcome these obstacles by identifying molecular targets to develop new therapeutic approaches to improve the quality of life of affected women. Once we put aside the paradigm of lesion-specific and cyclical inflammatory pain, further areas will open up and increase the treatment opportunities in a multimodal approach.

Author Contributions: R.V.V. and S.M. wrote the initial draft of the manuscript; R.V.V., E.T., J.S. and S.M. reviewed and edited the manuscript. All authors have read and agreed to the published version of the manuscript.

Funding: We acknowledge support from the German Research Foundation (DFG) and the Open Access Publication Fund of Charité—Universitätsmedizin Berlin.

Acknowledgments: The figure was created using BioRender.com.

Conflicts of Interest: The authors declare no conflict of interest.

References

1. Olive, D.L.; Pritts, E. Treatment of endometriosis. *N. Engl. J. Med.* **2001**, *345*, 266–275. [CrossRef] [PubMed]
2. Macer, M.L.; Taylor, H.S. Endometriosis and infertility. A review of the pathogenesis and treatment of endometriosis-associated infertility. *Obstet. Gynecol. Clin. N. Am.* **2012**, *39*, 535–549. [CrossRef] [PubMed]
3. Wei, Y.; Liang, Y.; Lin, H.; Dai, Y.; Yao, S. Autonomic nervous system and inflammation interaction in endometriosis-associated pain. *J. Neuroinflam.* **2020**, *17*, 80. [CrossRef]
4. Simoens, S.; Hummelshoj, L.; D'Hooghe, T. Endometriosis: Cost estimates and methodological perspective. *Hum. Reprod. Update* **2007**, *13*, 395–404. [CrossRef] [PubMed]
5. Nnoaham, K.E.; Hummelshoj, L.; Webster, P.; d'Hooghe, T.; de Cicco Nardone, F.; de Cicco Nardone, C.; Jenkinson, C.; Kennedy, S.H.; Zondervan, K.T.; World Endometriosis Research Foundation Global Study of Women's Health consortium. Impact of endometriosis on quality of life and work productivity: A multicenter study across ten countries. *Fertil. Steril.* **2011**, *96*, 366.e8–373.e8. [CrossRef]
6. Maddern, J.; Grundy, L.; Castro, J.; Brierley, S.M. Pain in endometriosis. *Front. Cell. Neurosci.* **2020**, *14*, 1–16. [CrossRef] [PubMed]
7. Cramer, D.W.; Missmer, S.A. The epidemiology of endometriosis. *Obstet. Gynecol. Clin. N. Am.* **2003**, *30*, 1–19. [CrossRef] [PubMed]
8. Milingos, S.; Protopapas, A.; Drakakis, P.; Liapi, A.; Loutradis, D.; Kallipolitis, G.; Milingos, D.; Michalas, S. Laparoscopic management of patients with endometriosis and chronic pelvic pain. *Ann. N. Y. Acad. Sci.* **2003**, *997*, 269–273. [CrossRef]
9. Abesadze, E.; Sehouli, J.; Mechsner, S.; Chiantera, V. Possible role of the posterior compartment peritonectomy, as a part of the complex surgery, regarding recurrence rate, improvement of symptoms and fertility rate in patients with endometriosis, long-term follow-up. *J. Minim. Invasive Gynecol.* **2019**, *27*, 1103–1111. [CrossRef] [PubMed]
10. Leyendecker, G.; Herbertz, M.; Kunz, G.; Mall, G. Endometriosis results from the dislocation of basal endometrium. *Hum. Reprod.* **2002**, *17*, 2725–2736. [CrossRef]
11. Bulun, S.E.; Yilmaz, B.D.; Sison, C.; Miyazaki, K.; Bernardi, L.; Liu, S.; Kohlmeier, A.; Yin, P.; Milad, M.; Wei, J. Endometriosis. *Endocr. Rev.* **2019**, *40*, 1048–1079. [CrossRef]
12. Ibrahim, M.G.; Sillem, M.; Plendl, J.; Taube, E.T.; Schüring, A.; Götte, M.; Chiantera, V.; Sehouli, J.; Mechsner, S. Arrangement of myofibroblastic and smooth muscle-like cells in superficial peritoneal endometriosis and a possible role of transforming growth factor beta 1 (TGFβ1) in myofibroblastic metaplasia. *Arch. Gynecol. Obstet.* **2019**, *299*, 489–499. [CrossRef] [PubMed]
13. Liang, Y.; Xie, H.; Wu, J.; Liu, D.; Yao, S. Villainous role of estrogen in macrophage-nerve interaction in endometriosis. *Reprod. Biol. Endocrinol.* **2018**, *16*, 122. [CrossRef] [PubMed]
14. Gruber, T.M.; Mechsner, S. Pathogenesis of endometriosis: The origin of pain and subfertility. *Cells* **2021**, *10*, 1381. [CrossRef] [PubMed]
15. Greene, R.; Stratton, P.; Cleary, S.D.; Ballweg, M.L.; Sinaii, N. Diagnostic experience among 4334 women reporting surgically diagnosed endometriosis. *Fertil. Steril.* **2009**, *91*, 32–39. [CrossRef]

16. Dückelmann, A.M.; Taube, E.; Abesadze, E.; Chiantera, V.; Sehouli, J.; Mechsner, S. When and how should peritoneal endometriosis be operated on in order to improve fertility rates and symptoms? The experience and outcomes of nearly 100 cases. *Arch. Gynecol. Obstet.* **2021**, *304*, 143–155. [CrossRef] [PubMed]
17. Ballweg, M.L. Impact of endometriosis on women's health: Comparative historical data show that the earlier the onset, the more severe the disease. *Best Pract. Res. Clin. Obstet. Gynaecol.* **2004**, *18*, 201–218. [CrossRef]
18. Carlyle, D.; Khader, T.; Lam, D.; Vadivelu, N.; Shiwlochan, D.; Yonghee, C. Endometriosis pain management: A review. *Curr. Pain Headache Rep.* **2020**, *24*, 49. [CrossRef]
19. Bazot, M.; Daraï, E. Diagnosis of deep endometriosis: Clinical examination, ultrasonography, magnetic resonance imaging, and other techniques. *Fertil. Steril.* **2017**, *108*, 886–894. [CrossRef]
20. Hogg, C.; Horne, A.W.; Greaves, E. Endometriosis-associated macrophages: Origin, phenotype, and function. *Front. Endocrinol.* **2020**, *11*, 7. [CrossRef] [PubMed]
21. Velho, R.V.; Halben, N.; Chekerov, R.; Keye, J.; Plendl, J.; Sehouli, J.; Mechsner, S. Functional changes of immune cells: Signal of immune tolerance of the ectopic lesions in endometriosis? *Reprod. Biomed. Online* **2021**, *43*, 319–328. [CrossRef] [PubMed]
22. Haas, D.; Chvatal, R.; Reichert, B.; Renner, S.; Shebl, O.; Binder, H.; Wurm, P.; Oppelt, P. Endometriosis: A premenopausal disease? Age pattern in 42,079 patients with endometriosis. *Arch. Gynecol. Obstet.* **2012**, *286*, 667–670. [CrossRef] [PubMed]
23. Terman, G.; Bonica, J. Spinal mechanisms and their modulation. In *Bonica's Management of Pain*; Loeser, J., Butler, S., Chapman, C., Turk, D., Eds.; Lippincott Williams & Wilkins: Philadelphia, PA, USA, 2001.
24. Wang, G.; Tokushige, N.; Russell, P.; Dubinovsky, S.; Markham, R.; Fraser, I.S. Hyperinnervation in intestinal deep infiltrating endometriosis. *J. Minim. Invasive Gynecol.* **2009**, *16*, 713–719. [CrossRef] [PubMed]
25. Coxon, L.; Horne, A.W.; Vincent, K. Pathophysiology of endometriosis-associated pain: A review of pelvic and central nervous system mechanisms. *Best Pract. Res. Clin. Obstet. Gynaecol.* **2018**, *51*, 53–67. [CrossRef] [PubMed]
26. Bayliss, W.M. On the origin from the spinal cord of the vaso-dilator fibres of the hind-limb, and on the nature of these fibres. *J. Physiol.* **1901**, *26*, 173–209. [CrossRef]
27. Arnold, J.; Vercellino, G.F.; Chiantera, V.; Schneider, A.; Mechsner, S.; de Arellano, M.L.B. Neuroimmunomodulatory alterations in non-lesional peritoneum close to peritoneal endometriosis. *Neuroimmunomodulation* **2013**, *20*, 9–18. [CrossRef] [PubMed]
28. Van der Kleij, H.P.M.; Forsythe, P.; Bienenstock, J. Autonomic neuroimmunology. In *Encyclopedia of Neuroscience*; Academic Press: London, England, 2009; pp. 1003–1008.
29. Chiu, I.M.; von Hehn, C.A.; Woolf, C.J. Neurogenic inflammation and the peripheral nervous system in host defense and immunopathology. *Nat. Neurosci.* **2012**, *15*, 1063–1067. [CrossRef]
30. Bacci, M.; Capobianco, A.; Monno, A.; Cottone, L.; Di Puppo, F.; Camisa, B.; Mariani, M.; Brignole, C.; Ponzoni, M.; Ferrari, S.; et al. Macrophages are alternatively activated in patients with endometriosis and required for growth and vascularization of lesions in a mouse model of disease. *Am. J. Pathol.* **2009**, *175*, 547–556. [CrossRef] [PubMed]
31. Anaf, V.; Chapron, C.; El Nakadi, I.; De Moor, V.; Simonart, T.; Noël, J.C. Pain, mast cells, and nerves in peritoneal, ovarian, and deep infiltrating endometriosis. *Fertil. Steril.* **2006**, *86*, 1336–1343. [CrossRef]
32. Kirchhoff, D.; Kaulfuss, S.; Fuhrmann, U.; Maurer, M.; Zollner, T.M. Mast cells in endometriosis: Guilty or innocent bystanders? *Expert Opin. Ther. Targets* **2012**, *16*, 237–241. [CrossRef] [PubMed]
33. Kempuraj, D.; Papadopoulou, N.; Stanford, E.J.; Christodoulou, S.; Madhappan, B.; Sant, G.R.; Solage, K.; Adams, T.; Theoharides, T.C. Increased numbers of activated mast cells in endometriosis lesions positive for corticotropin-releasing hormone and urocortin. *Am. J. Reprod. Immunol.* **2004**, *52*, 267–275. [CrossRef] [PubMed]
34. Vallvé-Juanico, J.; Houshdaran, S.; Giudice, L.C. The endometrial immune environment of women with endometriosis. *Hum. Reprod. Update* **2019**, *25*, 565–592. [CrossRef] [PubMed]
35. Rocha, M.G.; e Silva, J.C.; Ribeiro da Silva, A.; Candido Dos Reis, F.J.; Nogueira, A.A.; Poli-Neto, O.B. TRPV1 expression on peritoneal Endometriosis Foci is associated with chronic pelvic pain. *Reprod. Sci.* **2011**, *18*, 511–515. [CrossRef] [PubMed]
36. Liu, J.; Liu, X.; Duan, K.; Zhang, Y.; Guo, S.-W. The expression and functionality of transient receptor potential vanilloid 1 in ovarian endometriomas. *Reprod. Sci.* **2012**, *19*, 1110–1124. [CrossRef]
37. Nie, J.; Liu, X.; Guo, S.-W. Immunoreactivity of oxytocin receptor and transient receptor potential vanilloid type 1 and its correlation with dysmenorrhea in adenomyosis. *Am. J. Obstet. Gynecol.* **2010**, *202*, 346.e1–346.e8. [CrossRef] [PubMed]
38. Arnold, J.; Barcena de Arellano, M.L.; Rüster, C.; Vercellino, G.F.; Chiantera, V.; Schneider, A.; Mechsner, S. Imbalance between sympathetic and sensory innervation in peritoneal endometriosis. *Brain. Behav. Immun.* **2012**, *26*, 132–141. [CrossRef]
39. Ferrero, S.; Haas, S.; Remorgida, V.; Camerini, G.; Fulcheri, E.; Ragni, N.; Straub, R.H.; Capellino, S. Loss of sympathetic nerve fibers in intestinal endometriosis. *Fertil. Steril.* **2010**, *94*, 2817–2819. [CrossRef]
40. Nance, D.M.; Sanders, V.M. Autonomic innervation and regulation of the immune system (1987–2007). *Brain. Behav. Immun.* **2007**, *21*, 736–745. [CrossRef]
41. Sanders, V.M.; Kasprowicz, D.J.; Kohm, A.P.; Swanson, M. Neurotransmitter receptors on lymphocytes and other lymphoid cells. In *Psychoneuroimmunology, 1st. ed.*; Ader, R., Felten, D., Cohen, N., Eds.; Academic Press: New York, NY, USA, 2001; pp. 161–196.
42. Baerwald, C.; Graefe, C.; von Wichert, P.; Krause, A. Decreased density of beta-adrenergic receptors on peripheral blood mononuclear cells in patients with rheumatoid arthritis. *J. Rheumatol.* **1992**, *19*, 204–210.
43. Heijnen, C.J.; Rouppe van der Voort, C.; Wulffraat, N.; van der Net, J.; Kuis, W.; Kavelaars, A. Functional α1-adrenergic receptors on leukocytes of patients with polyarticular juvenile rheumatoid arthritis. *J. Neuroimmunol.* **1996**, *71*, 223–226. [CrossRef]

44. Kohm, A.P.; Sanders, V.M. Norepinephrine: A messenger from the brain to the immune system. *Immunol. Today* **2000**, *21*, 539–542. [CrossRef]
45. Straub, R.H. Autoimmune disease and innervation. *Brain. Behav. Immun.* **2007**, *21*, 528–534. [CrossRef]
46. Yan, D.; Liu, X.; Guo, S.W. Neuropeptides substance p and calcitonin gene related peptide accelerate the development and fibrogenesis of endometriosis. *Sci. Rep.* **2019**, *9*, 1–22. [CrossRef] [PubMed]
47. de Arellano, M.L.B.; Mechsner, S. The peritoneum—An important factor for pathogenesis and pain generation in endometriosis. *J. Mol. Med.* **2014**, *92*, 595–602. [CrossRef]
48. de Arellano, M.L.B.; Oldeweme, J.; Arnold, J.; Schneider, A.; Mechsner, S. Remodeling of estrogen-dependent sympathetic nerve fibers seems to be disturbed in adenomyosis. *Fertil. Steril.* **2013**, *100*, 801.e2–809.e2. [CrossRef]
49. Kolodkin, A.L. Semaphorin-mediated neuronal growth cone guidance. *Prog. Brain Res.* **1998**, *117*, 115–132.
50. Hui, D.H.F.; Tam, K.J.; Jiao, I.Z.F.; Ong, C.J. Semaphorin 3C as a therapeutic target in prostate and other cancers. *Int. J. Mol. Sci.* **2019**, *20*, 774. [CrossRef] [PubMed]
51. Richeri, A.; Chalar, C.; Martínez, G.; Greif, G.; Bianchimano, P.; Brauer, M.M. Estrogen up-regulation of semaphorin 3F correlates with sympathetic denervation of the rat uterus. *Auton. Neurosci.* **2011**, *164*, 43–50. [CrossRef]
52. Klatt, S.; Fassold, A.; Straub, R.H. Sympathetic nerve fiber repulsion: Testing norepinephrine, dopamine, and 17β-estradiol in a primary murine sympathetic neurite outgrowth assay. *Ann. N. Y. Acad. Sci.* **2012**, *1261*, 26–33. [CrossRef] [PubMed]
53. Scheerer, C.; Frangini, S.; Chiantera, V.; Mechsner, S. Reduced sympathetic innervation in endometriosis is associated to semaphorin 3C and 3F expression. *Mol. Neurobiol.* **2017**, *54*, 5131–5141. [CrossRef] [PubMed]
54. Godin, S.K.; Wagner, J.; Huang, P.; Bree, D. The role of peripheral nerve signaling in endometriosis. *FASEB BioAdv.* **2021**, *2021*, 00063. [CrossRef]
55. Aredo, J.; Heyrana, K.; Karp, B.; Shah, J.; Stratton, P. Relating chronic pelvic pain and endometriosis to signs of sensitization and myofascial pain and dysfunction. *Semin. Reprod. Med.* **2017**, *35*, 88–97. [CrossRef] [PubMed]
56. Hoffman, D. Central and peripheral pain generators in women with chronic pelvic pain: Patient centered assessment and treatment. *Curr. Rheumatol. Rev.* **2015**, *11*, 146–166. [CrossRef] [PubMed]
57. Vilotti, S.; Marchenkova, A.; Ntamati, N.; Nistri, A. B-type natriuretic peptide-induced delayed modulation of TRPV1 and P2X3 receptors of mouse trigeminal sensory neurons. *PLoS ONE* **2013**, *8*, e81138.
58. Davenport, A.J.; Neagoe, I.; Bräuer, N.; Koch, M.; Rotgeri, A.; Nagel, J.; Laux-Biehlmann, A.; Machet, F.; Coelho, A.M.; Boyce, S.; et al. Eliapixant is a selective P2X3 receptor antagonist for the treatment of disorders associated with hypersensitive nerve fibers. *Sci. Rep.* **2021**, *11*, 1–13.
59. Waldhoer, M.; Bartlett, S.E.; Whistler, J.L. Opioid receptors. *Annu. Rev. Biochem.* **2004**, *73*, 953–990. [CrossRef]
60. Toll, L.; Bruchas, M.R.; Calo', G.; Cox, B.M.; Zaveri, N.T. Nociceptin/orphanin FQ receptor structure, signaling, ligands, functions, and interactions with opioid systems. *Pharmacol. Rev.* **2016**, *68*, 419–457. [CrossRef]
61. Totorikaguena, L.; Olabarrieta, E.; Matorras, R.; Alonso, E.; Agirregoitia, E.; Agirregoitia, N. Mu opioid receptor in the human endometrium: Dynamics of its expression and localization during the menstrual cycle. *Fertil. Steril.* **2017**, *107*, 1070.e1–1077.e1. [CrossRef]
62. Chatzaki, E.; Margioris, A.N.; Makrigiannakis, A.; Castanas, E.; Georgoulias, V.; Gravanis, A. Kappa opioids and TGFbeta1 interact in human endometrial cells. *Mol. Hum. Reprod.* **2000**, *6*, 602–609. [CrossRef]
63. Hatzoglou, A.; Gravanis, A.; Margioris, A.N.; Zoumakis, E.; Castanas, E. Identification and characterization of opioid-binding sites present in the Ishikawa human endometrial adenocarcinoma cell line. *J. Clin. Endocrinol. Metab.* **1995**, *80*, 418–423.
64. Zhu, Y.; Pintar, J.E. Expression of opioid receptors and ligands in pregnant mouse uterus and placenta. *Biol. Reprod.* **1998**, *59*, 925–932. [CrossRef]
65. Matsuzaki, S.; Canis, M.; Vaurs-Barrière, C.; Boespflug-Tanguy, O.; Dastugue, B.; Mage, G. DNA microarray analysis of gene expression in eutopic endometrium from patients with deep endometriosis using laser capture microdissection. *Fertil. Steril.* **2005**, *84*, 1180–1190. [CrossRef] [PubMed]
66. Matsuzaki, S.; Canis, M.; Pouly, J.L.; Botchorishvili, R.; Déchelotte, P.J.; Mage, G. Differential expression of genes in eutopic and ectopic endometrium from patients with ovarian endometriosis. *Fertil. Steril.* **2006**, *86*, 548–553. [CrossRef]
67. Matsuzaki, S.; Canis, M.; Pouly, J.L.; Botchorishvili, R.; Déchelotte, P.J.; Mage, G. Both GnRH agonist and continuous oral progestin treatments reduce the expression of the tyrosine kinase receptor B and mu-opioid receptor in deep infiltrating endometriosis. *Hum. Reprod.* **2007**, *22*, 124–128. [CrossRef]
68. Marcu, I.; Gee, A.; Lynn, B. Cannabinoids and chronic pelvic pain in women: Focus on endometriosis. *J. Endometr. Pelvic Pain Disord.* **2021**, *13*, 155–165. [CrossRef]
69. Tanaka, K.; Mayne, L.; Khalil, A.; Baartz, D.; Eriksson, L.; Mortlock, S.A.; Montgomery, G.; McKinnon, B.; Amoako, A.A. The role of the endocannabinoid system in aetiopathogenesis of endometriosis: A potential therapeutic target. *Eur. J. Obstet. Gynecol. Reprod. Biol.* **2020**, *44*, 87–94. [CrossRef] [PubMed]
70. Muller, C.; Morales, P.; Reggio, P.H. Cannabinoid ligands targeting TRP channels. *Front. Mol. Neurosci.* **2018**, *11*, 487. [CrossRef] [PubMed]
71. Bouaziz, J.; Bar On, A.; Seidman, D.S.; Soriano, D. The clinical significance of endocannabinoids in endometriosis pain management. *Cannabis Cannabinoid Res.* **2017**, *2*, 72–80. [CrossRef]

72. Small-Howard, A.L.; Shimoda, L.M.N.; Adra, C.N.; Turner, H. Anti-inflammatory potential of CB1-mediated cAMP elevation in mast cells. *Biochem. J.* **2005**, *388*, 465–473. [CrossRef] [PubMed]
73. Leconte, M.; Nicco, C.; Ngô, C.; Arkwright, S.; Chéreau, C.; Guibourdenche, J.; Weill, B.; Chapron, C.; Dousset, B.; Batteux, F. Antiproliferative effects of cannabinoid agonists on deep infiltrating endometriosis. *Am. J. Pathol.* **2010**, *177*, 2963–2970. [CrossRef]
74. Bilgic, E.; Guzel, E.; Kose, S.; Aydin, M.C.; Karaismailoglu, E.; Akar, I.; Usubutun, A.; Korkusuz, P. Endocannabinoids modulate apoptosis in endometriosis and adenomyosis. *Acta Histochem.* **2017**, *119*, 523–532. [CrossRef] [PubMed]
75. Sanchez, A.M.; Cioffi, R.; Viganò, P.; Candiani, M.; Verde, R.; Piscitelli, F.; Di Marzo, V.; Garavaglia, E.; Panina-Bordignon, P. Elevated systemic levels of endocannabinoids and related mediators across the menstrual cycle in women with endometriosis. *Reprod. Sci.* **2016**, *23*, 1071–1079. [CrossRef]
76. Luschnig, P.; Schicho, R. Cannabinoids in gynecological diseases. *Med. Cannabis Cannabinoids* **2019**, *2*, 14–21. [CrossRef] [PubMed]
77. Sanchez, A.M.; Vigano, P.; Mugione, A.; Panina-Bordignon, P.; Candiani, M. The molecular connections between the cannabinoid system and endometriosis. *Mol. Hum. Reprod.* **2012**, *18*, 563–571. [CrossRef] [PubMed]
78. Dmitrieva, N.; Nagabukuro, H.; Resuehr, D.; Zhang, G.; McAllister, S.L.; McGinty, K.A.; Mackie, K.; Berkley, K.J. Endocannabinoid involvement in endometriosis. *Pain* **2010**, *151*, 703. [CrossRef] [PubMed]
79. Armour, M.; Sinclair, J.; Chalmers, K.J.; Smith, C.A. Self-management strategies amongst Australian women with endometriosis: A national online survey. *BMC Complement. Altern. Med.* **2019**, *19*, 1–8. [CrossRef] [PubMed]
80. Burney, R.O.; Lathi, R.B. Menstrual bleeding from an endometriotic lesion. *Fertil. Steril.* **2009**, *91*, 1926–1927. [CrossRef] [PubMed]
81. Králíčková, M.; Vetvicka, V. Immunological aspects of endometriosis: A review. *Ann. Transl. Med.* **2015**, *3*, 153.
82. Tran, L.V.P.; Tokushige, N.; Berbic, M.; Markham, R.; Fraser, I.S. Macrophages and nerve fibres in peritoneal endometriosis. *Hum. Reprod.* **2009**, *24*, 835–841. [CrossRef] [PubMed]
83. Schulke, L.; Berbic, M.; Manconi, F.; Tokushige, N.; Markham, R.; Fraser, I.S. Dendritic cell populations in the eutopic and ectopic endometrium of women with endometriosis. *Hum. Reprod.* **2009**, *24*, 1695–1703. [CrossRef] [PubMed]
84. Bulun, S.E. Endometriosis. *N. Engl. J. Med.* **2009**, *360*, 268–279. [CrossRef]
85. Scheerer, C.; Bauer, P.; Chiantera, V.; Sehouli, J.; Kaufmann, A.; Mechsner, S. Characterization of endometriosis-associated immune cell infiltrates (EMaICI). *Arch. Gynecol. Obstet.* **2016**, *294*, 657–664. [CrossRef]
86. Galli, S.J.; Grimbaldeston, M.; Tsai, M. Immunomodulatory mast cells: Negative, as well as positive, regulators of immunity. *Nat. Rev. Immunol.* **2008**, *8*, 478–486. [CrossRef] [PubMed]
87. Binda, M.M.; Donnez, J.; Dolmans, M.M. Targeting mast cells: A new way to treat endometriosis. *Expert Opin. Ther. Targets* **2017**, *21*, 67–75. [CrossRef] [PubMed]
88. Berbic, M.; Fraser, I.S. Regulatory T cells and other leukocytes in the pathogenesis of endometriosis. *J. Reprod. Immunol.* **2011**, *88*, 149–155. [CrossRef]
89. Crispim, P.C.A.; Jammal, M.P.; Murta, E.F.C.; Nomelini, R.S. Endometriosis: What is the influence of immune cells? *Immunol. Investig.* **2020**, *50*, 372–388. [CrossRef] [PubMed]
90. Capobianco, A.; Rovere-Querini, P. Endometriosis, a disease of the macrophage. *Front. Immunol.* **2013**, *4*, 1–14. [CrossRef]
91. Nie, M.F.; Xie, Q.; Wu, Y.H.; He, H.; Zou, L.J.; She, X.L.; Wu, X.Q. Serum and ectopic endometrium from women with endometriosis modulate macrophage M1/M2 polarization via the Smad2/Smad3 pathway. *J. Immunol. Res.* **2018**, *2018*, 6285813. [CrossRef] [PubMed]
92. Laganà, A.S.; Salmeri, F.M.; Ban Frangež, H.; Ghezzi, F.; Vrtačnik-Bokal, E.; Granese, R. Evaluation of M1 and M2 macrophages in ovarian endometriomas from women affected by endometriosis at different stages of the disease. *Gynecol. Endocrinol.* **2020**, *36*, 441–444. [CrossRef]
93. Sugamata, M.; Ihara, T.; Uchiide, I. Increase of activated mast cells in human endometriosis. *Am. J. Reprod. Immunol.* **2005**, *53*, 120–125. [CrossRef]
94. Paula, R.; Oliani, A.H.; Vaz-Oliani, D.C.; D'Ávila, S.C.; Oliani, S.M.; Gil, C.D. The intricate role of mast cell proteases and the annexin A1-FPR1 system in abdominal wall endometriosis. *J. Mol. Histol.* **2015**, *46*, 33–43. [CrossRef] [PubMed]
95. Kolaczkowska, E.; Kubes, P. Neutrophil recruitment and function in health and inflammation. *Nat. Rev. Immunol.* **2013**, *13*, 159–175. [CrossRef] [PubMed]
96. Burns, K.A.; Thomas, S.Y.; Hamilton, K.J.; Young, S.L.; Cook, D.N.; Korach, K.S. Early endometriosis in females is directed by immune-Mediated estrogen receptor a and IL-6 cross-Talk. *Endocrinology* **2018**, *159*, 103–118. [CrossRef]
97. Wang, X.-M.; Ma, Z.-Y.; Song, N. Inflammatory cytokines IL-6, IL-10, IL-13, TNF-α and peritoneal fluid flora were associated with infertility in patients with endometriosis. *Eur. Rev. Med. Pharmacol. Sci.* **2018**, *22*, 2513–2518.
98. Riccio, L.D.G.C.; Santulli, P.; Marcellin, L.; Abrão, M.S.; Batteux, F.; Chapron, C. Immunology of endometriosis. *Best Pract. Res. Clin. Obstet. Gynaecol.* **2018**, *50*, 39–49. [CrossRef] [PubMed]
99. Wang, F.; Wang, H.; Jin, D.; Zhang, Y. Serum miR-17, IL-4, and IL-6 levels for diagnosis of endometriosis. *Medicine* **2018**, *97*, e10853. [CrossRef]
100. McKinnon, B.D.; Bertschi, D.; Bersinger, N.A.; Mueller, M.D. Inflammation and nerve fiber interaction in endometriotic pain. *Trends Endrocrinol. Metab.* **2015**, *26*, 1–10. [CrossRef]
101. Zhou, J.; Chern, B.S.M.; Barton-Smith, P.; Phoon, J.W.L.; Tan, T.Y.; Viardot-Foucault, V.; Ku, C.W.; Tan, H.H.; Chan, J.K.Y.; Lee, Y.H. Peritoneal fluid cytokines reveal new insights of endometriosis subphenotypes. *Int. J. Mol. Sci.* **2020**, *21*, 3515. [CrossRef] [PubMed]

Article

Peritoneal Modulators of EZH2-miR-155 Cross-Talk in Endometriosis

Sarah Brunty [1,†], Kristeena Ray Wright [1,†], Brenda Mitchell [2] and Nalini Santanam [1,*]

1. Department of Biomedical Sciences, Joan C. Edwards School of Medicine, Marshall University, Huntington, WV 25755, USA; binion2@live.marshall.edu (S.B.); kristeena.ray@gmail.com (K.R.W.)
2. Department of Obstetrics and Gynecology, Joan C. Edwards School of Medicine, Marshall University, Huntington, WV 25755, USA; dawleyb@marshall.edu
* Correspondence: santanam@marshall.edu
† These authors contributed equally to this work.

Abstract: Activation of trimethylation of histone 3 lysine 27 (H3K27me3) by EZH2, a component of the Polycomb repressive complex 2 (PRC2), is suggested to play a role in endometriosis. However, the mechanism by which this complex is dysregulated in endometriosis is not completely understood. Here, using eutopic and ectopic tissues, as well as peritoneal fluid (PF) from IRB-approved and consented patients with and without endometriosis, the expression of PRC2 complex components, JARID2, miR-155 (known regulators of EZH2), and a key inflammatory modulator, FOXP3, was measured. A higher expression of EZH2, H3K27me3, JARID2, and FOXP3 as well as miR-155 was noted in both the patient tissues and in endometrial PF treated cells. Gain-or-loss of function of miR-155 showed an effect on the PRC2 complex but had little effect on JARID2 expression, suggesting alternate pathways. Chromatin immunoprecipitation followed by qPCR showed differential expression of PRC2 complex proteins and its associated binding partners in JARID2 vs. EZH2 pull down assays. In particular, endometriotic PF treatment increased the expression of *PHF19* ($p = 0.0474$), a gene silencer and co-factor that promotes PRC2 interaction with its targets. Thus, these studies have identified the potential novel crosstalk between miR-155-PRC2 complex-JARID2 and PHF19 in endometriosis, providing an opportunity to test other epigenetic targets in endometriosis.

Keywords: endometriosis; epigenetics; EZH2; microRNA

1. Introduction

Endometriosis is defined by the presence of endometrial tissue in ectopic locations, typically in or around the peritoneal cavity [1,2]. While the exact prevalence of endometriosis is likely underrepresented, most sources cite that a minimum of 10% of women in their reproductive years have this disease [3–5]. Primarily described as a hormonal disorder, the pathogenesis of endometriosis has also been linked to immunological/inflammatory, genetic, and environmental factors. More recently, the role of epigenetics in the development and progression of this disorder has been investigated [6–12]. Epigenetic mechanisms are heritable changes to one's phenotype that are not associated with a change in nucleotide sequence and include DNA methylation, post-translational modifications to histone proteins, and often microRNAs [13,14].

In addition to heterochromatin-like protein 1 (HP-1), polycomb (PcG) and trithorax (TrxG) complexes are at the heart of epigenetics. Responsible for maintaining gene repression and activity, respectively [15], the latter two complexes function antagonistically to establish epigenetic regulation [15]. Polycomb repressive complex 1 (PRC1), polycomb repressive complex 2 (PRC2), and Pho repressive complex (PhoRC) all form the PcG complexes, with the former two typically being the subject of extensive epigenetic research. The Polycomb Repressive Complex 2 (PRC2) consists of four core proteins, RbAp46/48, Embryonic Ectoderm Development (EED), Suppressor of Zeste 12 (SUZ12), and Enhancer of Zeste Homolog 2 (EZH2), the catalytic subunit of the PRC2 complex. These components work together to regulate chromatin structure via tri-methylation of lysine 27 on histone 3 (H3K27me3) [16,17], which is also known to interact with PRC1. EED binds the histone site while EZH2 methylates it, with the help of SUZ12 [18]. This modification leads to the formation of closed chromatin structure (heterochromatin) and thus marks transcriptional repression, as further demonstrated by the presence of other co-factors [19–21].

There is very little known about the mechanistic role of PRC2 complex and how it is regulated in the endometriosis disease process. While an in vivo study showed heightened expression of EZH2 and trimethylation of H3K27 in secretory endometrium and endometriotic lesions [22,23], another cell culture study showed that inhibition of PGE2 receptors EP3 and EP4 occur concurrently with decreased EZH2 expression [24], supporting a role for PRC2 in endometriosis-associated pain.

It has been shown that the PRC2 complex (specifically EZH2) is, at least partly, regulated by Jumonji and AT-Rich Interaction Domain Containing 2 (JARID2) [25], a member of the largest family of histone demethylases, the jumonji family, where all but JARID2 contain the catalytic JmjC domain responsible for histone demethylation [26,27]. Research has found that JARID2 is a cofactor for PRC2 [28]. Additionally, its methylation by the PRC2 complex at K116 is part of a regulatory mechanism that controls the PRC2 enzymatic activity where the methylated JARID2 binds to the EED component of the PRC2 complex. This is required for efficient deposition of H3K27me3 during cell differentiation and fine-tunes the PRC2 activity [29]. JARDI2 is thought to be crucial in the development and progression of cancer. This is due to its cross-talk with EZH2 and PRC2 activity in embryonic stem cells (ESC), as JARID2 is necessary for proper ESC differentiation [25,30,31].

JARID2 is suggested to be modulated by few mechanisms. For example, iron oxidation, which occurs due to increased reactive oxygen species generation and known to be present in excess in women with endometriosis, blocks the catalytic activity of JARID2 [32]. JARID2 is also a common target of microRNAs some of which have been identified by our laboratory to be differentially expressed (miR-30b, miR-30c, miR-10a, miR-29a, miR-26a, miR-148a, miR-181a, miR-30e) in endometriotic lesions compared to control tissues [33]. Palma et al. showed in acute lymphoid leukemia that miR-155-5p induced cell death via a network of mechanisms, including regulation of cyclinD1 by JARID2 [34]. Other such studies support the possibility that miR-155-5p could have been evolved to regulate PRC2 by tweaking JARID2 expression [35]. Interestingly, miR-155-5p is an established promoter of inflammation via regulation of macrophages and cytokines [35–37]. Thus, targeting this demethylase (JARID2) via modulators such as microRNAs, could be a novel method of treatment for endometriosis.

miR-155 is highly expressed in regulatory T-cells (Tregs), where it is targeted by transcription factor forkhead box P3 (FOXP3) [38]. Though limited in evidence, FOXP3 also plays a role in the inflammatory aspect of endometriosis, which correlates with miR-155-5p being a promoter of inflammation. The prevalence of FOXP3$^+$ Tregs in an endometriotic environment during secretory phase prevent leukocyte recruitment to the sites of endometriosis [39]. Additionally, peritoneal fluid (PF) from women with endometriosis has a higher concentration of FOXP3-expressing TCD4$^+$ CD25^{high} cells than the PF of control patients [40,41]. Other studies have also shown that FoxP3 is an inducer of miR-155 [42].

It is important to note that FOXP3 also has an indirect relationship with the EZH2 component of PRC2. Overexpression of the FOXP3 protein not only lessened the proliferative effects of EZH2, but also enhanced degradation of the EZH2 protein in breast cancer models [43]. Conversely, there is evidence that trimethylation of H3K27 by EZH2 is capable of silencing FOXP3 promoter regions, therefore leading to aberrant Treg cell differentiation and function [44]. These studies suggest a complex interplay between epigenetic mediators, PRC2 complex, miR-155-5p, JARID2 and the inflammatory mediator FOXP3. In this study, it is hypothesized that the imbalance in this crosstalk triggers inflammatory responses and possibly nociception in endometriosis. This current study investigated the crosstalk between these mediators in endometriotic patient tissues and in an endometriosis cell model.

2. Results

2.1. PRC2 Complex and JARID2 mRNA and Protein Expression in Endometriotic Tissues

The endogenous expression of PRC2 complex proteins in endometriotic tissues were first determined. qPCR was used to determine the mRNA expression of PRC2 components SUZ12, EED, and EZH2 in eutopic tissue from women with no endometriosis (EuN, $n = 5$) or women with endometriosis (EuE, $n = 10$) and ectopic tissue from women with endometriosis (EcE, $n = 6$) (Figure 1A). When compared to the EuN tissues, expression of all three PRC2 protein complex (*SUZ12*, *EED* and *EZH2*) and *JARID2*, was higher in both the eutopic (EuE) and ectopic (EcE) tissue from endometriosis patients. Compared to EuN tissues, *SUZ12* levels increased close to 2-fold for EcE but was not significant, however there was a significant increase in *EED* expression by 5.07-fold in EuE ($p = 0.0153$) and 7.13-fold ($p = 0.0067$) in EcE. *EZH2* expression was also increased 2.35-fold in the EuE and 3.10-fold in the EcE but did not reach significance. Expression for *JARID2* increased over 2-fold in EcE tissues, but this was not significant.

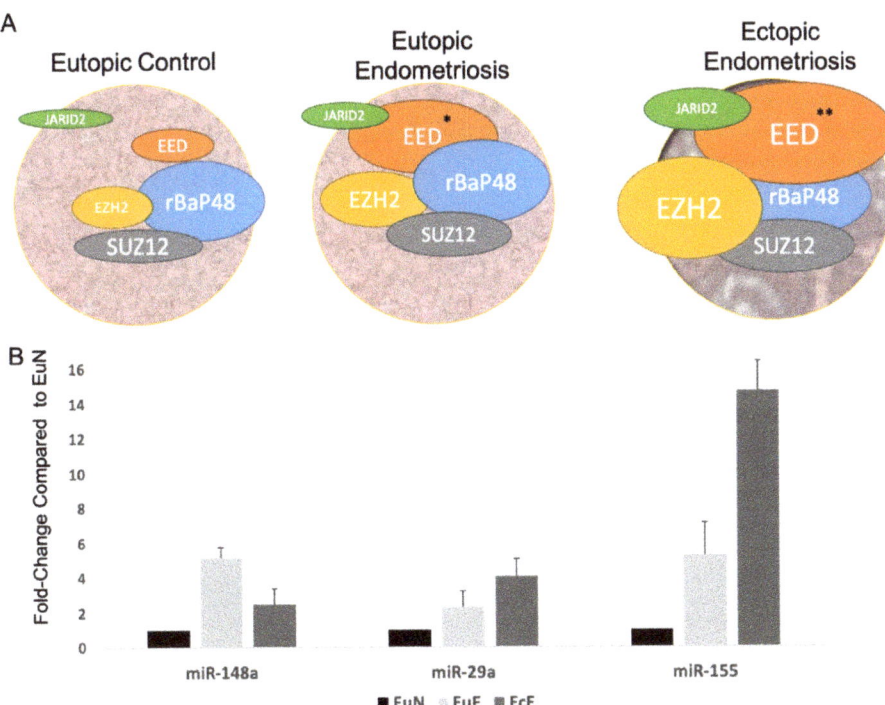

Figure 1. mRNA expression of PRC2 complex and JARID2 and miRNAs that target JARID2 in endometriotic tissues. (**A**) Relative mRNA expression of polycomb repressor complex 2 (PRC2) elements and *JARID2* in eutopic tissues from control women, EuN ($n = 5$), or eutopic and ectopic tissues from women with endometriosis, EuE ($n = 10$) and EcE tissues ($n = 6$). In general, these elements were upregulated in both eutopic and ectopic endo tissues compared to control tissue with *EED* showing significant upregulation in both the eutopic ($p = 0.0153$) and ectopic ($p = 0.0067$). *JARID2* expression was higher in EcE. * $p < 0.05$, ** $p < 0.01$ when compared to EuN tissues. (**B**) Compared to control tissues ($n = 7$), expression of miR-148a, miR-29a, and miR-155 (miRNAs that target JARID2) were all higher in endo tissues (both eutopic and ectopic, $n = 8$).

Protein expression was also determined using the automated Western blotting system, WES. While EZH2 showed a significant increase of >7 fold ($p = 0.0219$) in EcE tissues compared to EuN, no significant difference was seen in expression of H3K27me3 or JARID2 (Figure S1). This lack of change in JARID2 expression might be attributed to its altered regulation.

2.2. miRNAs Targeting JARID2 in Endometriotic Tissues

The expression levels of miRNAs that regulate JARID2 was next determined in the patient tissues. miRNA qPCR assays were used to measure expression of miR-148a, miR-29a, and miR-155, which, among others, target JARID2 (Targetscan 7.1 and Ingenuity Pathway Analysis Qiagen, Germantown, MD, USA). Interestingly, all three miRNAs were overexpressed in both EuE and EcE tissues compared to EuN tissues (Figure 1B). Both miR-148a and miR-155 showed an over 5-fold increase in expression for the EuE tissues and were also shown to be induced more than 2.5–14-fold, respectively on EcE, while miR-29a expression increased 2–4-fold with levels higher in EuE and EcE tissues.

2.3. PRC2 Complex mRNA and Protein Expression in PF Treated Endometrial Cells

Peritoneal cavity is one of the major sites for endometriotic lesions in women with endometriosis [45,46]. These patients also exhibit larger volumes of PF rich in inflammatory and nociceptive molecules [47,48]. Current theories propose a dynamic role for PF in modulating the growth of endometriotic lesions, which might be epigenetically regulated by the altered expression of certain miRNAs previously shown in endometriosis [49,50]. Whether PF from patients with and without endometriosis differentially regulated the PRC2 complex proteins in endometrial cells was determined. For this, human endometrial cells were exposed to 1% PF from women with ($n = 13$) or without endometriosis ($n = 12$) for 48 h followed by the measurement of both mRNA and protein expression of PRC2 complex proteins using similar techniques as described for the endometriotic tissues. Cells treated with both 1% control or endo PF had increased *SUZ12, EED,* and *EZH2* mRNA expression but none were shown to be statistically significant (Figure 2A). When protein expression was determined using the automated Western Blotting system, WES, EZH2 showed no significant difference in expression levels when compared to the media control. While H3K27me3 did show an upregulation of over 2-fold for endo PF treated cells, this was not significant. (Figure 2B,C).

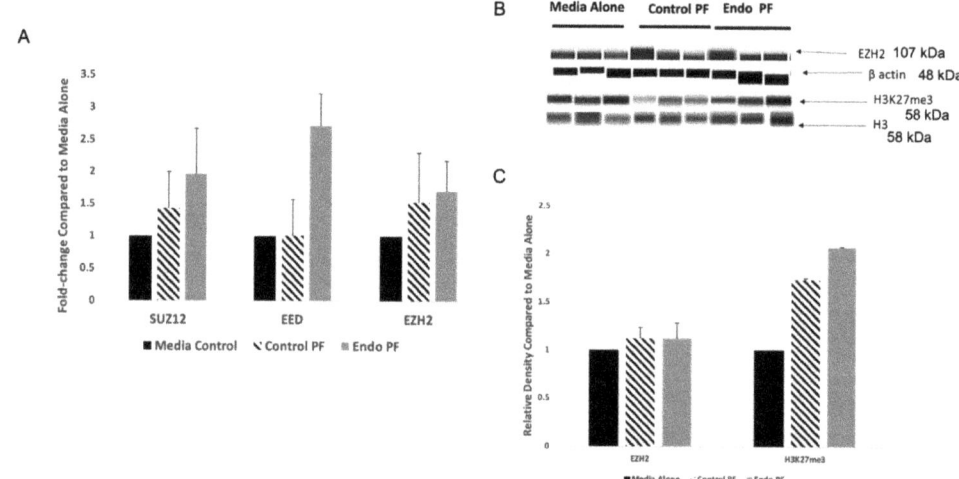

Figure 2. mRNA and protein expression of PRC2 complex proteins in PF treated endometrial cells. (**A**) mRNA expression of *SUZ12, EED,* and *EZH2* in cells treated with control PF ($n = 12$) and endo PF ($n = 13$), relative to expression in a media control

($p > 0.05$). (**B**) Representative WES images and densitometric analysis for EZH2, and H3K27me3 in PF-treated cells. (**C**) Relative protein expression of EZH2, and H3K27me3 in PF-treated cells was calculated in relation to a media control and presented as a ratio in which media alone is 1. Densities of protein bands obtained were normalized to β-actin or H3. It is to be noted that molecular weights of protein bands in automated WES system differs from the traditional Western blotting, due to differences in technology.

2.4. JARID2 and miRNAs Targeting It in PF Treated Endometrial Cells

The expression of JARID2 in the peritoneal fluid treated endometrial cells was also examined. While both the control and endo PF treated cells showed an increase in mRNA expression of *JARID2* when compared to media alone, neither was shown to be significant (Figure 3A). Analysis of protein expression of JARID2 showed a significant upregulation of expression when cells were treated with endo PF of 3.61-fold ($p = 0.0027$) and by about 2-fold compared to control PF ($p = 0.0096$) treated cells (Figure 3B,C).

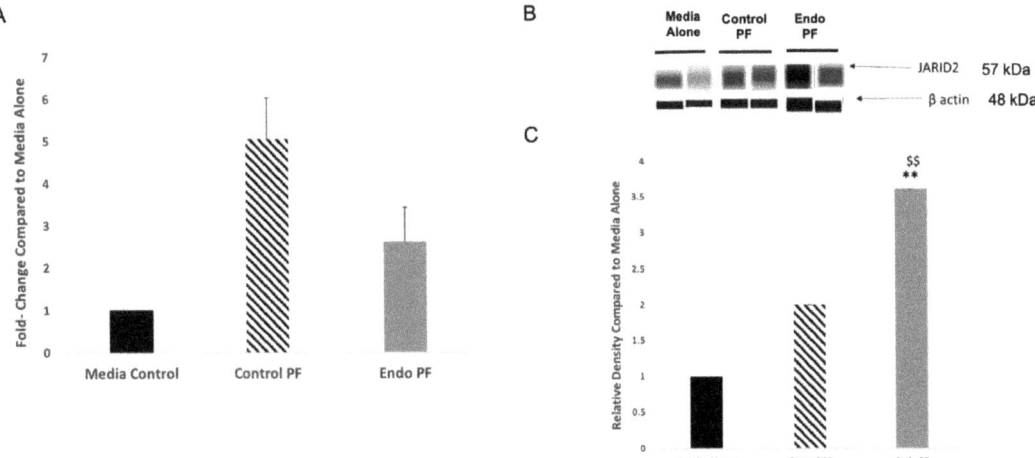

Figure 3. mRNA and protein expression of JARID2 in PF treated endometrial cells. (**A**) mRNA expression of JARID2 in cells treated with control PF ($n = 12$) and endo PF ($n = 13$), relative to expression in a media control ($n = 6$) ($p > 0.05$). (**B**) Representative WES images and densitometric analysis for JARID2 in PF-treated cells. (**C**) Relative protein expression of JARID2 in PF-treated cells was calculated in relation to a media control and presented as a ratio in which media alone is 1. Significant upregulation of JARID2 of 3.61-fold was seen in the endo PF treated cells when compared to media alone cells ($p = 0.0027$) and by about 2-fold compared to control PF ($p = 0.0096$) treated cells. ** significant difference ($p < 0.01$) when compared to media alone. $$ Significant difference ($p < 0.05$) in mean compared to control PF. Densities of the protein bands obtained were normalized to β-actin or H3. It is to be noted that molecular weights of protein bands in automated WES system differs from the traditional Western blotting, due to differences in technology.

Next, it was assessed if the addition of the PF to the endometrial cells changed the expression levels of the miRNAs that regulates JARID2 levels. miR-148a and miR-29a showed a decrease in expression in both control and endo PF treated endometrial cells, while miR-29a showed a decrease in expression for the control PF treated cells but a slight increase in the endo PF treated cells. Surprisingly, but consistent with what was observed earlier in the EcE tissues, miR-155 showed an increase in expression in both control and endo PF treated cells, but no results were shown to be statistically significant. (Figure 4). This increase in miR-155 might have lowered the JARID2 expression.

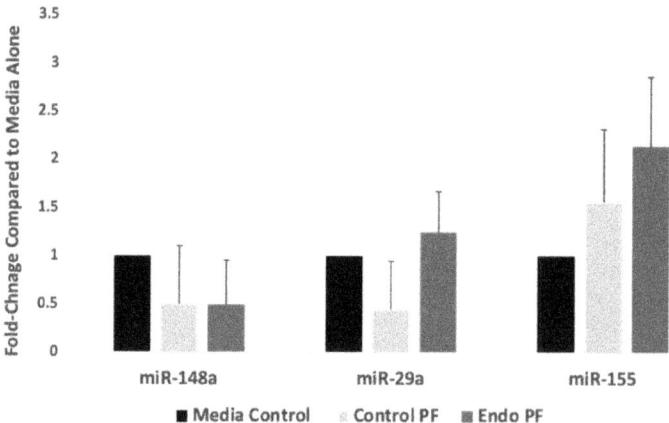

Figure 4. Expression of miRNAs that target JARID2 in PF treated endometrial cells. Compared to media control cells ($n = 4$), expression of miR-148a was shown to be lower in the endo PF treated cells while miR-155 and miR-29a was increased in expression but none were significant. control PF ($n = 12$), endo PF ($n = 13$).

2.5. FOXP3 mRNA and Protein Expression in Endometrial Tissues and PF Treated Endometrial Cells

With the knowledge that FOXP3 is a regulator of miR-155, the expression levels of FOXP3 in the endometrial tissues and in the PF treated endometrial cells were determined. qPCR showed that while the tissues from patients with endometriosis (EuE and EcE) were slightly upregulated compared to EuN, there was no significance between the expressions (Figure 5A). Relative protein expressions of FOXP3 are shown in Figure 5B. No significant difference was seen between the mean density of endo tissue and control tissue bands.

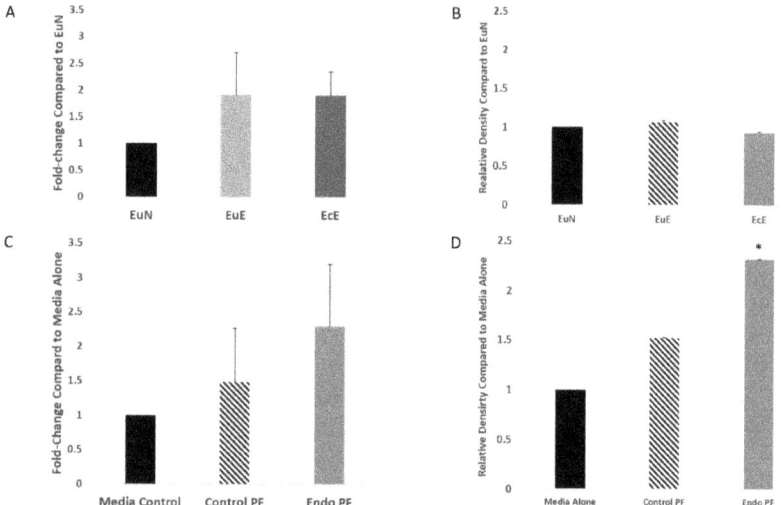

Figure 5. mRNA and protein expression of FOXP3 in patient tissues and PF treated cells. (**A**) Relative mRNA expression of *FOXP3* in EuN ($n = 5$), EuE ($n = 10$), and EcE ($n = 6$). Upregulation of the *FOXP3* mRNA expression in the endometriotic patient tissues was observed but was not significant; (**B**) Relative protein expression of FOXP3 in EuE and EcE was calculated in relation to EuN. Down-regulation of EuE and EcE were seen when compared to EuN. For all comparisons made,

$p > 0.05$. (**C**) mRNA expression of FOXP3 in cells treated with control PF ($n = 12$) and endo PF ($n = 13$), relative to expression in a media control ($p > 0.05$). (**D**) Relative protein expression of FOXP3 in PF-treated cells was calculated in relation to a media control and presented as a ratio, in which media alone or EuN is 1. FOXP3 expression was 2.32-fold higher in endo PF ($p = 0.0493$) than in control media alone treated cells. * $p < 0.05$. Densities of the protein bands obtained were normalized to β-actin or H3.

FOXP3 mRNA expression in the endo PF treated cells were shown to be increased in expression but was not significant (Figure 5C). For protein expression using the automated Western blotting system, WES, FOXP3 was increased in cells treated with both control and endo PF, but a statistically significant change in expression was only shown with endo PF treatment (2.32-fold, $p = 0.0493$) (Figure 5D).

2.6. miR-155 Regulates PRC2 Complex and FOXP3

Since JARID2 and FOXP3 are targets of miR-155 and miR-155 was upregulated in endometriotic tissues and PF treated cells, it was investigated if modulating miR-155 levels using a mimic or inhibitor will alter these target genes. To test this, the expression of JARID2, PRC2 complex and FOXP3 were determined in endometrial cells transfected with a miR-155 mimic or inhibitor (antagonist). Transfection efficiency of miR-155 is shown in Figure 6A. In cells transfected with the mimic, treatment with control PF increased the expression of miR-155 by over 3-fold, compared to when treated with the inhibitor, where the expression decreased below 0.50-fold. In contrast, in cells transfected with the mimic, treatment with endo PF increased miR-155 expression by 1.5-fold but decreased below 0.50-fold after treatment in cells transfected with the inhibitor. Upon PF treatment of the cells transfected with the miR-155 mimic, there was minimal effect on *JARID2* mRNA expression ($p > 0.05$), but seemed to increase *FOXP3* expression in cells treated with control PF and even more so in cells treated with endo PF. In contrast, PF treatment of miR-155 inhibitor transfected cells had no major effect on *JARID2* or *FOXP3* mRNA expression (Figure 6B,C).

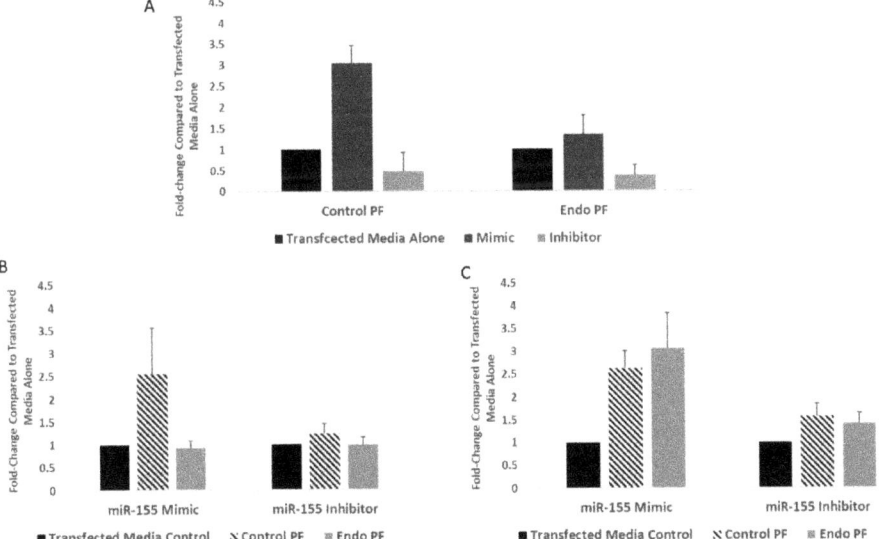

Figure 6. Key mRNA levels in cells transfected with a miR-155 mimic and inhibitor. (**A**) Levels of miR-155 showing transfection efficiency. (**B**) Transfection with a miR-155 mimic had little effect on *JARID2* expression in PF-treated cells ($p > 0.05$), (**C**) but seemed to increase *FOXP3* expression in cells treated with control PF. Compared to control media, the miR-155 inhibitor had no major effect on *JARID2* or *FOXP3* expression in PF treated cells.

Western blotting analysis showed that overexpression of miR-155 resulted in significantly lower JARID2 protein expression in control PF-treated cells compared to endo PF-treated cells ($p = 0.0106$). Neither EZH2 nor H2K27me3 protein expression showed any significant up or downregulation in cells overexpressing miR-155 (Figure 7A). In contrast, while both JARID2 and EZH2 showed an upregulation in protein expression in the endo PF treatment groups, when miR-155 was inhibited, no significance was achieved. The protein expression of H3K27me3 in the control PF-treated cells in miR-155 inhibited cells, was significantly upregulated when compared to both the transfected media alone cells and the endo PF-treated cells ($p = 0.0105$ and 0.0138, respectively) (Figure 7B). In miR-155 overexpressing cells, both control and endo PF significantly increased FOXP3 protein expression when compared to transfected media alone ($p = 0.0005$ and 0.0079, respectively). In contrast no significant difference in FOXP3 protein expression was seen in cells transfected with an miR-155 inhibitor (Figure 7C).

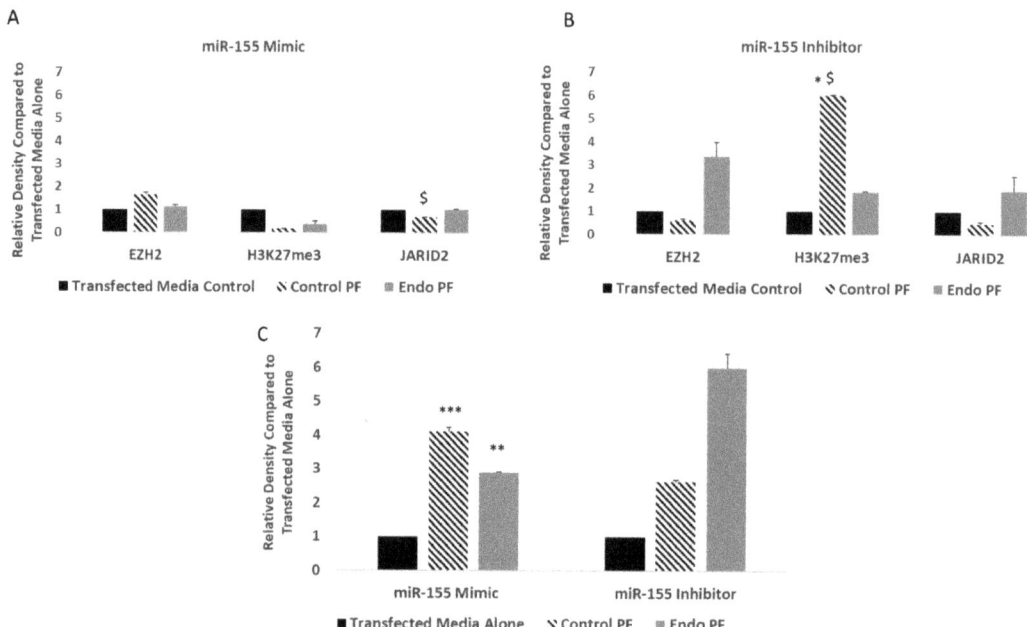

Figure 7. Expression of key targets in cells transfected with miR-155 mimic and inhibitor. (**A**) Transfection with a miR-155 mimic resulted in significantly lower JARID2 expression in control PF-treated cells ($n = 6$) compared to endo PF-treated cells ($n = 6$) ($p = 0.0106$). No significant difference in expression was seen in EZH2 or H3K27me3. (**B**) Transfection with a miR-155 inhibitor resulted in higher H3K27me3 for the control PF-treated cells when compared to transfected media and endo PF-treated cells ($p = 0.0105$, 0.0138, respectively). Relative expression of EZH2 and JARID2 showed no significant increase or decrease in any of the treated groups. (**C**) Transfection with an miR-155 mimic showed significant upregulation of FOXP3 in both control and endo PF-treated cells ($p = 0.0005$, 0.0079) when compared to transfected media alone. Though FOXP3 was induced by 3 or 6-fold in control or endo PF treated cells transfected with miR-155 inhibitor, no significance was observed. * $p < 0.05$, ** $p < 0.01$, and *** $p < 0.005$ compared to transfected media alone, $ Significant difference ($p < 0.05$) in mean compared to endo PF. Density of protein bands obtained was normalized to β-actin or H3.

2.7. ChIP Using JARID2 or EZH2 Antibody Reveals Other Co-Factors of PRC2 Complex

In order to delineate the alterations in the binding partners of EZH2 in the PF treated cells, ChIP was performed using either JARID2 or EZH2 antibodies followed by ChIP-qPCR promoter array of genes associated with polycomb and trithorax complexes in cells treated with or without PF. Table 1A provides a list of focused gene panel involved in polycomb and trithorax complex activity, that were differentially expressed in endo PF treated cells when compared to control PF after IP by either JARID2 or EZH2 antibodies. The enrichment of EZH2 after JARID2 IP was lower in endo PF-treated cells compared to control cells. However, EZH1, a polycomb enzyme which is responsible for mono-, di-, or tri-methylation of H3K27, showed an enrichment after JARID2 IP in endo treated cells when compared to control PF treated cells but this enrichment was not significant. In contrast, the enrichment of JARID2 after EZH2 IP was over 5-fold higher in endo PF treated cells compared to control PF treated cells. ARID1A, a subunit of the SWI/SNF complex, with an antagonistic relationship with EZH2 [51], showed enrichment after both JARID2 IP and even higher after EZH2 IP.

Table 1. ChIP-qPCR of PRC2 complex proteins in PF-treated cells. Chromatin Immunoprecipitation (ChIP) was used to analyze interactions between JARID2 and EZH2 and genes associated with the polycomb and trithorax complexes, normalized to IgG. **A.** Fold change values represent the ratio of enrichment/binding of JARID2 or EZH2 to various genes in endo PF-treated cells ($n = 3$) to enrichment in control PF treated cells ($n = 3$). Genes with a p-value < 0.05 are shown as bold and italicized. EZH1 and EZH2 are also shown but did not have a significant p-value for either JARID2 or EZH2 when comparing the two cell treatments. **B.** Fold change values representing the ratio of enrichment/binding in EZH2 precipitated cells ($n = 3$) to enrichment in JARID2 precipitated cells ($n = 3$) for both cell treatments. p-values < 0.05 are shown as bold and italicized along with EZH1, EZH2, and JARID2 which did not show significant p-values for either treatment.

A		JARID2		EZH2	
Symbol	Gene Name	Fold Change (Endo PF/Control PF)	p-Value	Fold Change (Endo PF/Control PF)	p-Value
ARID1A	AT rich interactive domain 1A (SWI-like)	3.39	*0.0117*	10.65	0.1342
ASXL2	Additional sex combs like 2 (*Drosophila*)	4.51	0.2999	8.88	*0.0395*
CXXC1	CXXC finger protein 1	3.70	*0.0139*	8.56	0.1014
DNMT3B	DNA (cytosine-5-) methyltransferase 3 beta	1.13	0.8213	4.25	*0.0165*
EZH1	Enhancer of zeste homolog 1 (*Drosophila*)	1.4713	0.7986	12.11	0.259
EZH2	Enhancer of zeste homolog 2 (*Drosophila*)	0.3789	0.5621	12.79	0.2746
INO80	INO80 homolog (*S. cerevisiae*)	1.50	0.6214	3.76	*0.0182*
JARID2	Jumonji, AT rich interactive domain 2	2.92	0.2653	5.05	*0.0498*
PHF1	PHD finger protein 1	4.55	*0.0316*	13.31	0.1494
PHF19	PHD finger protein 19	0.2890	0.2152	4.76	0.1622

B		Control PF		Endo PF	
Symbol	Gene Name	Fold Change (JARID2/EZH2)	p-Value	Fold Change (JARID2/EZH2)	p-Value
DNMT3B	DNA (cytosine-5-) methyltransferase 3 beta	2.49	*0.0164*	0.66	0.385
E2F6	E2F transcription factor 6	4.52	*0.00027*	0.51	0.4839
EZH1	Enhancer of zeste homolog 1 (*Drosophila*)	0.91	0.9143	0.34	0.3762
EZH2	Enhancer of zeste homolog 2 (*Drosophila*)	3.59	0.3551	0.68	0.6713
JARID2	Jumonji, AT rich interactive domain 2	1.6	0.6838	0.92	0.8731
MTF2	Metal response element binding transcription factor 2	15.63	*0.0234*	0.67	0.6671
PHF19	PHD finger protein 19	1.96	0.3848	0.12	0.1440
SMARCA5	SWI/SNF related, matrix associated, actin dependent regulator of chromatin, subfamily a, member 5	8.13	*0.039*	0.73	0.7004

When comparing the genes involved in polycomb and trithorax complex activity, pulled down by the two antibodies, (Table 1B), JARID2 IP compared to EZH2 IP showed upregulation of 4 genes with p-values < 0.05 in control PF treated cells. While no significant p-values were seen for any genes in the endo PF treated cells, when JARID2/EZH2 ratio was calculated, all but 7 genes were shown to be downregulated in these cells suggesting that ChIP by EZH2 in endo PF treated cells has more of an effect on the pull-down expression of these genes compared to JARID2. Any p-values > 0.05 may be due in part to the smaller sample size tested.

2.8. PHF19, a Key Co-Factor in the miR-155-JARID2-EZH2 Crosstalk in Endometriosis

The polycomb-like proteins, PHF1 and PHF19 are critical components of PRC2 complex, both of which showed enrichment after EZH2 IP in the endo PF treated cells (fold change, 13.31 and 4.76-fold, respectively). Both these proteins are shown to work with the PRC2 complex in the manner similar to JARID2 in which they form subcomplexes with PRC2 core components and modulate the enzymatic activity of PRC2 and its recruitment [52,53]. Interestingly, PHF19 is also shown to interact with miR-155 to bring the PRC2 complex to its target [54]. In order to validate the ChIP findings, mRNA expression of *PHF19* was determined in the PF treated endometrial cells using qPCR. mRNA analysis revealed that *PHF19* was upregulated in endometrial cells treated with both control and endo PF when compared to media alone cells with the expression of *PHF19* reaching almost 11.5-fold in the endo PF treated cells ($p = 0.0474$), suggesting that PHF19 may be working along with miR-155 to bring the PRC2 complex to its target and promote endometriosis (Figure 8).

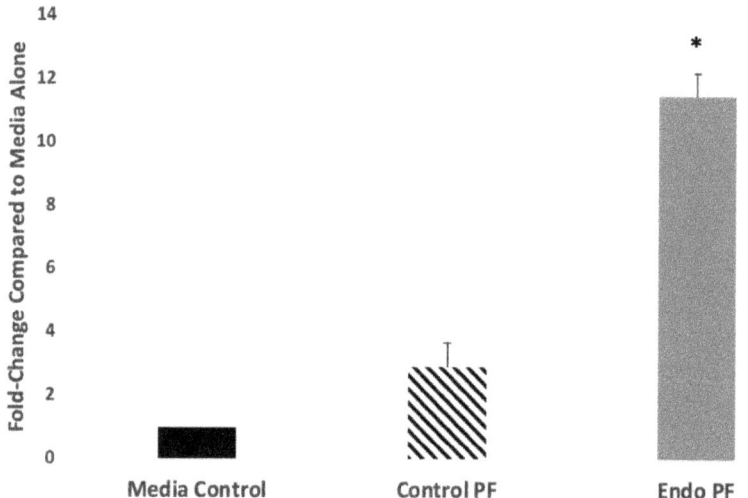

Figure 8. mRNA expression of PHF19 in endometrial cells treated with PF. When Ishikawa endometrial cells were treated with endo PF, expression of *PHF19* was shown to increase 11.50-fold relative to media alone treated cells ($p = 0.0474$). * $p < 0.05$ compared to media alone.

2.9. Promoter Methylation of Inflammatory Genes

To assess changes in promoter methylation patterns in PF treated cells, a global DNA methylation array of genes involved in inflammation and autoimmunity was performed. The heat map in Figure S2A presents a range (from 0 to 100) of "M", the fraction of input genomic DNA containing 2+ methylated CpG sites in the targeted region of a gene. Genes that were shown to be impacted by DNA methylation by having significant *p*-values (<0.05) (Figure S2B) were C-C Motif Chemokine Ligand 25 (CCL25), Cluster of Differentiation 8a (CD8A), CCAAT Enhancer Binding Protein Beta (CEBPB), Dipeptidyl peptidase 4 (DPP4), forkhead box P3 (FOXP3), interleukin-4 receptor (IL4R), Jun Proto-Oncogene, AP-1 Transcription Factor Subunit (JUN), Mitogen-activated protein kinase 14 (MAPK14), MHC class I polypeptide-related sequence B (MICB), and transforming growth factor beta 1 (TGFB1). All genes had an increased methylation pattern in cells treated with endo PF compared to the media control. The exception was MAPK14, which decreased in methylation in the endo PF treated cells. FOXP3 M values were 54.02% in endo PF treated cells ($p < 0.0001$), 26.54% in control PF treated cells ($p = 0.0151$), and 0.23% in media control. Bisulfite sequencing will be used in the future to better understand the methylation patterns of sample DNA.

3. Discussion

Our laboratory has been studying mechanisms leading to endometriosis and pain experienced by endometriosis patients [55–58]. This study stemmed from our previous investigations into the miRNA profile of endometriosis tissues and PF treated cells [33]. Nineteen percent of differentially expressed miRNAs in endo tissues targeted JARID2. Despite the global downregulation seen in the micronome of endometriotic tissues [33], miRNAs that targeted JARID2 were highly expressed in the eutopic tissues of endometriosis patients who also experienced pain as a symptom. The overexpression of miR-148a, miR-29a [33], and miR-155 in endo tissues (Figure 1B) seemed to further support this theory. As shown in Figure 1A, there was an increased expression of PRC2 complex proteins such as *EED* (0.0067), as well as a noticeable trend in overexpression of corresponding genes in ectopic tissues from endometriosis patients, particularly in *EZH2*. This correlates with the findings of Colon-Caraballo and colleagues [8,23] and supports the characterization of EZH2 as a contributor to transcriptional repression and progression of the disease.

Although miR-155 was not originally identified based on the micronome array ($p > 0.05$), its relationship with JARID2 has recently drawn the attention of researchers in the field of inflammatory diseases [34,35]. miR-155 seems to play a key intermediate that regulates the crosstalk between JARID2 and PRC2 complex. miR-155 also plays a role in inflammation by working with FOXP3 to promote an inflammatory environment, since it has been shown that FOXP3 induces miR-155 expression [38,42]. Hence, miR-155 is a potential therapeutic target. This study explored the role of miR-155 in endometriosis by studying its interactions with the PRC2 complex, JARID2 and FOXP3. Endometrial cells were transfected with a miR-155 mimic or antagonist and then exposed to endo or control PF treatments. All PRC2 complex proteins examined showed an increase in expression in endo PF treated cells when compared to media alone treated cells. However, the cells transfected with a miR-155 mimic showed a downregulation of PRC2 complex proteins when exposed to either control or endo PF. The effect of gain- or- loss- of function of miR-155 on *JARID2* expression was interesting. miR-155 mimic transfected cells treated with control PF showed an increase in *JARID2* expression, while endo PF showed no change in expression. When transfected with the miR-155 inhibitor, no statistical difference in expression was seen in cells treated with control or endo PF. These results were unexpected and suggest that the miR-155 regulation of JARID2 is not sufficient to alter its expression. Hence, other transcription factors and/or epigenetic mediators could play a role in its aberrant expression in endometriosis.

FOXP3 showed a significant increase in expression in both control and endo PF treated cells when transfected with a miR-155 mimic (Figure 7C), which paralleled the results seen for mRNA expression (Figure 6C). Such interactions between miR-155 and FOXP3 has been observed earlier. In diffuse B-cell lymphoma (DLBCL), high FOXP3 expression was correlated with a poor prognosis in patients and when miR-155 was silenced in these cells, there was a parallel decrease in FOXP3 levels [59]. In breast cancer, it was found that FOXP3 and miR-155 work together to down regulate ZEB2, resulting in reduced invasion [42].

Methylation of the FOXP3 promoter could be partly responsible for pain that women with endometriosis may experience based on the trend of increased methylation in cells treated with PF from endo patients, particularly those reporting pain (Figure S2). This has been seen in both biliary atresia and prostatitis [60,61]. Bamidele and colleagues looked at the interaction of EZH2 and FOXP3 in inflammatory bowel disease and found that a mutation in FOXP3 disrupted EZH2 recruitment and its co-repressive function. They also showed that IL-6 voided the FOXP3-EZH2 interaction and that this destabilized interaction may drive the gastrointestinal inflammation [62]. This disruption in interaction may also be true in endometriosis, since we and others have shown that IL-6 is increased in patients with endometriosis [55,63]. While *FOXP3* mRNA expression in endo PF-treated cells trended to be higher than that of cells treated with control PF, there was no statistical significance observed between the two treatments. These results suggest that FOXP3 is working alongside miR-155 to modulate the expression of EZH2.

EZH2 mRNA expression in cells treated with both control and endo PF were higher when compared to media alone cells, but there was no statistical difference seen. However, an upregulation was seen in H3K27me3 in cells treated with endo PF. This is also significant as H3K27me3 is the downstream target of EZH2 and performs the transcriptional repression in cells [64]. The benefit of studying the PRC2 complex proteins in tissues and treated cells gave us the ability to compare short-term (in vitro) and long-term (in vivo) effects of peritoneal fluid on endometrial cells. This difference is likely to contribute to explaining the disparities in the observed results.

ChIP-qPCR was used to better understand the regulatory roles of JARID2 and EZH2 and their cross-interactions in endometriosis. By observing how it binds to regulatory elements of various genes, a sense of how the mechanisms described above differ between PF from patients with and without endometriosis was gained. The data presented in Table 1 showed that the pull-down expression of JARID2 by EZH2 IP was by over 5-fold higher in cells treated with endo PF compared to control PF. It is interesting to note that, while not significant, JARID2 IP has a fold-change greater than 1 for EZH1, while for EZH2 it is less than 1 for endo PF treated cells. This suggests that the JARID2 interaction with EZH2 may not be as strong as it is with EZH1, which can also methylate H3K27 to contribute to transcriptional repression. Although it is typically associated with active domains, EZH1 can actually achieve repressive results similar to EZH2 via additional histone modifications [65–67]. It is interesting to note that when comparing genes after immunoprecipitations by the two antibodies (JARID2 and EZH2) in the two PF (endo or control PF) treated cells (Table 1B), the endo PF treated cells showed a trend of having a fold-change less than 1 when comparing JARID2 vs. EZH2 IP. This suggests that EZH2 in endo PF treated cells is having more of an effect on the expression of all genes in the array (PRC2 complex core, alternate and binding partners) when compared to JARID2 further supporting a role for EZH2 in endometriosis.

One gene that should be noted and that was shown to have higher fold-change post EZH2 IP in endo PF treated cells vs. control PF treated cells was PHF19. PHF19 is a gene silencer and co-factor that can bind H3K36me3, which allows it to act as a recruiter for the PCR2 complex [68,69]. PHF19 also promotes tumorigenesis by the enhancement of the deposition of H3K27me3 and when PHF19 is depleted, this led to a loss of H3K27me3 domains [70]. This suggests that another mechanism which may be at play in transcriptional repression involves PHF19. PHF19 has also been deemed to play a role in the switch from proliferative to invasive states in melanoma cells [71]. Thus there are studies suggesting targeting PHF19 as an alternate strategy to inhibit EZH2 [72]. This study found that *PHF19* mRNA expression was significantly upregulated in cells treated with endo PF (Figure 8). This may suggest that miR-155 and PHF19 may be working together to bring the PRC2 complex to its targets in endometriosis. Putting these results together with miR-155 transfection studies, this study suggests that while miR-155 and PHF19 may be the main helper in regulating the PRC2 complex in endometriosis, JARID2 may be taking up the slack when miR-155 is inhibited.

The findings presented here, as summarized in Figure 9, provide potential mechanisms that may be at play in endometriosis patients. This study shows that in the presence of endometrial PF, all the components of the PRC2 complex, along with JARID2, FOXP3 and miR-155 are increased in expression when compared to control PF. Gain-or loss-of function of miR-155 showed an effect on PRC2 complex proteins but not on JARID2 levels. This suggested that other epigenetic regulators may be involved. ChiP-qPCR pull-down studies using JARID2 or EZH2 antibodies in PF treated cells showed alterations in epigenetic proteins associated with either of these complexes. In addition to the known binding partners such as EZH1, DNMT3B etc, the expression of PHF19 (a PRC2 complex co-factor) was highly upregulated in EZH2 compared to JARID2 pull-down assay. This finding, in addition to what is known in the literature [54,69,70,72], it is presumable that in women with endometriosis, FOXP3/miR-155, in conjunction with PHF19, co-localizes with the PRC2 complex to promote its interaction and function with its targets. This leads to the increased H3K27me3 deposition thus modulating gene transcription. In contrast, this complex has a reverse effect on JARID2, thus preventing its association with the PRC2 complex, unless miR-155 is altered. This novel crosstalk among key epigenetic regulators leads to an increase in inflammation and growth of endometriotic lesions. This opens the door for testing newer targets in addition to the EZH2 inhibitors and miRNA mimics/antagonists currently being tested in endometriosis. For example, although histone demethylase inhibitors are thought to be ineffective against JARID2 due to its lack of true demethylase activity, additional investigations into the role of JARID2 in endometriosis could uncover alternate options to therapeutically regulate it, such as dihydroartemisinin which has been used in prostate cancer [73]. Additionally, the role for PHF19 as the master-regulator of the miR-155-PRC2 complex-JARID2 crosstalk is also a viable candidate for therapy and should be further explored in endometriosis.

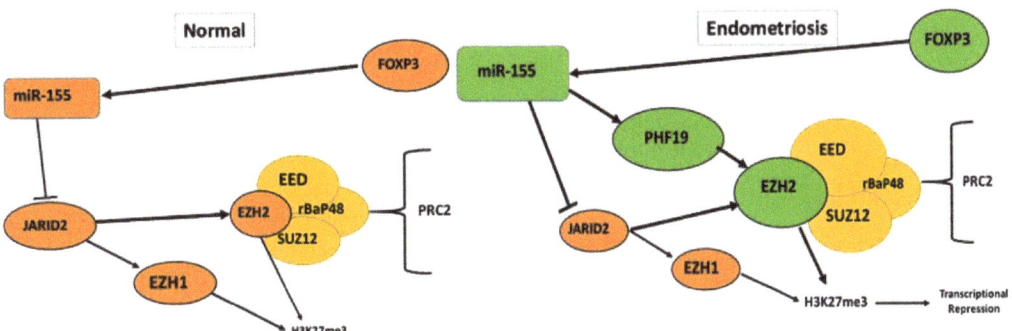

Figure 9. Proposed schematic of the epigenetic crosstalk playing a role in endometriosis. Mechanism proposed in normal women vs. women with endometriosis. Arrows indicate activation or general targeting while "T" bars indicate inhibition.

4. Materials and Methods

4.1. Human Subject Participants

Women ages 18 to 60 years, undergoing tubal ligation or having non-endometriosis disorders (controls, n = 12) or patients with endometriosis ("endo", laparoscopically diagnosed followed by pathological confirmation and/or patients with symptoms, n = 14) were recruited from Obstetrics-Gynecology clinic at Cabell Huntington Hospital, Joan C Edwards School of Medicine, Marshall University, in Huntington, WV, USA. This HIPAA compliant study was approved by the Institutional Review Board of the Marshall University School of Medicine and was carried out per the principles of the Declaration of Helsinki. All patients were consented prior to the study. The inclusion criteria included women ages 18–60 years old, with normal menstrual cycles and otherwise in normal health (except for pain and endometriosis) who have not been on any hormonal medication for at least one month before sample collection. Exclusion criteria included subjects with current medical illnesses such as diabetes, cardiovascular disease, hyperlipidemia, hypertension, systemic lupus erythematosis or rheumatologic disease, positive HIV/AIDS, active infection. Subjects were asked to stop multivitamins that contain high levels of antioxidants and anti-inflammatory medications prior to sample collection.

In this study, majority of the samples where from endo patients diagnosed with stage I/II and only one at stage IV. Pathological confirmation for endo patients classified the patients as mostly belonging to the peritoneal or uterine serosa pathology. All women completed a gynecologic/infertility history form, a pre-operative quality of life questionnaire and assessment of pain using a visual analog scale for assessment of endometriosis associated pain (dysmenorrhea, non-menstrual pelvic pain, dyspareunia, and dyschesia) (adapted from the validated International Pelvic Pain Society's Pelvic Assessment Form). Date of their last menstrual period was used to assess their cycle time.

4.2. RNA and Protein Isolation in Peritoneal Fluid-Treated Cells

Peritoneal fluid (PF) (devoid of blood contamination) was collected on ice from all women during laparoscopic surgery. Peritoneal fluid was spun at $2000 \times g$ to remove any cellular debris. The supernatant was used immediately for studies or stored in a $-80\ °C$ freezer for future use. To establish a cell model of the peritoneal environment, Ishikawa cells, a human (39-year-old woman) established endometrial epithelial cell line (Cat No: 99040201, Sigma-Aldrich, St. Louis, MO, USA), were cultured in T75 flasks in complete media (DMEM/F12, 10% FBS, 1% Pen/Strep, 1% L-glutamine). These cells were used because they express characteristics similar to those of mature endometrial epithelial cells [74–76]. Approximately 70% confluent cells were treated with 1% PF from patients for 48 h in a DMEM/F12 media containing 1% charcoal-stripped FBS. Patient peritoneal fluid (PF) groups were control PF (fluid from women without endometriosis) and endo PF (fluid from women with endometriosis). The concentrations of PF chosen were based on our previous published studies [33,55]. At the end of the 48-h treatment, cells were collected using Qiazol Lysis reagent (Cat No: 79306, Qiagen, Gaithersburg, MD, USA) and RNA was isolated using the Qiagen miRNeasy Mini Kit (Cat No: 217004, Qiagen, Gaithersburg, MD, USA). The quantity and quality of RNA were measured in the NanoDrop 2000 spectrophotometer. Cell lysates for measuring proteins, were prepared in RIPA buffer containing protease inhibitors (Cat No: P2714, Sigma-Aldrich, St. Louis, MO, USA) and protein concentrations were measured using a modified Lowry protocol [77].

4.3. Endometrial Tissue Collection and RNA/Protein Isolation

Endometrial (eutopic) tissues from control patients (EuN), eutopic tissues from endometriosis (peritoneal endometriosis, "endo") patients (EuE), and ectopic endometriotic tissues (EcE) from endo patients were removed during laparoscopy/laparotomy by a qualified physician. Biopsy fragments were immediately placed in RNA*later* solution (Cat No: 76104, Qiagen, Gaithersburg, MD, USA) and subsequently stored in a freezer at $-80\ °C$. RNA extraction from 100 mg of tissue (eutopic and ectopic) was carried out using Qiazol Lysis Reagent (Cat No: 79306, Qiagen, Gaithersburg, MD, USA). Tissues were homogenized using zirconium oxide beads in a Bullet Blender® homogenizer (SKU: BBX24, Next Advance, Troy, NY, USA) and RNA was isolated using the Qiagen miRNeasy Mini Kit following the manufacturer's recommendations (Cat No: 217004, Qiagen, Gaithersburg, MD, USA). The quantity and quality of RNA were measured using the NanoDrop 2000 spectrophotometer (Cat No: ND2000, Thermo Scientific, Waltham, MA, USA). Protein lysates from 50 mg of tissue was homogenized in RIPA buffer prior to protein estimation by a modified Lowry method [77].

4.4. mRNA and miRNA Expression in Tissues and PF-Treated Endometrial Cells

RNA (which includes miRNA) isolated from the tissues and treated cells were used. cDNA synthesis from 1 µg of each sample was performed using iScript cDNA synthesis kit (Cat No: 1708890, Biorad, Hercules, CA, USA). mRNA expression was analyzed in the cDNA samples using SYBR Green (Cat No: 1725270, Biorad, Hercules, CA, USA) and the primers listed in Table S1. 18S was used for normalization of mRNA expression. For determining miRNA expression, cDNA synthesis from 2 µg of each sample was performed using miScript II RT Kit (Cat No: 218161, Qiagen, Gaithersburg, MD, USA). Following cDNA synthesis, the expression of miR-29a, miR-148a, and miR-155 in tissues and PF-treated cells were determined using the appropriate Qiagen Primer Assay Kit, as per the manufacturer's instructions. A primer assay for RNU6 was used as housekeeping for miRNA expression.

4.5. Protein Expression in PF-Treated Cells and Patient Tissues

Total protein was measured using a modified Lowry method. Protein (7 µg for cells and 5 µg for tissues) was run on the automated Western blotting system, WES [78] (Cat No: 004-600, Protein Simple, San Jose, CA, USA). The primary anti-rabbit antibodies for EZH2 (1:50, Cat No: 5426S), FOXP3 (1:25, Cat No: 12632S), JARID2 (1:50, Cat No: 13594S), and H3K27me3 (1:25, Cat No: 9733S) (Cell Signaling, Danvers, MA, USA), anti-rabbit β-actin (1:100, Cat no: 4970S, Cell Signaling, Danvers, MA, USA), and anti-rabbit H3 (1:100, Cat No: 39451, Active Motif, Carlsbad, CA, USA) were used to measure expression levels within the samples. HRP-conjugated rabbit secondary antibody provided in the WES kit was used. Plates (12-230 kDa and 25 capillary) were run using default settings and results analyzed using the Compass for WES software (Version 5.0.1). Band area given by the software was used and normalized to β-actin or H3. Results were expressed as a ratio in which media alone (for cell treatments) or EuN (for patient tissues) was considered to be 1. It is important to note that proteins examined using the automated Western Blotting system, WES, will have different expected molecular weights compared to traditional Western blotting, due to differences in technology.

4.6. Cell Transfection with miR-155 Mimic/Inhibitor

Cells were transfected using SiPORT™ NeoFX™ transfection agent (Cat No: AM4510, Ambion, Austin, TX, USA) as recommended by the manufacturer. In short, the SiPORT™ NeoFX™ was diluted in Opti-MEM® Reduced Serum Media (Cat No: 31985062, Invitrogen, Carlsbad, CA, USA) and incubated for 10 min at room temperature. miR-155 mimic (Pre-miR™), inhibitor (Anti-miR™), positive control (anti-let-7c) (Cat no: 4392431, Thermo Scientific, Waltham, MA, USA), and negative control (Negative control #1) (Cat No: AM17010, Thermo Scientific, Waltham, MA, USA) were diluted in cell media (DMEM/F12, 10% FBS, 1% Pen/Strep, 1% L-glutamine) to a final concentration of 30 nM and then combined with the transfection agent and incubated for 10 min at room temperature. Transfection mixtures were added to 6-well plates and overlaid with cell suspensions. Cells were then incubated for 24 h prior to treatment with peritoneal fluid from control and endometriosis patients, as previously described. Transfection efficiency was tested by collecting cells in Qiazol and assessing miRNA expression using the miR-155 primer assay. RNA was isolated using the miRNeasy Mini Kit following the manufacturer's recommendations (Cat No: 217004, Qiagen, Gaithersburg, MD, USA). RT-qPCR was used (as previously described) to determine the expression of key downstream targets such as, JARID2 and FOXP3.

Western blots were performed in the traditional manner. Total protein was measured using a modified Lowry method. Protein (35 µg) was separated on a 4–20% Tris-HCl gradient gel (Cat No: 4561096, Biorad, Hercules, CA, USA) and transferred onto nitrocellulose membranes. After washing with Tris-buffered saline with Tween 20 (TBST), the membranes were blocked in 5% bovine serum albumin or 5% milk in TBST for 1 h, then incubated at 4 °C overnight with anti-rabbit antibody against JARID2 (Cat No: 13594S), FOXP3 (Cat No: 12632S), EZH2 (Cat No; 5426S), and H3K27me3 (Cat No: 9733S) (1:1000, Cell Signaling, Danvers, MA, USA) and anti-mouse against β-actin (1:4000, Cat No: A5316, Sigma-Aldrich, St. Louis, MO, USA). Anti-rabbit antibody against H4/H3 was diluted 1:20,000 (Cat No: 07-108, Sigma-Aldrich, St. Louis, MO, USA). Dilutions for primary antibodies varies from that used for WES due to the different methods used. The membranes were washed and incubated with HRP-linked anti-rabbit or anti-mouse secondary antibody (1:6000, Cat No: A6154, A4416, Sigma-Aldrich, St. Louis, MO, USA) for one hour at room temperature. After washing, membranes were developed in HRP Substrate (Cat No: WBKLS05000, Millipore, Temecula, CA, USA) and imaged using the ChemiDoc system (Cat No: 1708265, Biorad, Hercules, CA, USA). Densitometric levels of protein bands were quantified and normalized to β-actin or H3. Results were expressed as a ratio in which media alone was 1.

4.7. EpiTect Methylation Array

An EpiTect Methyl II Complete PCR Array (Cat No: 335005, Qiagen, Gaithersburg, MD, USA) was used to examine the levels of methylation in genes involved in inflammation and autoimmunity, in PF treated Ishikawa endometrial cells. Cells were treated as previously described and collected. DNA was isolated from the cells and DNA quantity and quality of RNA were measured using the NanoDrop 2000 spectrophotometer (Cat No: ND2000, Thermo Scientific, Waltham, MA, USA). Protocol provided by the manufacturer was followed. Input DNA was obtained and aliquoted into four equal portions and subjected to mock, methylation sensitive, methylation-dependent, and double restriction endonuclease digestion. After digestion, the enzyme reactions were used for qPCR using Sybrgreen. Analysis was performed using algorithm provided by Qiagen/SA Biosciences (Gaithersburg, MA, USA). A heat map was created from the data provided using Prism software (Version 9.0.0) (GraphPad, Inc., La Jolla, CA, USA).

4.8. Chromatin Immunoprecipitation (ChIP)

Chromatin Immunoprecipitation (ChIP) was performed using the Chromatrap ChIP-Seq kit (Cat No: 500189, Porvair, Ashland, VA, USA) using either JARID2 or EZH2 antibodies. Approximately 70% confluent Ishikawa cells were treated with 1% PF from patients for 48 h in a DMEM/F12 media containing 1% charcoal-stripped FBS. Proteins were cross-linked by adding formaldehyde (0.75% by volume) and allowing for a 10-min incubation at room temperature. Glycine (0.5M) was added and incubated for an additional 10 min. Cells were twice rinsed with PBS, collected in 1 mL PBS and pelleted by centrifugation. All other buffer and components used were obtained from the kit. Protocol v1.5 of the manufacturer's instructions was followed (Porvair, Ashland, VA, USA). Cells were suspended in 800 µL of hypotonic buffer before being centrifuged and the nuclear pellet was separated and resuspended in 400 µL of pre-warmed lysis buffer. Sonication was performed using a Covaris ME220 (SKU: 500506, Woburn, MA, USA). Each sample was aliquoted into 3 different tubes prior to sonication. Each tube was sonicated for 100 s and sheering efficiency was verified using an agarose gel as a smear of DNA fragments between 100–500 bp in length. ChIP-grade anti-JARID2 antibody (Cat No: 13594, Cell Signaling, Danvers, MA, USA) and EZH2 (Cat No: 5246S, Cell Signaling, Danvers, MA, USA) was used for antibody precipitation. DNA concentration was determined by NanoDrop 2000 spectrophotometer. The Human Polycomb & Trithorax Complexes EpiTect ChIP qPCR Array (Cat No: 334211 GH-506A, Qiagen, Gaithersburg, MA, USA) consisting of primers for genes belonging to the polycomb and trithorax complexes (core, alternate, and additional components), as well as polycomb co-factors such as PHD finger protein 19 (PHF19) and heterochromatin (CBX) proteins was run for all samples. Percent enrichment and further statistical analysis was calculated using algorithm provided by Qiagen/SA Biosciences (Gaithersburg, MA, USA).

4.9. Statistical Analysis

Prism software (Version 9.0.0, GraphPad, Inc., La Jolla, CA, USA) was used for analysis of all the non-array qPCR and WES data obtained from human tissue and cell culture studies. All values were expressed as mean ± standard error of the mean (SEM). A one-way ANOVA followed by Tukey's post hoc test was used to detect any significant p-values. p Values less than 0.05 were considered to be significant.

Supplementary Materials: The following are available online at https://www.mdpi.com/article/10.3390/ijms22073492/s1.

Author Contributions: Conceptualization, S.B., K.R.W. and N.S.; methodology, S.B., K.R.W. and N.S.; software, S.B., K.R.W.; validation, S.B., K.R.W. and N.S.; formal analysis, S.B. and K.R.W.; investigation, S.B., K.R.W. and N.S.; resources, B.M.; data curation, S.B., K.R.W. and N.S.; writing—original draft preparation, S.B. and K.R.W.; writing—review and editing, S.B., K.R.W., B.M. and N.S.; visualization,

S.B., K.R.W. and N.S.; supervision, B.M.; project administration, S.B., K.R.W., B.M. and N.S.; funding acquisition, S.B. and N.S. All authors have read and agreed to the published version of the manuscript.

Funding: Funding for S.B. was provided by PhRMA Grant 218218 Pre-Doctoral Fellowship for Pharmacology/Toxicology. NS was partially supported by NCRR/NCATS (NIH) through grant UL1TR000117 (UK-CCTS-Marshall) and NIGMS under grant number P20GM103434 (WV-INBRE).

Institutional Review Board Statement: The study was conducted according to the guidelines of the Declaration of Helsinki and approved by the Institutional Review Board (or Ethics Committee) of Marshall University School of Medicine (Protocol IRBNET3: 114954-25 and date of approval = 13 May 2020).

Informed Consent Statement: Informed consent was obtained from all subjects involved in the study.

Data Availability Statement: Data sharing not applicable.

Acknowledgments: The authors would like to thank Sandra White and Morgan Ruley for coordinating patient sample collection. The authors would like to thank Robert Nerhood and David Jude (Department of OB-GYN, MUSOM) for their continuous support. We also thank Philippe Georgel for his intellectual contributions to this study.

Conflicts of Interest: The authors declare no conflict of interest.

References

1. Burney, R.O.; Giudice, L.C. Pathogenesis and pathophysiology of endometriosis. *Fertil. Steril.* **2012**, *98*, 511–519. [CrossRef]
2. Giudice, L.C. Clinical practice. Endometriosis. *N. Engl. J. Med.* **2010**, *362*, 2389–2398. [CrossRef] [PubMed]
3. Ciarmela, P.; Critchley, H.; Christman, G.M.; Reis, F.M. Pathogenesis of endometriosis and uterine fibroids. *Obs. Gynecol. Int.* **2013**, *2013*, 656571. [CrossRef] [PubMed]
4. Platteeuw, L.; D'Hooghe, T. Novel agents for the medical treatment of endometriosis. *Curr. Opin. Obstet. Gynecol.* **2014**, *26*, 243–252. [CrossRef] [PubMed]
5. Rowlands, I.J.; Abbott, J.A.; Montgomery, G.W.; Hockey, R.; Rogers, P.; Mishra, G.D. Prevalence and incidence of endometriosis in Australian women: A data linkage cohort study. *BJOG* **2020**. [CrossRef]
6. Guo, S.W. Epigenetics of endometriosis. *Mol. Hum. Reprod.* **2009**, *15*, 587–607. [CrossRef] [PubMed]
7. Nasu, K.; Kawano, Y.; Tsukamoto, Y.; Takano, M.; Takai, N.; Li, H.; Furukawa, Y.; Abe, W.; Moriyama, M.; Narahara, H. Aberrant DNA methylation status of endometriosis: Epigenetics as the pathogenesis, biomarker and therapeutic target. *J. Obstet. Gynaecol. Res.* **2011**, *37*, 683–695. [CrossRef]
8. Colon-Caraballo, M.; Monteiro, J.B.; Flores, I. H3K27me3 is an Epigenetic Mark of Relevance in Endometriosis. *Reprod. Sci.* **2015**, *22*, 1134–1142. [CrossRef]
9. Stephens, L.; Whitehouse, J.; Polley, M. Western herbal medicine, epigenetics, and endometriosis. *J. Altern. Complem. Med.* **2013**, *19*, 853–859. [CrossRef]
10. Brunty, S.; Mitcell, B.; Bou-Zgheib, N.; Santanam, N. Endometriosis and ovarian cancer risk, an epigenetic connection. *Ann. Transl. Med.* **2020**. [CrossRef]
11. Koninckx, P.; Kennedy, S.; Barlow, D. Pathogenesis of endometriosis: The role of peritoneal fluid. *Gynecol. Obs. Investig.* **1999**, *47* (Suppl. 1), 23–33. [CrossRef] [PubMed]
12. Guo, S.W. Genesis, genes and epigenetics of endometriosis-associated infertility. *Nat. Rev. Endocrinol.* **2019**, *15*, 259–260. [CrossRef]
13. Bird, A. Perceptions of epigenetics. *Nature* **2007**, *447*, 396–398. [CrossRef] [PubMed]
14. Deichmann, U. Epigenetics: The origins and evolution of a fashionable topic. *Dev. Biol.* **2016**, *416*, 249–254. [CrossRef]
15. Steffen, P.A.; Ringrose, L. What are memories made of? How Polycomb and Trithorax proteins mediate epigenetic memory. *Nat. Rev. Mol. Cell Biol.* **2014**, *15*, 340–356. [CrossRef] [PubMed]
16. Cao, R.; Wang, L.; Wang, H.; Xia, L.; Erdjument-Bromage, H.; Tempst, P.; Jones, R.S.; Zhang, Y. Role of histone H3 lysine 27 methylation in Polycomb-group silencing. *Science* **2002**, *298*, 1039–1043. [CrossRef] [PubMed]
17. Kuzmichev, A.; Nishioka, K.; Erdjument-Bromage, H.; Tempst, P.; Reinberg, D. Histone methyltransferase activity associated with a human multiprotein complex containing the Enhancer of Zeste protein. *Genes Dev.* **2002**, *16*, 2893–2905. [CrossRef]
18. Geisler, S.J.; Paro, R. Trithorax and Polycomb group-dependent regulation: A tale of opposing activities. *Development* **2015**, *142*, 2876–2887. [CrossRef]
19. Fuks, F. DNA methylation and histone modifications: Teaming up to silence genes. *Curr. Opin. Genet. Dev.* **2005**, *15*, 490–495. [CrossRef]
20. Vire, E.; Brenner, C.; Deplus, R.; Blanchon, L.; Fraga, M.; Didelot, C.; Morey, L.; Van Eynde, A.; Bernard, D.; Vanderwinden, J.M.; et al. The Polycomb group protein EZH2 directly controls DNA methylation. *Nature* **2006**, *439*, 871–874. [CrossRef]
21. Kondo, Y. Epigenetic cross-talk between DNA methylation and histone modifications in human cancers. *Yonsei Med. J.* **2009**, *50*, 455–463. [CrossRef]

22. Colon-Caraballo, M.; Torres-Reveron, A.; Soto-Vargas, J.L.; Young, S.L.; Lessey, B.; Mendoza, A.; Urrutia, R.; Flores, I. Effects of histone methyltrasnferase inhibition in endometriosis. *Biol. Reprod.* **2018**, *99*, 293–307. [CrossRef]
23. Seguinot-Tarafa, I.; Luna, N.; Suarez, E.; Appleyard, C.B.; Flores, I. Inhibition of Histone Methyltransferase EZH2 Suppresses Endometriotic Vesicle Development in a Rat Model of Endometriosis. *Reprod. Sci.* **2020**, *27*, 1812–1820. [CrossRef]
24. Arosh, J.A.; Lee, J.; Starzinski-Powitz, A.; Banu, S.K. Selective inhibition of prostaglandin E2 receptors EP2 and EP4 modulates DNA methylation and histone modification machinery proteins in human endometriotic cells. *Mol. Cell. Endocrinol.* **2015**, *409*, 51–58. [CrossRef] [PubMed]
25. Li, G.; Margueron, R.; Ku, M.; Chambon, P.; Bernstein, B.E.; Reinberg, D. Jarid2 and PRC2, partners in regulating gene expression. *Genes Dev.* **2010**, *24*, 368–380. [CrossRef] [PubMed]
26. Klose, R.J.; Kallin, E.M.; Zhang, Y. JmjC-domain-containing proteins and histone demethylation. *Nat. Rev. Genet.* **2006**, *7*, 715–727. [CrossRef]
27. Kooistra, S.M.; Helin, K. Molecular mechanisms and potential functions of histone demethylases. *Nat. Rev. Mol. Cell Biol.* **2012**, *13*, 297–311. [CrossRef] [PubMed]
28. Dong, H.; Liu, S.; Zhang, X.; Chen, S.; Kang, L.; Chen, Y.; Ma, S.; Fu, X.; Liu, Y.; Zhang, H.; et al. An Allosteric PRC2 Inhibitor Targeting EED Suppresses Tumor Progression by Modulating the Immune Response. *Cancer Res.* **2019**, *79*, 5587–5596. [CrossRef] [PubMed]
29. Sanulli, S.; Justin, N.; Teissandier, A.; Ancelin, K.; Portoso, M.; Caron, M.; Michaud, A.; Lombard, B.; Da Rocha, S.T.; Offer, J.; et al. Jarid2 Methylation via the PRC2 Complex Regulates H3K27me3 Deposition during Cell Differentiation. *Mol. Cell* **2015**, *57*, 769–783. [CrossRef]
30. Pasini, D.; Cloos, P.A.; Walfridsson, J.; Olsson, L.; Bukowski, J.P.; Johansen, J.V.; Bak, M.; Tommerup, N.; Rappsilber, J.; Helin, K. JARID2 regulates binding of the Polycomb repressive complex 2 to target genes in ES cells. *Nature* **2010**, *464*, 306–310. [PubMed]
31. Landeira, D.; Fisher, A.G. Inactive yet indispensable: The tale of Jarid2. *Trends Cell Biol.* **2011**, *21*, 74–80. [CrossRef]
32. Niu, Y.; DesMarais, T.L.; Tong, Z.; Yao, Y.; Costa, M. Oxidative stress alters global histone modification and DNA methylation. *Free Radic. Biol. Med.* **2015**, *82*, 22–28. [CrossRef]
33. Wright, K.R.; Mitchell, B.; Santanam, N. Redox regulation of microRNAs in endometriosis-associated pain. *Redox Biol.* **2017**, *12*, 956–966. [CrossRef]
34. Palma, C.A.; Al Sheikha, D.; Lim, T.K.; Bryant, A.; Vu, T.T.; Jayaswal, V.; Ma, D.D. MicroRNA-155 as an inducer of apoptosis and cell differentiation in Acute Myeloid Leukaemia. *Mol. Cancer* **2014**, *13*, 79. [CrossRef]
35. Escobar, T.M.; Kanellopoulou, C.; Kugler, D.G.; Kilaru, G.; Nguyen, C.K.; Nagarajan, V.; Bhairavabhotla, R.K.; Northrup, D.; Zahr, R.; Burr, P.; et al. miR-155 activates cytokine gene expression in Th17 cells by regulating the DNA-binding protein Jarid2 to relieve polycomb-mediated repression. *Immunity* **2014**, *40*, 865–879. [CrossRef]
36. Yao, Y.; Li, G.; Wu, J.; Zhang, X.; Wang, J. Inflammatory response of macrophages cultured with Helicobacter pylori strains was regulated by miR-155. *Int. J. Clin. Exp. Pathol.* **2015**, *8*, 4545–4554.
37. Jablonski, K.A.; Gaudet, A.D.; Amici, S.A.; Popovich, P.G.; Guerau-de-Arellano, M. Control of the Inflammatory Macrophage Transcriptional Signature by miR-155. *PLoS ONE* **2016**, *11*, e0159724. [CrossRef] [PubMed]
38. Kohlhaas, S.; Garden, O.A.; Scudamore, C.; Turner, M.; Okkenhaug, K.; Vigorito, E. Cutting edge: The Foxp3 target miR-155 contributes to the development of regulatory T cells. *J. Immunol.* **2009**, *182*, 2578–2582. [CrossRef]
39. Berbic, M.; Fraser, I.S. Regulatory T cells and other leukocytes in the pathogenesis of endometriosis. *J. Reprod. Immunol.* **2011**, *88*, 149–155. [CrossRef] [PubMed]
40. Podgaec, S.; Rizzo, L.V.; Fernandes, L.F.; Baracat, E.C.; Abrao, M.S. CD4(+) CD25(high) Foxp3(+) cells increased in the peritoneal fluid of patients with endometriosis. *Am. J. Reprod. Immunol.* **2012**, *68*, 301–308. [CrossRef] [PubMed]
41. Olkowska-Truchanowicz, J.; Bocian, K.; Maksym, R.B.; Bialoszewska, A.; Wlodarczyk, D.; Baranowski, W.; Zabek, J.; Korczak-Kowalska, G.; Malejczyk, J. CD4(+) CD25(+) FOXP3(+) regulatory T cells in peripheral blood and peritoneal fluid of patients with endometriosis. *Hum. Reprod.* **2013**, *28*, 119–124. [CrossRef] [PubMed]
42. Brown, C.Y.; Dayan, S.; Wong, S.W.; Kaczmarek, A.; Hope, C.M.; Pederson, S.M.; Arnet, V.; Goodall, G.J.; Russell, D.; Sadlon, T.J.; et al. FOXP3 and miR-155 cooperate to control the invasive potential of human breast cancer cells by down regulating ZEB2 independently of ZEB1. *Oncotarget* **2018**, *9*, 27708–27727. [CrossRef] [PubMed]
43. Shen, Z.; Chen, L.; Yang, X.; Zhao, Y.; Pier, E.; Zhang, X.; Yang, X.; Xiong, Y. Downregulation of Ezh2 methyltransferase by FOXP3: New insight of FOXP3 into chromatin remodeling? *Biochim. Biophys. Acta* **2013**, *1833*, 2190–2200. [CrossRef] [PubMed]
44. Xiong, Y.; Khanna, S.; Grzenda, A.L.; Sarmento, O.F.; Svingen, P.A.; Lomberk, G.A.; Urrutia, R.A.; Faubion, W.A., Jr. Polycomb antagonizes p300/CREB-binding protein-associated factor to silence FOXP3 in a Kruppel-like factor-dependent manner. *J. Biol. Chem.* **2012**, *287*, 34372–34385. [CrossRef] [PubMed]
45. Barcena de Arellano, M.L.; Mechsner, S. The peritoneum—An important factor for pathogenesis and pain generation in endometriosis. *J. Mol. Med.* **2014**, *92*, 595–602. [CrossRef] [PubMed]
46. Carpinello, O.J.; Sundheimer, L.W.; Alford, C.E.; Taylor, R.N.; DeCherney, A.H. Endometriosis. In *Endotext*; Feingold, K.R., Anawalt, B., Boyce, A., Chrousos, G., de Herder, W.W., Dungan, K., Grossman, A., Hershman, J.M., Hofland, H.J., Kaltsas, G., et al., Eds.; MDText.com.Inc: South Dartmouth, MA, USA, 2000.

47. Bedaiwy, M.A.; Falcone, T.; Sharma, R.K.; Goldberg, J.M.; Attaran, M.; Nelson, D.R.; Agarwal, A. Prediction of endometriosis with serum and peritoneal fluid markers: A prospective controlled trial. *Hum. Reprod.* **2002**, *17*, 426–431. [CrossRef]
48. Jorgensen, H.; Hill, A.S.; Beste, M.T.; Kumar, M.P.; Chiswick, E.; Fedorcsak, P.; Isaacson, K.B.; Lauffenburger, D.A.; Griffith, L.G.; Qvigstad, E. Peritoneal fluid cytokines related to endometriosis in patients evaluated for infertility. *Fertil. Steril.* **2017**, *107*, 1191–1199.e2. [CrossRef] [PubMed]
49. Braza-Boils, A.; Salloum-Asfar, S.; Mari-Alexandre, J.; Arroyo, A.B.; Gonzalez-Conejero, R.; Barcelo-Molina, M.; Garcia-Oms, J.; Vicente, V.; Estelles, A.; Gilabert-Estelles, J.; et al. Peritoneal fluid modifies the microRNA expression profile in endometrial and endometriotic cells from women with endometriosis. *Hum. Reprod.* **2015**, *30*, 2292–2302. [CrossRef]
50. Braza-Boils, A.; Gilabert-Estelles, J.; Ramon, L.A.; Gilabert, J.; Mari-Alexandre, J.; Chirivella, M.; Espana, F.; Estelles, A. Peritoneal fluid reduces angiogenesis-related microRNA expression in cell cultures of endometrial and endometriotic tissues from women with endometriosis. *PLoS ONE* **2013**, *8*, e62370.
51. Bitler, B.G.; Aird, K.A.; Zhang, R. Epigenetic synthetic lethality in ovarian clear cell carcinoma: EZH2 and ARID1A mutations. *Mol. Cell. Oncol.* **2016**, *3*, e1032476. [CrossRef] [PubMed]
52. Dong, C.; Nakagawa, R.; Oyama, K.; Yamamoto, Y.; Zhang, W.; Dong, A.; Li, Y.; Yoshimura, Y.; Kamiya, H.; Nakayama, J.I.; et al. Structural basis for histone variant H3tK27me3 recognition by PHF1 and PHF19. *Elife* **2020**, *9*, e58675. [CrossRef]
53. Li, H.; Liefke, R.; Jiang, J.; Kurland, J.V.; Tian, W.; Deng, P.; Zhang, W.; He, Q.; Patel, D.J.; Bulyk, M.L.; et al. Polycomb-like proteins link the PRC2 complex to CpG islands. *Nature* **2017**, *549*, 287–291. [CrossRef] [PubMed]
54. Ji, Y.; Fioravanti, J.; Zhu, W.; Wang, H.; Wu, T.; Hu, J.; Lacey, N.E.; Gautam, S.; Le Gall, J.B.; Yang, X.; et al. miR-155 harnesses Phf19 to potentiate cancer immunotherapy through epigenetic reprogramming of CD8(+) T cell fate. *Nat. Commun.* **2019**, *10*, 2157. [CrossRef]
55. Ray, K.; Fahrmann, J.; Mitchell, B.; Paul, D.; King, H.; Crain, C.; Cook, C.; Golovko, M.; Brose, S.; Golovko, S.; et al. Oxidation-sensitive nociception involved in endometriosis-associated pain. *Pain* **2015**, *156*, 528–539. [CrossRef] [PubMed]
56. Ray, K.L.; Mitchell, B.L.; Santanam, N. Power over pain: A brief review of current and novel interventions for endometriosis-associated pain. *J. Endometr. Pelvic Pain Disord.* **2014**, *6*, 163–173. [CrossRef]
57. Rong, R.; Ramachandran, S.; Santanam, N.; Murphy, A.A.; Parthasarathy, S. Induction of monocyte chemotactic protein-1 in peritoneal mesothelial and endometrial cells by oxidized low-density lipoprotein and peritoneal fluid from women with endometriosis. *Fertil. Steril.* **2002**, *78*, 843–848. [CrossRef]
58. Santanam, N.; Kavtaradze, N.; Murphy, A.; Dominguez, C.; Parthasarathy, S. Antioxidant supplementation reduces endometriosis-related pelvic pain in humans. *Transl. Res.* **2013**, *161*, 189–195. [CrossRef]
59. Zhang, J.; Wei, B.; Hu, H.; Liu, F.; Tu, Y.; Zhao, M.; Wu, N. Preliminary study on decreasing the expression of FOXP3 with miR-155 to inhibit diffuse large B-cell lymphoma. *Oncol. Lett.* **2017**, *14*, 1711–1718. [CrossRef]
60. Li, K.; Zhang, X.; Yang, L.; Wang, X.X.; Yang, D.H.; Cao, G.Q.; Li, S.; Mao, Y.Z.; Tang, S.T. Foxp3 promoter methylation impairs suppressive function of regulatory T cells in biliary atresia. *Am. J. Physiol. Gastrointest. Liver Physiol.* **2016**, *311*, G989–G997. [CrossRef]
61. Chen, J.; Zhan, C.; Zhang, L.; Zhang, L.; Liu, Y.; Zhang, Y.; Du, H.; Liang, C.; Chen, X. The Hypermethylation of Foxp3 Promoter Impairs the Function of Treg Cells in EAP. *Inflammation* **2019**, *42*, 1705–1718. [CrossRef]
62. Bamidele, A.O.; Svingen, P.A.; Sagstetter, M.R.; Sarmento, O.F.; Gonzalez, M.; Neto, M.B.B.; Kugathasan, S.; Lomberk, G.; Urrutia, R.A.; Faubion, W.A. Disruption of FOXP3-EZH2 Interaction Represents a Pathobiological Mechanism in Intestinal Inflammation. *Cell. Mol. Gastroenterol.* **2019**, *7*, 55–71. [CrossRef] [PubMed]
63. Li, S.; Fu, X.; Wu, T.; Yang, L.; Hu, C.; Wu, R. Role of Interleukin-6 and Its Receptor in Endometriosis. *Med. Sci. Monit.* **2017**, *23*, 3801–3807. [CrossRef] [PubMed]
64. Muller, J.; Hart, C.M.; Francis, N.J.; Vargas, M.L.; Sengupta, A.; Wild, B.; Miller, E.L.; O'Connor, M.B.; Kingston, R.E.; Simon, J.A. Histone methyltransferase activity of a Drosophila Polycomb group repressor complex. *Cell* **2002**, *111*, 197–208. [CrossRef]
65. Mochizuki-Kashio, M.; Aoyama, K.; Sashida, G.; Oshima, M.; Tomioka, T.; Muto, T.; Wang, C.; Iwama, A. Ezh2 loss in hematopoietic stem cells predisposes mice to develop heterogeneous malignancies in an Ezh1-dependent manner. *Blood* **2015**, *126*, 1172–1183. [CrossRef] [PubMed]
66. Shen, X.; Liu, Y.; Hsu, Y.J.; Fujiwara, Y.; Kim, J.; Mao, X.; Yuan, G.C.; Orkin, S.H. EZH1 mediates methylation on histone H3 lysine 27 and complements EZH2 in maintaining stem cell identity and executing pluripotency. *Mol. Cell* **2008**, *32*, 491–502. [CrossRef]
67. Son, J.; Shen, S.S.; Margueron, R.; Reinberg, D. Nucleosome-binding activities within JARID2 and EZH1 regulate the function of PRC2 on chromatin. *Genes Dev.* **2013**, *27*, 2663–2677. [CrossRef]
68. Qin, S.; Guo, Y.; Xu, C.; Bian, C.; Fu, M.; Gong, S.; Min, J. Tudor domains of the PRC2 components PHF1 and PHF19 selectively bind to histone H3K36me3. *Biochem. Biophys. Res. Commun.* **2013**, *430*, 547–553. [CrossRef]
69. Brien, G.L.; Gambero, G.; O'Connell, D.J.; Jerman, E.; Turner, S.A.; Egan, C.M.; Dunne, E.J.; Jurgens, M.C.; Wynne, K.; Piao, L.; et al. Polycomb PHF19 binds H3K36me3 and recruits PRC2 and demethylase NO66 to embryonic stem cell genes during differentiation. *Nat. Struct. Mol. Biol.* **2012**, *19*, 1273–1281. [CrossRef]
70. Ren, Z.; Ahn, J.H.; Liu, H.; Tsai, Y.H.; Bhanu, N.V.; Koss, B.; Allison, D.F.; Ma, A.; Storey, A.J.; Wang, P.; et al. PHF19 promotes multiple myeloma tumorigenicity through PRC2 activation and broad H3K27me3 domain formation. *Blood* **2019**, *134*, 1176–1189. [CrossRef]

71. Ghislin, S.; Deshayes, F.; Middendorp, S.; Boggetto, N.; Alcaide-Loridan, C. PHF19 and Akt control the switch between proliferative and invasive states in melanoma. *Cell Cycle* **2012**, *11*, 1634–1645. [CrossRef] [PubMed]
72. Brien, G.L.; Jerman, E.; Campbell, M.; Adrian, B.P. Abstract A28: Targeting PCL3/PHF19 as an alternative therapeutic strategy to EZH2 inhibition in PRC2-deregulated cancers. *Cancer Res.* **2013**, *73* (Suppl. 13), A28.
73. Paccez, J.D.; Duncan, K.; Sekar, D.; Correa, R.G.; Wang, Y.; Gu, X.; Bashin, M.; Chibale, K.; Libermann, T.A.; Zerbini, L.F. Dihydroartemisinin inhibits prostate cancer via JARID2/miR-7/miR-34a-dependent downregulation of Axl. *Oncogenesis* **2019**, *8*, 14. [CrossRef] [PubMed]
74. Nishida, M.; Kasahara, K.; Kaneko, M.; Iwasaki, H.; Hayashi, K. Establishment of a new human endometrial adenocarcinoma cell line, Ishikawa cells, containing estrogen and progesterone receptors. *Nihon Sanka Fujinka Gakkai Zasshi* **1985**, *37*, 1103–1111. [PubMed]
75. Bulun, S.E.; Cheng, Y.H.; Yin, P.; Imir, G.; Utsunomiya, H.; Attar, E.; Innes, J.; Julie Kim, J. Progesterone resistance in endometriosis: Link to failure to metabolize estradiol. *Mol. Cell. Endocrinol.* **2006**, *248*, 94–103. [CrossRef]
76. Cho, S.; Mutlu, L.; Zhou, Y.; Taylor, H.S. Aromatase inhibitor regulates let-7 expression and let-7f-induced cell migration in endometrial cells from women with endometriosis. *Fertil. Steril.* **2016**, *106*, 673–680. [CrossRef]
77. Lowry, O.H.; Rosebrough, N.J.; Farr, A.L.; Randall, R.J. Protein measurement with the Folin phenol reagent. *J. Biol. Chem.* **1951**, *193*, 265–275. [CrossRef]
78. Harris, V.M. Protein detection by Simple Western analysis. *Methods Mol. Biol.* **2015**, *1312*, 465–468. [PubMed]

MDPI
St. Alban-Anlage 66
4052 Basel
Switzerland
Tel. +41 61 683 77 34
Fax +41 61 302 89 18
www.mdpi.com

International Journal of Molecular Sciences Editorial Office
E-mail: ijms@mdpi.com
www.mdpi.com/journal/ijms

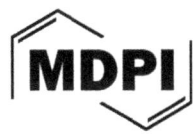

www.ingramcontent.com/pod-product-compliance
Lightning Source LLC
LaVergne TN
LVHW070640100526
838202LV00013B/847